Psychosocial Aspects of Pediatric Oncology

Psychosocial Aspects of Pediatric Oncology

Editors

Shulamith Kreitler

University of Tel-Aviv, Israel, and
Psychooncology Unit, Tel-Aviv Medical Center, Israel

Myriam Weyl Ben Arush

Meyer Children's Hospital, Rambam Medical Center, Haifa, Israel

John Wiley & Sons, Ltd

Other Wiley Editorial Offices

John Wiley & Sons Inc., 111 River Street, Hoboken, NJ 07030, USA

Jossey-Bass, 989 Market Street, San Francisco, CA 94103-1741, USA

Wiley-VCH Verlag GmbH, Boschstr. 12, D-69469 Weinheim, Germany

John Wiley & Sons Australia Ltd, 33 Park Road, Milton, Queensland 4064, Australia

John Wiley & Sons (Asia) Pte Ltd, 2 Clementi Loop #02-01, Jin Xing Distripark, Singapore
129809

John Wiley & Sons Canada Ltd, 22 Worcester Road, Etobicoke, Ontario, Canada M9W
1L1

Wiley also publishes its books in a variety of electronic formats. Some content that appears
in print may not be available in electronic books.

British Library Cataloguing in Publication Data

A catalogue record for this book is available from the British Library

ISBN 0 471 49939 0

Typeset in 10/12pt Times by Dobbie Typesetting Ltd, Tavistock, Devon
Printed and bound in Great Britain by TJ International Ltd, Padstow, Cornwall
This book is printed on acid-free paper responsibly manufactured from sustainable forestry
in which at least two trees are planted for each one used for paper production.

In memory of Gabriel

Contents

List of Contributors

BERGMAN, JONATHAN — *David Geffen School of Medicine, UCLA Pediatric Pain Program, Department of Pediatrics, #22-464 MDCC, UCLA School of Medicine, 10833 Le Conte Avenue, Los Angeles, CA 90095-1752, USA*

ELHASID, RONIT — *Pediatric Hematology Oncology Department, Meyer Children's Hospital, Rambam Medical Center, Bat Galim Street, Haifa 31096, ISRAEL*

GROOTENHUIS, MARTHA A. — *Emma Kinderziekenhuis, Academic Medical Center, Psychosocial Department, University of Amsterdam, Meibergdreef 9, 1105 AZ Amsterdam, THE NETHERLANDS*

HAIN, RICHARD D.W. — *Department of Child Health, University of Wales College of Medicine, Llandough Hospital, Penlan Road, Cardiff CF64 2XX, Wales, UNITED KINGDOM*

IZRAELI, SHAI — *Department of Pediatric Hemato-Oncology, Safra Children Hospital, Sheba Medical Center, Tel-Hashomer 52621, ISRAEL*

JENNEY, MERIEL E.M. — *Department of Paediatric Oncology, Llandough Hospital, Penlan Road, Penarth CF64 2XX, Wales, UNITED KINGDOM*

KREITLER, MICHAL M. — *Psychooncology Unit, Tel-Aviv Medical Center, 6 Weitzman Street, Tel-Aviv 64239, ISRAEL*

KREITLER, SHULAMITH — *Department of Psychology, Tel-Aviv University, Tel-Aviv 69978, ISRAEL*

KRIVOY, ELENA — *Pediatric Hematology Oncology Department, Meyer Children's Hospital, Rambam Medical Center, Bat Galim Street, Haifa 31096, ISRAEL*

LAST, BOB F. — *Emma Kinderziekenhuis, Academic Medical Center, Psychosocial Department, University of Amsterdam, Meibergdreef 9, 1105 AZ Amsterdam, THE NETHERLANDS*

MAHAJAN, AMITA   *Department of Paediatric Oncology, Llandough*
                         Hospital, Penlan Road, Penarth CF64 2XX, Wales,
                         UNITED KINGDOM

MEITAR, DAFNA   *Department of Behavioral Science, Sackler School*
                         of Medicine, Tel-Aviv University, Tel-Aviv,
                         ISRAEL

MULHERN, RAYMOND K.   *Division of Behavioral Medicine, St. Jude Chil-*
                         dren's Research Hospital, 332 North Lauderdale,
                         Memphis, Tennessee 38105-2794, USA

MYERS, CYNTHIA D.   *David Geffen School of Medicine, UCLA Pediatric*
                         Pain Program, Department of Pediatrics, #22-464
                         MDCC, UCLA School of Medicine, 10833 Le
                         Conte Avenue, Los Angeles, CA 90095-1752, USA

OPPENHEIM, DANIEL   *Department of Pediatrics and Unit of Psycho-*
                         Oncology, Institut Gustave Roussy, 94805 Villejuif,
                         FRANCE

PHIPPS, SEAN   *Division of Behavioral Medicine, St. Jude*
                         Children's Research Hospital, 332 North
                         Lauderdale, Memphis, Tennessee 38105-2794, USA

POSTOVSKY, SERGEY   *Pediatric Hematology Oncology Department,*
                         Meyer Children's Hospital, Rambam Medical
                         Center, Bat Galim Street, Haifa 31096, ISRAEL

RECHAVI, GIDEON   *Department of Pediatric Hemato-Oncology, Safra*
                         Children Hospital, Sheba Medical Center, Tel-
                         Hashomer 52621, ISRAEL

SEACORD, DEBRA   *Neuropsychiatric Institute, University of California*
                         Los Angeles, Los Angeles 90024-1759, CA, USA

SEGEV-SHOHAM, ELSA   *Pediatric Oncology Unit, Haemek Medical Center,*
                         Afula, ISRAEL

SKEEN, JANE E.   *Paediatric Haematology/Oncology, Level 7,*
                         Starship Children's Hospital, Private Bag 92024,
                         Auckland, NEW ZEALAND

STUBER, MARGARET L.   *Neuropsychiatric Institute, University of California*
                         Los Angeles, Los Angeles 90024-1759, CA, USA

TADMOR, CIPORAH S.   *Pediatric Hematology Oncology Department,*
                         Rambam Medical Center, Bat Galim Street, Haifa
                         31096, ISRAEL

TOURNAY, ANNE

Division of Pediatric Neurology, University of California at Irvine, 101 The City Drive South, Bldg 2, 3rd Floor, Orange, CA 92868, USA

WEBSTER, M. LOUISE

Paediatric Consultation Liaison Psychiatry Team, Starship Children's Hospital, Private Bag 92024, Auckland, NEW ZEALAND

WEYL BEN ARUSH, MYRIAM

Pediatric Hematology Oncology Department, Meyer Children's Hospital, Rambam Medical Center, Technion Faculty of Medicine, Bat Galim Street, Haifa 31096, ISRAEL

WHITE, HOLLY

Division of Behavioral Medicine, St. Jude Children's Research Hospital, 332 North Lauderdale, Memphis, Tennessee 38105-2794, USA

WOLFE, JOANNE

Pediatric Advanced Care Team, Children's Hospital Boston and the Dana-Farber Cancer Institute, Harvard School of Medicine, 44 Binney Street, Boston, MA 02115, USA

ZELTZER, LONNIE K.

David Geffen School of Medicine, UCLA Pediatric Pain Program, Department of Pediatrics, #22-464 MDCC, UCLA School of Medicine, 10833 Le Conte Avenue, Los Angeles, CA 90095-1752, USA

Foreword

The past twenty-five years have seen a remarkable increase in research and education in the psychosocial aspects of cancer, including the founding of a sub-specialty – psycho-oncology. Most of this work has addressed adult psychosocial care. However, only patchy attention has been given to the problems of children and their families. And, surely, it has been far less than appropriate, given the emotional pain that accompanies life-threatening illness in children. It is a great contribution, therefore, that the editors of this book have undertaken to collect our current knowledge and research in pediatric psychosocial oncology and publish a cohesive and comprehensive textbook that addresses these issues in the care of children with cancer.

They have drawn upon an international group of experts who have summarized the current information on a range of critically important topics. Co-editorship by a pediatric oncologist and a psycho-oncologist is an added strength, which follows the principle of full integration of psychological care into medical care. The book will benefit both the primary oncology team members and psycho-oncologists and mental health professionals working in pediatric cancer. Greater attention needs to be given to this area, and this work will raise awareness of the issues for public and professional audiences. It is a publication to inform stakeholders like parents, families and advocacy groups, thereby creating a stronger case for expanded psychosocial resources in healthcare policy decisions.

As a grandparent who has recently lost a lovely, three-year-old grandson to cancer (to whom the editors have kindly dedicated this work), I can attest to the importance of this book from dual viewpoints: professionally, as founder of the International Psycho-oncology Society, and personally, as a grieving grandmother. I commend the editors for this global view of children's emotional needs and guidelines for their management in the context of life-threatening illness. The contributors to this volume have elucidated the goal that, over time, no child's distress related to illness should go unrecognized and untreated.

Jimmie C. Holland, MD
Attending Psychiatrist, Department of Psychiatry & Behavioral Sciences
Wayne E. Chapman Chair in Psychiatric Oncology
Memorial Sloan-Kettering Cancer Center, New York
and Professor of Psychiatry, Department of Psychiatry
Weill Medical College of Cornell University, New York

PART ONE
MEDICAL ASPECTS

1

Cancer in Children – an Introduction

SHAI IZRAELI AND GIDEON RECHAVI

Department of Pediatric Hemato-Oncology, Safra Children Hospital,
Sheba Medical Center, Tel-Hashomer, Israel
Tel Aviv University Medical School, Tel Aviv, Israel

Approximately one of every 450 children will develop cancer by adulthood, and despite the remarkable cure rate cancer is still the leading cause of death in children after the neonatal period. In this introduction we shall highlight some unique medical aspects of childhood cancer that are especially pertinent to pediatric psycho-oncology. For more details about specific diseases the reader is referred to the available textbooks in pediatric oncology.

The characteristic cancers of children are different from those encountered in adults. Typically they arise in tissues and organs that develop most rapidly during embryogenesis and the postnatal period. Indeed, it is likely that most cancers in children result from unfortunate developmental 'accidents', often occurring in utero. In contrast, the typical 'adult' malignancies arise in epithelial cells covering the surface of ducts and body cavities that are exposed for prolonged periods of time to a large variety of environmental carcinogens. Colon cancer, for example, is the end stage of a slow multistep transition from normal tissue through benign polyps to malignant invasive carcinomas. Colon cancer may be prevented by either modifying diet or by treatment with drugs such as aspirin which affects the tumorigenic response of the colonic mucosa to carcinogens, or by removal of benign polyps. Unlike cancers in adults, most cancers in children cannot be prevented, are not preceded by obvious pre-malignant lesions and are not amenable to early diagnosis. Indeed, several international trials of massive screening for pre-malignant lesions or early stages of neuroblastoma, a childhood cancer of the sympathetic nervous system, have proved futile. These issues are relevant when dealing with the parents of a child with cancer, who are, naturally, overwhelmed by guilt and

Psychosocial Aspects of Pediatric Oncology. Edited by S. Kreitler and M. Weyl Ben Arush
© 2004 John Wiley & Sons Ltd: ISBN 0 471 49939 0

self-blame. It is important to explain to the parents that in the best of our knowledge cancers in children are not caused by wrongdoing of the child or his/her parents, nor could they have been diagnosed earlier (except, of course, in cases of a clear medical neglect).

Most of the tumors arise spontaneously although there are rare familial hereditary cancer syndromes. For example, retinoblastoma, a malignant tumor of the retina, is often hereditary. A child with hereditary retinoblastoma is likely to develop tumors in the other eye and later may also be diagnosed with osteosarcoma, a malignant bone tumor. Most of these children are cured and their chances of passing the hereditary trait are 50%. Families with hereditary cancer syndromes require therefore special lifelong attention and present the health care community with new challenges. One of these big challenges is caused by modern genetic diagnostic techniques which enable identification of individuals carrying a cancer-predisposing mutation while they are still healthy. This medically helpful knowledge may also add a significant psychosocial burden to the patients and their families.

Another high risk group is identical twins. An identical twin of a child with leukemia has 25% risk of developing the same leukemia before the age of 7 years. After the first decade of life the risk is no more than 1%, thus proving that this phenomenon is not genetic. The mystery has been solved recently. As leukemia is commonly an 'accident' during embryonic development, pre-leukemic cells can circulate from one embryonic twin to the other through their common vascular channels. Other than these examples, in most instances there is no substantial basis for the fear that other young members of the family will develop cancer as well. Moreover, the rate of cancer in the offspring of childhood cancer survivors is not significantly higher than in the normal population. Thus, in the majority of instances we can safely reassure the families that the cancer will not spread in the family.

The most common malignancy in children involves the lymphoid system, especially acute lymphoblastic leukemia (ALL). During embryonic develop-ment and early childhood the normal lymphoid system has to develop rapidly and acquire the capability of mounting specific immune responses against an enormous variety of foreign antigens. For efficient diversification of the various immune receptors, lymphoid cells possess an unusual type of genetic instability that predispose them to rare genetic accidents leading to acute leukemia. ALL is most common in young children but occurs throughout childhood.

The nervous system is another rapidly developing organ that also involves substantial fine-tuned diversification and differentiation during embryogenesis and early childhood. The frequency of tumors of the nervous system is almost equal to ALL and together these malignancies are responsible for more than half of the cancers in children. Many of these tumors are relatively slow-growing gliomas, often implying living through childhood with slowly progressing brain tumors. A large fraction of childhood brain tumors have an embryonic and more aggressive phenotype. These include medullo-blastoma, a cancer of the cerebellum, retinoblastoma, and neuroblastoma, a malignant tumor of the peripheral sympathetic nervous system. Embryonic tumors outside the nervous system such as Wilm's tumor of the kidney, hepatoblastoma and various tumors of the gonads are also typical to children.

The third most common type of malignancy of children is a diverse group of tumors of the musculoskeletal and the soft tissues. These sarcomas can arise at any age and have specific molecular, pathological and clinical characteristics. Many of those occur more frequently during adolescence, a period of robust musculoskeletal development.

Pediatric oncology is one of the greatest medical success stories of the last four decades. The cure rate of childhood cancer has increased from about 25% in the 1960s to more than 75% in the 1990s. This remarkable progress has occurred in almost all types of childhood malignancies and is due to the exquisite sensitivity of these malignancies to chemotherapy and to the series of carefully conducted collaborative empirical clinical trials in Europe and the USA.

The paradigm of this success is childhood ALL, a uniformly fatal disease in the 1960s that has become curable in almost 80% of the children today. The treatment 'protocol' of childhood ALL consists of 2–3 years of therapy utilizing up to 10 chemotherapeutic drugs given in various combinations. Intensive remission induction and consolidation therapies, lasting up to half a year, are followed by prolonged less intensive maintenance therapy. During the first half-year the child requires frequent hospitalizations for administration of drugs or for combating infectious complications of chemotherapy. The child can attend kindergarten or school and function almost normally during the rest of the therapy.

A specific problem associated with ALL and relevant to the topic of this textbook is the need for prevention therapy to the central nervous system (CNS). Early trials with chemotherapy failed because of recurrence of the leukemia in the CNS. Apparently due to the poor penetration of most chemotherapeutic drugs to the CNS it serves as a 'sanctuary' haven for leukemic cells. Cure of ALL became a reality only when routine irradiation of the brain was added to systemic chemotherapy. This success has proven to be a mixed blessing as the exposure of the brain of young children to a hefty dose of radiation resulted in severe long-term intellectual, behavioral and other neurological impairments. Modern treatment of ALL includes cranial radiation in modest doses to less than 20% of the children and the mainstay of prophylactic therapy to the CNS consists mainly of a combination of systemic and intrathecal methotrexate. While this approach has been proven to be less toxic than irradiation, its long-term neurological implications still need to be studied.

The treatment of solid tumors combines usually at least two modalities. Local control is achieved through surgery or radiotherapy. Because of the severe long-term toxicities of radiating growing tissues, surgery is preferred when possible. Modern pediatric surgical oncology has become much less mutilating. Thus in most instances bone and soft tissue sarcomas can be removed by limb-sparing surgery. Still in many instances, such as brain tumors, Hodgkin's disease and inoperable sarcomas, irradiation is unavoidable. It is critically important that irradiation is delivered in centers specializing in treatment of children because of many specific considerations unique to these patients that are required for minimizing long-term side effects and conservation of symmetric growth and development.

The most significant progress in the treatment of childhood solid tumors occurred when the concept of 'adjuvant chemotherapy' was introduced. The model tumor was osteosarcoma. Even when the tumor was localized to the limb and the limb was amputated the long-term survival was no more than 20%. Since all deaths were caused by distant metastases the unavoidable conclusion was that micro-metastases were present in most of the patients with localized tumors at the time of diagnosis. The administration of 'adjuvant chemotherapy' – chemotherapy that is delivered with the intention of destroying those unseen micro-metastases, has led to the current 70% survival rates. Typically these patients today are treated first with chemotherapy, followed by surgical removal of the tumor with sparing of the limb, and another period of intensive chemotherapy. The concept of adjuvant chemotherapy has also been adopted by the adult oncologists for chemotherapy-sensitive tumors such as breast cancer.

The recent decade has witnessed remarkable development in molecular biology and diagnostics. Techniques allowing the visualization and quantifications of genes and gene products have enabled molecular classification of tumors and adjustment of therapy to the biological tumor subtype. Again, pediatric oncology has shown the way. Thus, for example, the identification of the BCR-ABL fusion gene in a child with leukemia or the detection of multiple copies of the NMYC oncogene in a child with neuroblastoma lead to their classification as high-risk patients and to assignment to especially intensive treatments that include bone marrow transplantation. The identification of specific molecular abnormalities has also raised hopes for development of cancer-specific, less toxic therapies. While some of these therapies have already been introduced for adult malignancies, none has been developed for childhood cancer. The harsh, sad reality is that developing new drugs for a rare disease such as childhood cancer has not been a top priority of the pharmaceutical industry.

While childhood cancer is a relatively rare disease, its high cure rate is having significant impact in developed societies. Currently, one in every 900 young (less than 45-year-old) Americans has been cured from childhood cancer. It is estimated that within 20 years this rate will increase to more than one in every 400. Unlike adult cancer, occurring mostly in the post-retirement age, children cured from cancer are expected to live many more productive years. Thus the quality of life of childhood cancer survivors and the late effects of the cancer and its treatment have become a major focus of modern pediatric oncology and are particularly relevant for the field of psycho-oncology.

Although children tolerate the acute toxicities of chemotherapy better than adults, growing children are more vulnerable to the delayed effects of cancer therapy such as the effects on growth, the endocrine system, fertility, the myocardium, the neuropsychological function and the occurrence of secondary cancers. Moreover, because children tolerate chemotherapy better than adults they often receive far greater dose-intensity and are therefore more likely to develop late sequelae. Of the different therapeutic modalities, irradiation is associated with the highest rates of late effects in children.

Most relevant for this textbook are the late neuropsychological sequelae of childhood cancer therapy. Long-term neurological impairments are associated with leukemia and brain tumors, the two most common malignancies of children. Learning difficulties have been most commonly attributed to cranial irradiation and are related to the dose and the age at the time of irradiation. For example, cranial irradiation with 3600 cGy of children with brain tumors who are younger than 36 months is universally associated with marked decreases in IQ. Newer therapeutic protocols are attempting to delay radiation and lower the dose in young children.

Although radiation doses in children with ALL are significantly lower than those used for children with brain tumors, they are still likely to have long-term neuropsychological sequelae. These effects are mainly in attention capacities and other nonverbal cognitive processing skills and not in the global IQ. These deficits correlate with focal findings in magnetic resonance imaging (MRI) of the brain and neurophysiological studies. As with brain tumors the extent and timing of the deficits are related to the radiation dose and the age at the time of radiation. Girls less than 5 years old are most vulnerable. At the extreme end of the spectrum of neurological toxicity is progressive necrotizing leukoencephalopathy, a rare and devastating complication, occurring mainly in patients who have received a combination of higher dose radiotherapy and intrathecal methotrexate. Although significantly less neurological impairment is seen in children with ALL treated with intrathecal therapy only, it is premature to conclude that no neuropsychological deficits are expected. Indeed, minor abnormalities in brain imaging are commonly detected and the long-term significance of these changes is presently unknown.

It is impossible to write an introduction to a book on the psychology of children without referring to adolescence. Surviving normal adolescence is a challenge to children, their parents and educators and provides the livelihood of pediatric psychologists. Cancer in this life period is extraordinarily more challenging. Adolescents tend to delay bringing medical problems to attention and are less compliant with therapy. For example, it has been clearly shown that adolescents with ALL tend to be less adherent to the oral chemotherapy regimen during the maintenance period and that their prognosis directly correlates with their degree of compliance. There are also some unique medical issues such as preservation of fertility, and a large list of psychosocial issues. Because of these issues the need for a specific discipline for adolescent and young adult oncology is being considered now in the USA and Europe.

The final issue relates to the topic we all try to avoid. Despite the enormous success, one of every five children with cancer will die from the disease. The grim outlook for a particular child is often known soon after diagnosis. Yet studies have repeatedly shown that the prospect of dying is usually, if at all, addressed only very shortly before death. Even in the most hopeless cases, treatment is usually characterized by intensive attempts to cure and by ignoring the option of palliative care. This is one area where we, who deal with childhood cancer, can learn from our colleagues in the adult oncology field. Hospice and palliative care are new and much-needed concepts in pediatric oncology that, naturally, combine medical and psychosocial approaches. And after the death, there are bereaved parents, siblings and friends. They often cling to the pediatric oncology department and look for comfort and help. The 'End of Life' issue is a chapter in pediatric oncology waiting to be defined and written.

Pediatric oncology meets childhood psychology at the time of the diagnosis of these devastating diseases, during the difficulties associated with the toxicities of intensive chemotherapy, during the rehabilitation period, during the follow-up of the majority who are long-term survivors, and in the bereavement of those who have lost the most precious thing of all. Although the child is the one with the cancer, the pediatric oncology team interacts intensively with the siblings, parents, grandparents, friends, schoolteachers and more. It becomes a community affair in which the pediatric oncology team is in the center.

SUGGESTED READING

Smith, M.A., Gloeckler-Ries, L.A. (2002) Childhood cancer: incidence, survival and mortality. In Pizzo, P.A., Poplack, D.G. (Eds) *Principles and practice of pediatric oncology* (4th edn). Baltimore: Lippincott Williams & Wilkins, pp. 1–13.
Dreyer, Z.E., Blatt, J., Bleyer, A. (2002) Late effects of childhood cancer and its treatment. In Pizzo, P.A., Poplack, D.G. (Eds) *Principles and practice of pediatric oncology* (4th edn) Baltimore: Lippincott Williams & Wilkins, pp. 1431–1463.

2

Neuropsychological Aspects of Medical Treatments in Children with Cancer

RAYMOND K. MULHERN, HOLLY WHITE AND SEAN PHIPPS

Division of Behavioral Medicine, St. Jude Children's Research Hospital, Memphis, Tennessee, USA

INTRODUCTION

The present chapter will discuss primarily neuropsychological 'late effects' that are associated with childhood cancer and its treatment. The study of late effects presupposes that patients are long-term survivors, if not permanently cured, of their disease. Late effects are temporally defined as occurring after the successful completion of medical therapy, usually two or more years from the time of diagnosis, and it is generally assumed that late effects are chronic, if not progressive in their course. This definition serves to separate late effects from those effects of disease and treatment which are acute or subacute and time-limited such as chemotherapy-induced nausea and vomiting or temporary cognitive changes induced by cranial irradiation.

Our review will focus on the neuropsychological aspects of the medical treatment of childhood cancer by discussing current knowledge of brain damage among patients and how it is reflected in their cognitive abilities. We will direct these efforts toward the two most common forms of childhood cancer, acute lymphoblastic leukemia (ALL) and brain tumors. In addition, we will discuss neuropsychological implications for bone marrow (stem cell) transplantation because of its increasing prevalence in the treatment of childhood cancers. For each of these three topics, we will first provide the

Psychosocial Aspects of Pediatric Oncology. Edited by S. Kreitler and M. Weyl Ben Arush
© 2004 John Wiley & Sons Ltd: ISBN 0 471 49939 0

reader with a brief medical background followed by a review of the current literature. The literature review will provide an in-depth analysis of the types of cognitive impairments observed and known or suspected risk factors for impairments. Finally, we will close the chapter with a section that discusses interventions with the potential to prevent or minimize cognitive deficits acquired in the course of cancer treatment and their impact on the quality of life of pediatric cancer survivors.

Research interests in neuropsychological outcomes, as well as neurologic and other functional late effects, has shown an increase commensurate with improvements in effective therapy. For example, 30 years ago when few children were cured of ALL, questions relating to the ultimate academic or vocational performance of long-term survivors were trivial compared to the need for improved therapy. In contrast today, more than 80% of children diagnosed with ALL can be cured, and issues relating to their quality of life as long-term survivors have now received increased emphasis. There is at least comparable attention to neuropsychologic status in primary brain tumors and growing interest for children receiving transplants.

STEM CELL TRANSPLANTATION

Medical Issues

Stem cell or bone marrow transplant (SCT) has evolved over the past two decades from a heroic, experimental therapy of last resort, to a standard therapy for many high-risk leukemias, and the preferred first option after leukemic relapse (Sanders 1997, Santos 2000, Treleaven and Barrett 1998, Wingard 1997). Over 20 000 SCT procedures have been performed worldwide. The indications for SCT have widened to include a number of other malignant disorders, including lymphomas, solid tumors and even brain tumors, as well as a growing number of non-malignant disorders (Meller and Pinkerton 1998). The growth of bone marrow registries that allow for wider use of unrelated donor transplants, and developments in stem cell selection techniques that allow for haplotype transplants using parent donors, have greatly increased the availability of SCT as a viable treatment option for seriously ill children (Mehta and Powles 2000). At the same time, advances in supportive care have led to improved survival outcomes, and thus to rapidly growing numbers of long-term survivors of SCT.

Patients receiving SCT will receive conditioning with aggressive chemotherapy with or without total body irradiation (TBI) to eradicate active and residual malignant cells. Without SCT, conditioning would be fatal. The SCT procedure first involves harvesting bone marrow, the source of hematopoietic stem cells, from an identified suitable donor. This procedure, usually accomplished with the donor under general anesthesia, involves extracting marrow from the posterior iliac crests. The procedure is generally very safe and the donor usually leaves the hospital on the day of the harvest. The marrow may be processed prior to intravenous infusion into the patient. During the immediate post-transplant interval, the patient is at risk for a myriad of infections because of the immunosuppressive nature of the conditioning regimen and potential lack of engraftment. Graft versus host disease (GvHD) results when the patient rejects the donor's stem cells. GvHD may occur at varying levels of seriousness, graded 1 to 4 depending upon the number of organ systems involved (e.g., skin, gut, liver) and severity of symptoms (Sanders 1997). The treatment of GvHD usually includes steroids and cytotoxic agents.

Neuropsychological Issues

Beyond specific neurological complications, research has focused on the risk for global cognitive and academic deficits in pediatric survivors of SCT. The concern regarding potential cognitive declines resulting from SCT has been based, in part, on extrapolation from studies of ALL survivors who received CNS therapy, because, until recently, empirical data from pediatric SCT survivors have been limited (Phipps and Barclay 1996). Survivors of SCT are thought to be at risk for cognitive deficits as a result of their exposure to numerous potentially neurotoxic agents. Among the agents used in pre-transplant conditioning, TBI has been the primary focus of those assessing neurocognitive sequelae, but other cytotoxic conditioning agents, such as busulfan and other high-dose ablative chemotherapies are potentially neurotoxic as well (Chou et al. 1996, Miale, Sirithorn and Ahmed 1995, Peper et al. 1993). CNS toxicities are also associated with agents (e.g., cyclosporin) commonly used for the prophylaxis and/or treatment of GvHD; more speculative is the possibility of direct adverse effects of GvHD on the CNS (Coley et al. 1999, Pace et al. 1995, Padovan et al. 2001, Reese et al. 1991, Garrick 2000, Rouah et al. 1988).

The literature on neurocognitive outcomes in pediatric SCTs is only beginning to develop. The number of published studies is small, and they have frequently been limited by methodological difficulties, such as small sample size, or retrospective designs. The findings reported thus far have been somewhat contradictory, although a consensus is beginning to emerge. A few studies have indicated declines in cognitive or academic function following SCT, but a somewhat larger number of studies have reported normal neurodevelopment, with no evidence of declines in cognitive function (Cool 1996, Kramer et al. 1997, Smedler and Bolme 1995, Arvidson et al. 1999, Daniel-Llach et al. 1995, Pot-Mees 1989, Simms et al. 1999). Our interpretation is that many of the divergent findings in the literature may be related to age effects within and between cohorts, and that with due consideration of age effects, a relatively coherent picture of the neurocognitive late effects of SCT can be drawn.

The earliest published reports indicated no evidence of cognitive deficits following SCT. Kalieta *et al.* (1989) documented essentially normal development, 2–6 years post-SCT, in four children transplanted as infants: two with leukemia who were conditioned with single dose TBI (750 cGy), and two with aplastic anemia conditioned without TBI. Pot-Mees (1989) reported on a group of 43 children who were followed for a year post-SCT, and a subset of 23 for whom pre- and post-SCT cognitive evaluations were obtained. No significant changes were found in IQ scores post-SCT. The first study suggestive of possible post-SCT cognitive deficits was reported by Smedler *et al.* (1990). They divided their initial cohort of 32 survivors into three groups based on their age at SCT: <3 years; 3–11 years; and 12–17 years. They reported normal neurodevelopment post-SCT in the 12–17-year-old group. The 3–11 years age group showed some suggestions of difficulties, particularly in the area of perceptual and fine-motor skills. However, the youngest age group showed clear delays in sensorimotor development. Subsequent reports on a slightly larger cohort, continued to confirm this picture, and to point to TBI as the crucial determinant of adverse cognitive outcomes (Smedler and Bolme 1995, Smedler, Nilsson and Bolme 1995). Of 10 children transplanted at less than 3 years, all 8 who received TBI showed some evidence of developmental delay, whereas the 2 children who did not receive TBI showed normal development (Smedler, Nilsson and Bolme 1995).

The age-related findings reported by Smedler, Nilsson and Bolme (1995) presaged the later results from larger cohorts, and help to explain the apparent discrepant findings between the two largest prospective series of neurocognitive outcome in SCT survivors to date. Kramer and colleagues in a well-designed, prospective longitudinal study, reported on outcomes of 67 children assessed 1 year post-SCT, and a subset of 26 of these children who were re-assessed at 3 years post-SCT (Kramer *et al.* 1992, 1997). They reported a significant decline in IQ (a mean change of 6 points, or 0.4 standard deviation units) in their cohort at 1 year post-SCT. There were no further declines in the subset followed to 3 years post-SCT, but the deficits were maintained across time. In contrast, our group found no significant declines in global IQ or academic achievement in 102 survivors assessed at 1 year post-SCT, nor in a subset of 54 survivors followed 3 years post-SCT (Phipps *et al.* 1995, 2000). The discrepancies between these studies can be explained, in large part, by the differential age of the two cohorts. The Kramer *et al.* (1997) cohort had a mean age of 45 months, compared with 10 years in our cohort. Within our cohort (Phipps *et al.* 2000), the subset of children under 6 years showed declines comparable to those reported by Kramer's group (Kramer *et al.* 1997). In fact, our youngest patients (<3 years) showed an even greater decline than that reported by Kramer *et al.* (1997), and moreover, their cognitive function continued to decline through 3 years. In contrast to the report of Smedler *et al.* (1995), in neither the Kramer *et al.* (1997) nor the Phipps *et al.* (2000) studies was there any apparent effect of the use of TBI. In the Phipps *et al.* (2000) cohort, the TBI and no-TBI groups were large enough to detect relatively small effects, and none were apparent.

The findings from our cohort, in light of the previously published literature, led us to conclude that SCT, even with TBI, poses low to minimal risk for late cognitive and academic deficits in patients who are at least 6 years old at the time of transplant. For patients age 5 and under, and particularly for those younger than 3 years of age, the risk of cognitive impairment is increased, regardless of whether or not TBI is used in conditioning. The results of recently reported studies have continued to support this conclusion. Simms *et al.* (1998, 1999) reported on a cohort of 25 patients followed prospectively through 2 years post-SCT, and found normal cognitive function and academic achievement, with no evidence of decline over this timeframe. However, three of the four children in their cohort who were <3 years at the time of SCT showed substantial declines in developmental indices post-SCT. Likewise, Arvidson *et al.* (1999), and Daniel Llach *et al.* (2001), have reported similar normal functioning and absence of declines over time in SCT survivors.

Sources of Neuropsychological Deficits

Patients undergoing SCT are at risk for a number of adverse CNS events during the early post-SCT period, including cerebral hemorrhage, infectious complications such as viral encephalitis, metabolic encephalopathy, and other encephalopathies of unknown cause (Graus *et al.* 1996, Meyers *et al.* 1994, Marks 1998, Padovan *et al.* 1998, Patchell *et al.* 1985, Wiznitzer *et al.* 1984). Although the mortality associated with these complications is quite high, the surviving children are likely to recover with significant neurological impairments. Estimates of the frequency of neurological complications in SCT patients have ranged from 11% to as high as 70%, depending on survey methods (Graus *et al.* 1996, Meyers *et al.* 1994, Patchell *et al.* 1985). These surveys have generally involved only adult patients, or mixed adult/pediatric populations, and no surveys have been reported focusing solely on children. One of the earliest reports of late effects of SCT on the CNS indicated an incidence of leukoencephalopathy in 7% of patients, but this occurred only in those patients who had both previous CNS therapy and TBI (Thompson *et al.* 1986). More recent studies that have included diagnostic imaging have indicated the presence of abnormalities on MRI in nearly two-thirds of survivors (Coley *et al.* 1999, Padovan *et al.* 2001). The most common findings involve white matter lesions or mild cerebral atrophy. These abnormalities have not generally been associated with the use of TBI, but relate to the occurrence of graft versus host disease (GvHD), and, in particular, the use of corticosteroids and cyclosporin for the treatment of GvHD (Pace *et al.* 1995, Padovan *et al.* 2001, Coley *et al.* 1999a). In one study, the incidence of abnormalities in MRI exam (65%) was higher than the incidence of cognitive deficits, and there was no significant relationship between MRI findings and cognitive function (Padovan *et al.* 2001). Again, these studies have involved primarily adult patients.

ACUTE LYMPHOBLASTIC LEUKEMIA

Medical Issues

Approximately 20 000 children and adolescents under the age of 20 were diagnosed with cancer in 1999 (Steen and Mirro 2000). The most commonly diagnosed cancer in this age group is acute lymphoblastic leukemia (ALL), a malignant disorder of lymphoid cells found in the bone marrow that migrates to virtually every organ system, including the central nervous system (CNS), via the circulatory system. ALL accounts for one-fourth of all childhood cancers and 75% of all cases of childhood leukemia (Margolin and Poplack 1997). In the United States, approximately 3000 children are diagnosed with ALL each year with an incidence of three to four cases per 100 000 white children. ALL is more common among white than black children, and is also more common among boys than girls with a peak incidence at 4 years of age. Although genetic, environmental, viral, and immunodeficiency factors have been implicated in the pathogenesis of ALL, the precise causes of most cases of ALL remain largely unknown.

Presenting symptoms include fever, fatigue, pallor, anorexia, bone pain and bruising. Because the symptoms of ALL can mimic a number of non-malignant conditions, definitive diagnosis, usually made by bone marrow aspiration, is sometimes delayed. The duration of treatment varies from 30 to 36 months and, in the modern era, is usually restricted to intervention with combination chemotherapy, reserving cranial irradiation for patients who experience a CNS relapse. A better prognosis is associated with female gender, age at diagnosis between 2 and 10 years, a lower white blood cell count, and an earlier positive response to treatment. Treatment can be divided into four phases: remission induction, CNS preventative therapy, consolidation, and maintenance. The purpose of the remission induction phase is to rapidly eradicate leukemia cells from the bone marrow and circulatory system. CNS preventative therapy is necessary because the CNS is a sanctuary for occult leukemia. Traditionally, CNS therapy has included cranial radiation therapy (CRT) and intrathecal chemotherapy, usually with methotrexate or methotrexate combined with other drugs. However, because of the risks for CNS toxicity to be discussed later in this chapter, treatment is now usually restricted to intrathecal and systemic chemotherapy with equivalent success in the prevention of CNS relapses. Consolidation may be used to intensify therapy following remission induction. Maintenance therapy is required for a prolonged period because of the presences of undetectable levels of leukemia that, nevertheless, have the capacity to be fatal. After the completion of treatment, approximately 20% of those children who will eventually relapse will do so in the first year off therapy with a subsequent risk of relapse in the remaining patients of 2% to 3% per year for the next 3 to 4 years (Margolin and Poplack 1997).

Neuropsychological Issues

CNS preventative therapy is necessary because the CNS is a sanctuary for occult leukemia. Traditionally, CNS therapy has included CRT and intrathecal chemotherapy, usually with methotrexate (MTX) or MTX combined with other drugs. However, because of the risks for neurocognitive toxicity with CRT, treatment is now usually restricted to intrathecal and systemic chemotherapy with equivalent success in the prevention of CNS relapses. Recent reviews indicate that an overwhelming majority of studies that have investigated the neurocognitive morbidity of CRT in leukemia patients have found significant adverse effects (Moleski 2000, Roman and Sperduto 1995). The primary literature also confirms that children treated for ALL demonstrate significant intellectual declines in response to a myriad of approaches to CNS therapy (Brown, Madan-Swain and Pais 1992, Cetingul, Aydmok and Kantar 1999, Mulhern, Fairclough and Ochs 1991, Raymond-Speden *et al.* 2000, Waber *et al.* 2000). In general, recent reviews of this literature have concluded that children with intellectual decline understandably have increasing difficulty with academic achievement, that intellectual declines are usually more severe among children who are younger at the time of treatment and those who receive more aggressive therapy (i.e., more intensive chemotherapy or irradiation), and that these adverse effects of treatment are delayed but progressive (Mulhern, Phipps and Tyc 1999). The strongest evidence comes from longitudinally designed studies with internal control or comparison groups.

For example, the group at Children's Hospital of Los Angeles reported on 24 patients treated for ALL who had received CNS prophylactic therapy with 18 Gy CRT, intrathecal MTX, and intravenous MTX (Rubenstein, Varni and Katz 1990). Patients were assessed with IQ testing prior to beginning CNS therapy and at 1 and 4 years later. Although IQ scores remained stable at the 1-year interval, significant declines in Full-scale, Verbal, and Performance IQ scores were noted at the 4-year follow-up testing, with a mean loss of 6 to 7 IQ points. Furthermore, 12 of the 24 children had received special educational services at the final assessment with three of the 12 having repeated a grade prior to receiving special services. These results were disappointing because of the expectation that a reduction of the traditional CRT dose from 24 Gy to 18 Gy would minimize neurocognitive toxicity.

In a unique analysis across two institutional protocols at St. Jude Children's Research Hospital, patients who had received 24 Gy CRT and those who had been randomized to receive 18 Gy CRT or no CRT were compared over time with regard to their neurocognitive development (Mulhern, Fairclough and Ochs 1991). All patients also received intrathecal MTX and intravenous MTX therapy. With a median follow-up of 6.8 to 8.4 years for the groups, only small and non-significant changes in IQ values were noted with no significant differences between groups. However, 22–30% of all patients showed a clinically significant decline of Full-scale IQ over the study interval and scores on tests of arithmetic declined over time compared to normal expectations of same-age peers. Interestingly, one explanation for the lack of differences between CNS therapy groups were differences in parenteral MTX; the 18-Gy group had the lowest total dose, those in the 24-Gy group had approximately 1.5 times more, and those not receiving CRT received 10.7 times more MTX.

More recently, serial neurocognitive evaluations were performed on 30 children surviving ALL to 4 years post-diagnosis (Espy et al. 2001). Patients had received CNS treatment with chemotherapy only. Although IQ scores remained stable, arithmetic achievement declined significantly as well as patients' verbal fluency and visual–motor skills. These results recapitulated earlier reports that intrathecal and/or intravenous MTX were not benign to the CNS. For example, one cross-sectional study of 47 long-term survivors of ALL treated with chemotherapy only found statistically significant deficits in Performance IQ, as well as perceptual organization, and freedom from distractibility scores but no significant problems in academic achievement (Brown et al. 1998).

It is worth noting that at least one prospective study has failed to find IQ losses among patients treated without CRT at a 3-year follow-up (Copeland et al. 1996). Other types of chemotherapy, such as the use of dexamethasone instead of prednisone, in the treatment of children with ALL may also confer increased risk for neurocognitive impairment (e.g., Waber et al. 2000).

Mental Processing Deficits

Unfortunately, it is often difficult to separate the late neurocognitive effects of treatment (e.g., IQ loss, academic failure) from the effects of other, non-biological factors associated with childhood illness such as loss of social and environmental stimulation and missed school days (Brown and Madan-Swain 1993). It would also be preferable to identify early cognitive changes that predict later IQ loss. For these reasons, several studies have attempted to measure cognitive functioning using mental processing paradigms rather than relying on IQ and achievement testing that depend heavily on previously learned skills and information (Cousens *et al*. 1991, Lockwood, Bell and Colgrove 1999). The results have been mixed, presumably due to methodological variation and extreme within-sample variation. Despite these difficulties, recent findings are beginning to converge on specific cognitive processes that may underlie general cognitive impairments, typically summarized by the IQ score, observed in childhood ALL survivors. The majority of these cognitive processes fall under the umbrella of 'executive' or goal-directed cognitive processes. Executive functions are thought to be primarily mediated by control mechanisms in the frontal cortex, and include the ability to integrate multiple sources of information, keep track of multiple goals, ignore distracting information, and focus on new information or activities (Baddeley 1996, Shah and Miyake 1999). The focus of this section will be to discuss several relevant empirical studies of cognitive processes involving two aspects of executive functioning, attention and working memory, with the aim of constructing a coherent picture describing the intellectual impairments associated with chemotherapy/CRT in pediatric ALL survivors.

'Attention' is a broad term that refers to a group of interrelated cognitive processes, including the ability to be alert or orient to stimuli, selectively attend to stimuli while ignoring distracting information, sustain focused attention, and disengage and re-engage focus on new stimuli (Posner and Peterson 1990). 'Working memory' is another broad concept that can be loosely defined as the ability to hold task-relevant information in mind (or 'on-line') while simultaneously performing operations on that information (Shah and Miyake 1999). Working memory functions support higher cognitive functions (e.g., strategic, goal-directed activities), involving active maintenance (i.e., sustained attention), regulation, and control (i.e., selective attention) of information. Clearly, attention and working memory are not independent constructs. The inhibitory processes associated with selective attention are also required to keep irrelevant information from disrupting the task-relevant contents of working memory (Engle, Kane and Tulholski 1999).

Contemporary models of Attention Deficit Hyperactivity Disorder (ADHD) theorize that poor inhibitory control underlies working memory deficits, which in turn impair attention (Barkley, 1997). This theory of ADHD is consistent with popular models of executive functioning that suggest a high degree of overlap between attention, working memory, and other executive processes (Posner and Peterson 1990, Baddeley and Logie 1993). In practice, clinicians and researchers oftentimes make a distinction between executive cognitive processes, either for simplicity, or because many of the available tests to measure these constructs lend themselves to such a distinction. For consistency and clarity, we divided our review of late neurocognitive effects into sections on attentional deficits and working memory deficits.

Attentional Deficits

Studies of attention deficits in ALL survivors have used paradigms that range in complexity from simple detection tasks to more challenging tasks involving selective attention and task-switching. Brouwers *et al.* (1984) examined attentional functioning in long-term survivors of ALL who had been treated with intrathecal chemotherapy and CNS-directed radiation therapy. Using a simple alerted reaction time (SRT) task, Brouwers *et al.* compared the performance of 13 ALL patients with computed tomography (CT) scan abnormalities of the brain against 10 ALL patients with normal CT scans. The abnormal CT scan group was further subdivided into a cerebral atrophy group ($n = 8$) and an intracerebral calcifications group ($n = 5$). The SRT task required subjects to perform a simple reaction, such as a key press, in response to a stimulus, such as a light or a tone. In this task, the stimulus onset is preceded by an alerting/warning signal. This study revealed reaction-time impairments for patients with abnormal scans relative to patients with normal scans. Specifically, patients with abnormal scans reacted more slowly, and with more variability (especially at longer inter-stimulus intervals), than those with normal scans. The authors noted that response variability across inter-stimulus intervals was indicative of an attentional, rather than motor, impairment. In addition, task performance was most impaired for patients with intracerebral calcifications. These lesions tended to occur in basal ganglia and parietal regions, consistent with observed deficits in processing speed and sustained attention.

Attention deficits may affect cognitive functioning in others areas, as well. A study conducted by Brouwers and Poplack (1990) examined verbal and nonverbal memory in long-term survivors of ALL treated with combination CRT/intrathecal chemotherapy. As in Brouwers *et al.* (1984), children were divided into three groups, according to level of CT scan abnormality, and presented with two stories from the Wechsler Memory Scale (WMS) to assess verbal memory. The results indicated that those patients with normal CT scans outperformed patients with abnormal CT scans. As in the earlier study, patients with intracerebral calcifications showed greater impairment than patients with atrophy and patients with normal scans. When the authors correlated these and other memory and learning scores with the attentional impairments reported in Brouwers *et al.* (1984), they found that median reaction time correlated significantly with accuracy scores on all the verbal and nonverbal learning and memory tests. When attentional impairment was controlled statistically, group differences were greatly attenuated, especially in the verbal-linguistic domain. The authors concluded that attentional deficits are a major factor in the learning impairments and intellectual decline demonstrated by ALL patients.

Rodgers *et al.* (1999) used a clinical model of attention to examine attentional abilities in ALL survivors, divided into three primary processes:

Focus (encode, execute), Sustain, and Shift (Mirsky *et al.* 1991). The investigators studied a group of 19 long-term survivors of childhood ALL who were treated with combined CRT/chemotherapy, and a group of 19 sibling controls. Focus Encode was measured using the arithmetic and digit span subtests of the Wechsler Intelligence Scale for Children, and Focus Execute was examined using the speed of information processing subtest of the British Ability Scales and the coding subtest of the WISC-R. The VIGIL test battery was used to measure Sustain, and the Wisconsin Card Sort Test (WCST) was used to measure Shift. Rodgers *et al.* (1999) found that ALL survivors were impaired, relative to sibling controls, on the Focus elements (encode and execute). However, no significant group differences were found for the Sustain and Shift elements of attention. Although the measure of Shift was not impaired, the children in the ALL group had more difficulty maintaining an appropriate task set during the WCST relative to sibling controls. Specifically, children in the ALL group were more likely than controls to process each trial independently and were less able to execute strategy across trials. The investigators interpreted these findings as indicating that perhaps the ALL survivors, because of their slower processing speed, were unable to modify behavior in response to experimenter feedback.

Lockwood, Bell and Colegrove (1999) conducted a study of the long-term effects of CRT on attention functioning in survivors of childhood leukemia, using a different theoretical model of attention than that used in the Rodgers *et al.* (1999) study. Lockwood *et al.* (1999) separated attention into four components: Sensory Selection, Response Selection, Attentional Capacity, and Sustained Attention using Cohen's (1993) model. In this model, Sensory Selection refers to stimulus filtering, simple focusing, and automatic shifting of attention. Response Selection involves the inhibition and control of attention during goal-directed activity; this includes intentional, active switching. Attentional Capacity involves processing speed, temporal and spatial constraints, global resources, arousal, and motivation. Finally, Sustained Attention in Cohen's model of attention refers to the maintenance of attention and responses over time.

Lockwood *et al.* (1999) tested 56 survivors of childhood leukemia whose treatment had been randomly assigned to chemotherapy only or combined chemotherapy/CRT treatment. The investigators observed better performance for the chemotherapy alone group, relative to the chemotherapy/CRT group, on measures indicative of Sensory Selection and Attentional Capacity taken together, the results of Lockwood *et al.* (1999) and Rodgers *et al.* (1999) indicate that children treated with CRT tend to show greater impairments in speed of information processing and selective (focused) attention compared to children not treated with CRT. However, the results are less straightforward with regard to the presence of deficits in attentional shifting. Irradiated children in the Lockwood *et al.* (1999) study performed poorly on the

TRAILS B, a measure of Response Selection (Shift) that requires the participant to alternate between number searching and letter searching. These authors concluded that the CRT-treated children showed disrupted active mental shifting. In contrast, Rodgers *et al.* (1999) did not find support for deficits in Shift when using the Wisconsin Card Sort Test (WCST), despite the fact that the WCST has been found to correlate strongly with shifting ability as measured by tasks designed specifically to tap attention shifting (Miyake and Shah 1999). Indeed, Rodgers *et al.* (1999) found that ALL survivors had difficulty keeping task-relevant information in mind while performing the WCST. However, Rodgers *et al.* (1999) used a different aspect of WCST performance (perseverations score) as the basis for their conclusions. Hence, the apparent contradiction between the Rodgers *et al.* (1999) and Lockwood *et al.* (1999) studies might be an artifact of using different tests.

Working Memory Deficits

In addition to uncovering attentional deficits in survivors of ALL, empirical research has provided compelling evidence for working memory impairments in this population as well (e.g., Brouwers and Poplack 1990, Cousens *et al.* 1991, Hill *et al.* 1997). In fact, some researchers argue that working memory impairment is primarily responsible for the intellectual decline in ALL survivors (Schatz *et al.* 2000).

Rodgers *et al.* (1999) speculated that the attentional task-set disruption observed in their study occurred because ALL survivors were unable to modify their responding, perhaps because of relatively slow processing speed. While this argument does not directly implicate working memory, it does suggest that processing speed deficits underlie the failure to maintain task set. This is consistent with the recent model of cognitive deficits in ALL survivors proposed by Schatz *et al.* (2000). These researchers used statistical modeling to illustrate that IQ differences between ALL children treated with CRT versus non-irradiated controls were mediated by variations in working memory function, which in turn were partially accounted for by differences in processing speed. By this logic, the processing speed deficits observed in Rodgers *et al.* (1999) may have indirectly contributed to the failure to maintain task set by disrupting working memory, an interpretation that is consistent with the Schatz *et al.* (2000) theoretical framework of cognitive dysfunction in ALL survivors.

Schatz *et al.* (2000) published a study examining delayed neurocognitive deficits in long-term survivors of acute lymphoblastic leukemia (ALL). The results of this study revealed that survivors of ALL treated with cranial radiation therapy (CRT) were impaired on tasks of processing speed, IQ, and working memory, relative to matched healthy controls. The ALL survivors treated with chemotherapy alone did not differ from healthy controls on these

Table 2.1 Cognitive processing components of executive control skills

Cognitive process	Description	Representative task
Working memory	Ability to hold task-relevant information in mind while simultaneously performing operations on that information (e.g., Miyake and Shah 1999)	*Reading Span* (Daneman and Carpenter 1980)
Temporal tagging and updating	Temporally coding and updating information and replacing old information with new information (e.g., Jonides and Smith 1997)	*N-Back Task* (e.g., Jonides *et al.* 1997)
Sustained attention	Preparing to attend and sustaining alertness and vigilance over time (e.g., Posner and Peterson 1990)	*Connors' Continuous Performance Test (CPT)* (Connors 1995)
Selective attention	Selectively attending to relevant information while ignoring task-irrelevant information or responses (e.g., Posner and Peterson 1990)	*Stroop Color–Word Task* (Golden 1978)
Attention switching	Alternating between multiple tasks or mental sets (e.g., Monsell 1996)	*Number–Letter Task* (e.g., Rogers and Monsell 1995)

measures. IQ differences between the CRT group and control group were mediated by differences in working memory. However, processing speed only partially accounted for the working memory deficits observed in the CRT group. Based upon these findings, Schatz *et al.* proposed a developmental model in which CRT affects processing speed and working memory, processing speed moderates working memory declines, and working memory mediates intellectual impairment (IQ).

A summary of methods suggested to test for mental processing deficits is presented in Table 2.1.

Sources of Neuropsychological Deficits

Unfortunately, the treatment of ALL is associated with adverse effects on healthy tissue in the CNS that place survivors at significant risk for serious cognitive impairments (Moleski 2000, Roman and Sperduto 1995). Combined chemotherapy/CRT is generally associated with greater declines in intellectual and academic functioning than chemotherapy alone (Brown and Madan-Swain 1993, Cousens *et al.* 1988). Late effects of treatment-related CNS injury in ALL survivors may include diffuse and multifocal white matter abnormalities, demyelination, breakdown of the blood–brain barrier, microvascular occlusion, and calcifications in cortical gray matter and basal ganglia (Tsuruda *et al.* 1987, Corn *et al.* 1994). However, white matter injury is perhaps the principal factor in radiation- and chemotherapy-related CNS damage.

White matter is especially prone to radiation necrosis, and demyelination is frequently observed in the CNS following treatment (Burger and Boyko 1991). Chemotherapy, especially methotrexate, is also associated with white matter injury and subsequent leukoencephalopathy (Hudson, 1999). Leukoencephalopathy generally emerges as a late effect of treatment. The clinical course of this pathology is gradual, characterized by decreased alertness and, eventually, intellectual decline (Lee, Nauert and Glass 1986). Neuropathologically, multiple necrotic lesions in the periventricular white matter characterize leukoencephalopathy. As demyelination occurs, axons near the lesions become swollen without an inflammatory response. Patterns of white matter loss in animal models of treatment-related CNS injury suggest the involvement of vascular impairment in the demyelination process (Mildenberger *et al.* 1990).

The course of white matter injury during cancer treatment and its impact on neurocognitive function is further complicated by significant variance in white matter volume and distribution as a function of age and development. The development of myelin normally continues after birth into the third decade of life, and while the cerebral hemispheres are about 50% myelin, patterns of myelination differ across brain regions. The brain stem and cerebellar areas myelinate first, followed by the cerebral hemispheres, and finally, the anterior portions of the frontal lobes. Myelination of brain regions appears to parallel their functional maturation (Sowell *et al.* 1999). The interrelatedness of cognitive functions and the brain regions that support these functions is reflected in the rich connections between myelin in different brain areas; for example, frontal lobe white matter is linked extensively to posterior cortical and subcortical areas of the brain. White matter volumes vary from region to region. For example, the right frontal lobe is especially rich in myelin. For this reason, diffuse injury to white matter might disproportionately affect the cognitive processes of this region (e.g., attention, visuospatial ability). Hence, a global pathology of white matter can result in specific as well as non-specific impairments in cognitive function (Filley, 1998).

For example, the loss of myelin in ALL survivors might be associated with relatively specific cognitive impairments (e.g., selective attention deficits), as well as widely distributed functions in the brain, such as information processing speed. In a related study, de Groot *et al.* (2000) demonstrated that deficits in the speed of information processing correlated with the volume of white matter loss among older adults. New research findings are developing a link between white matter loss and neurocognitive outcome in survivors of pediatric cancer, as well (Mulhern *et al.* 1999).

Risk Factors for Neuropsychological Deficits

The well-documented findings of intellectual impairment in ALL survivors has prompted researchers to further investigate the risk factors that are associated with the development of cognitive dysfunction in long-term survivors of childhood leukemia. Variables include age, gender, socioeconomic status, baseline intelligence, age of diagnosis, therapeutic approach used to treat the cancer, and duration of therapy. When associated with a negative outcome, these variables are termed 'risk factors', and when linked to a positive outcome they are termed 'protective factors'. The identification of these factors will potentially aid clinicians in making important decisions regarding treatment planning and intervention.

Waber *et al.* (1990) examined the effects of age, gender, socioeconomic status (SES), and treatment modality on cognitive impairment in a group of children treated for ALL. This study utilized a control group with solid tumors to assess the risks associated with CNS prophylaxis. The preventative therapy for the ALL group included CNS-directed radiation therapy and intrathecal methotrexate. The solid tumor control group had radiation at the site of the tumor and systemic chemotherapy. These investigators measured intellectual and academic functioning in both groups of children by administering the Wechsler Intelligence Scale for Children-Revised (WISC-R), the Wide Range Academic Achievement Test-Revised (WRAT-R), and the Test of Reading Comprehension (TORC). The ALL group performed below average norms on all measures, while the solid brain tumor group performed above average on all measures. Group differences indicated that the ALL group was more cognitively impaired than the brain tumor group, and females in both groups were more impaired than males. In addition, the correlation between age, SES, and cognitive impairment within the ALL group differed as a function of gender. Specifically, early age of diagnosis and low SES were associated with more severe cognitive impairment in females, while these factors did not reliably correlate for males. The authors concluded that the major risk factor for CNS toxicity among children treated for ALL was gender; specifically, females were more impaired than males. Additionally, for females only, low SES and early age of diagnosis were predictive of greater impairment.

More recently, Waber *et al.* (1992) investigated the relationship of treatment modality and gender to neurocognitive outcome in ALL. This newer study failed to replicate the age of diagnosis effect on cognitive outcome demonstrated in the 1990 study. However, consistent with earlier findings, the investigators showed dose-related, gender-dependent effects of treatment on cognitive functioning in ALL survivors. Specifically, higher doses of chemotherapy (intravenous methotrexate) were associated with IQ decline, but only for females. Performance on measures of language-based academic skill and memory for digit strings did not differ as a function of gender. However, only the females demonstrated an overall decline in cognitive function, as measured by IQ. Systemic chemotherapy was also associated with lower IQ, but only for females. Hence, this study suggested that systemic, as well as CNS, chemotherapy should be evaluated as a risk factor for cognitive impairment, especially for females.

Brown, Madan-Swain and Pais (1992) investigated the effects of prophylactic chemotherapy and time on cognitive functioning in survivors of childhood ALL. These investigators compared four groups of children: ALL patients recently diagnosed, ALL patients 1-year post-diagnosis, ALL patients off-therapy, and healthy sibling controls. This design enabled the observation of the short-term and the cumulative effects of systemic and intrathecal chemotherapy on cognitive functioning. The results were consistent with late effects of chemotherapy. Specifically, longer intervals between treatment and neurocognitive testing were associated with a more severe cognitive outcome. Indeed, children in the 1-year post-diagnosis group were not significantly impaired relative to healthy sibling controls. In addition, the effects associated with chemotherapy alone were less severe than those associated with the combined CRT–chemotherapy therapeutic approach. However, chemotherapy alone was associated with simultaneous and spatial processing deficits, impairments presumably linked with impaired right-hemispheric dysfunction. This study underscores the importance of continuing neurocognitive evaluation for all survivors of ALL, including those treated with chemotherapy alone.

The type of cancer therapy (e.g., radiation therapy versus chemotherapy) is not the only aspect of treatment strategy that affects the neurocognitive outcome of ALL survivors. Intellectual functioning among ALL survivors is also influenced by the dose of CRT and the drug combination and route of administration (i.e., systemic vs. intrathecal) of chemotherapy. A recent study by Waber et al. (2000) found that two chemotherapeutic agents, dexamethasone and prednisone, were associated with different severities of neurocognitive outcome. While both of these drugs are glucocorticoid steroids, dexamethasone is more cytotoxic and CNS penetrating than prednisone. Because these characteristics enhance the clinical effectiveness of dexamethasone, this drug has recently been used in place of, or in addition to, prednisone in the treatment of ALL. Both dexamethasone and prednisone are toxic to neurons in the hippocampus, and have the potential to cause damage to the memory system. Consistent with the regions of neurotoxicity associated with these drugs, the adverse effects of these agents are associated with tasks that involve a high demand on memory and learning processes (Waber et al. 2000). However, children treated with dexamethasone showed greater cognitive deficits relative to children treated with prednisone. Hence, the lower incidence of relapse achieved with dexamethasone might be associated with more severe long-term cognitive dysfunction, a trade-off that should be considered when planning a therapeutic approach.

Age at diagnosis is another risk factor that has been studied extensively, in part because young children are generally at the greatest risk for traumatic events during development. This very young patient subgroup is at high risk for CNS disease, and therefore often requires aggressive prophylactic therapy to prevent relapse. Mulhern and colleagues conducted a cross-sectional study of 26 survivors of ALL treated in infancy and compared them to children surviving Wilm's tumor (Mulhern *et al.* 1992a). Overall, the patients treated for ALL performed significantly worse on testing of IQ, academic achievement, and memory than those treated for Wilm's tumor and had a higher incidence of special educational placement. There were trends noted for the severity of the neuropsychological deficits to be related to the dose of CRT used. A more recent study by Kaleita *et al.* (1999), investigated cognitive functioning among ALL survivors who had been treated with very high-dose chemotherapy during infancy. Fortunately, the investigators reported favorable neurological outcomes for these children at follow-up (mean age = 5.2 years). Kaleita *et al.* (1999) suggested that the neurocognitive outcome for ALL survivors treated during infancy is more favorable now than in the past. However, the authors acknowledge the possibility that late effects might emerge later in development. In summary, additional empirical research is necessary to clarify the role of risk factors in the neurocognitive outcome of ALL survivors.

BRAIN TUMORS

Medical Issues

Pediatric brain tumors are considerably more heterogeneous than ALL in that they vary by histology as well as location. Next to ALL, brain tumors are the second most frequently diagnosed malignancy of childhood and the most common pediatric solid tumor with an annual incidence of 2.2 to 2.5 per 100 000 (Heideman *et al.* 1997). The etiology of most pediatric brain tumors is unknown, although brain tumors can appear as a second malignancy following the treatment of ALL with cranial irradiation. Tumors are oftentimes characterized as being above (supratentorial) or below (infratentorial) the tentorium, a membrane that separates the cerebellum and brain stem from the rest of the brain. In approximate decreasing order of incidence, the most common tumors are supratentorial low-grade tumors, medulloblastoma, brain stem glioma, cerebellar astrocytomas, supratentorial high-grade tumors, and craniopharyngioma.

Among the more common symptoms of a brain tumor are morning headaches, nausea, and lethargy resulting from tumor obstruction of the ventricles and increased intracranial pressure. Problems with balance and cranial nerve findings are more common among patients with infratentorial tumors whereas seizures are more common among patients with supratentorial tumors. Computed tomography (CT) and/or magnetic resonance imaging are critical to the diagnosis of a pediatric brain tumors, although surgical resection or biopsy of tissue is usually necessary for definitive histological diagnosis. In addition to maximal safe surgical resection of the tumor, chemotherapy with or without cranial or craniospinal irradiation is indicated for malignant tumors (Heideman *et al.* 1997). Cranial irradiation is delivered once daily, five days each week for up to six weeks. The total dose delivered to the brain can be more than twice that given in the treatment of ALL.

Prognosis varies with the tumor type. For example, medulloblastoma, the most common malignant brain tumor in childhood, has a prognosis of approximately 65% long-term survival whereas children with intrinsic brain stem glioma have a prognosis of less than 10%. Although this chapter will focus on the neuropsychological toxicity of cranial irradiation, other potentially serious complications from irradiation (e.g., hormone deficiencies, growth retardation, second malignancies) are recognized in the literature as well as hearing loss from treatment with cisplatin chemotherapy.

Neuropsychological Issues

The quality of life in survivors of pediatric brain tumors was reported by Mostow *et al.* (1991) who studied 342 adults who had been treated for brain tumors before the age of 20 years and who had survived 5 years or more. When compared to their siblings, survivors were at significantly greater risk for unemployment, chronic health problems, and inability to operate a motor vehicle. Specific risk factors included male gender, supratentorial tumors, and treatment that included RT. Treatment at a younger age was associated with a greater risk of poor school achievement, never being employed, and never being married.

What, specifically, can account for the unacceptably high incidence of social and vocational problems among these survivors of pediatric brain tumors? An early review of intellectual outcomes among children treated for brain tumors included 22 studies of the neuropsychological status in 544 children surviving treatment for brain tumors (Mulhern *et al.* 1992b). A quantitative re-analysis of IQ data from 403 children investigated the impact of age, tumor location, and CRT. Although the mean IQ was 91.0, particular subgroups were clearly at greater risk. In particular, children who received CRT under the age of 4 years were very vulnerable to intellectual loss compared to older children (means, 73.4 vs. 87.0).

A comprehensive assessment of risk factors in children was conducted in a longitudinal design by Ellenberg *et al.* (1987). A total of 43 children with various brain tumors were followed with serial IQ testing. Univariate analyses found significantly lower IQs amongst those children who were younger at treatment, received a greater RT volume, and had cerebral (vs. posterior fossa) tumors. IQ deficits were greater with more time elapsed post-treatment. Multivariate analysis revealed that IQ at 1 month following diagnosis, age at treatment, and RT volume accounted for 80% of the variance in IQ scores 1 to 4 years later.

Jannoun and Bloom (1990) provided neuropsychological follow-up 3–20 years following irradiation in 62 children with a variety of brain tumors. Tumor location, RT volume (limited vs. full CRT), and patient gender had no discernible effect on IQ outcomes. The age of the patient at the time of treatment was the most powerful determinant of ultimate IQ with those under age 5 years at greatest risk (mean IQ = 72), those 6–11 years at intermediate risk (mean IQ = 93), and those older than 11 years functioning solidly in the normal range (mean IQ = 107). Although not statistically significant, children presenting with hydrocephalus had a 10-point decrement in IQ compared to those with normal pressure.

In the first randomized study comparing standard (36 Gy) and reduced (23.4 Gy) CRT in medulloblastoma, the Pediatric Oncology Group reported on the neuropsychological performance of 22 of 35 surviving eligible patients divided into four groups based upon CRT dose and age at CRT (younger or older than 9 years) (Mulhern *et al.* 1998). Although the numbers of patients in each of the four groups was small, there was a clear suggestion of both age and dose effects at the most recent testing: younger children with standard dose CRT had a median IQ of 70, younger children with reduced dose CRT had a median IQ of 85, older children with standard dose CRT had a median IQ of 83, and older children with reduced dose CRT had a median IQ of 92. Similar, although not necessarily statistically significant, differences between groups were found with regard to measures of attention and academic achievement. Overall, the authors conclude that the 35% dose reduction resulted in a measurable sparing of IQ for children diagnosed between the ages of 4 and 9 years of age.

A more recent study longitudinal study has been published by the Children's Cancer Group of 43 children who were survivors of average risk medulloblastoma treated with 23.4 Gy CRT and adjuvant chemotherapy at age 3 years or older (Ris *et al.* 2001). Overall, Full Scale IQ declined a mean of 17.4 points or 4.3 points per year, Verbal IQ declined a mean of 16.8 points or 4.2 points per year, and Nonverbal IQ declined a mean of 16 points or 4.0 points per year. Although no significant age effects were found for Full Scale IQ changes, children under the age of 7 years at CRT lost a mean of 20.8 points over the interval of observation, placing in question the notion that younger children benefit from lower doses of CRT. However, without an internal comparison group, no definitive answer could be drawn.

Another recent longitudinal study of children surviving treatment for medulloblastoma elucidates the changes in learning that underlie oftentimes noted declines in IQ in this group of children (Palmer *et al.* 2001). Forty-four children treated with CRT with or without chemotherapy received serial assessments of their FSIQ up to 12 years post-treatment. The mean IQ score of the sample was 83.6 at the most recent testing with a rate of decline from diagnosis estimated at 2.2 points per year with children younger than 8 years at CRT having a more rapid decline than older children (means, -3.2 vs. -1.2 points/year) and patients receiving CRT doses of 36 Gy or higher having a more rapid decline than those receiving lower CRT doses (-3.6 vs. -1.6 points/year). Importantly, the analysis of patient's performance using raw score values (uncorrected for age) demonstrated a positive learning slope which was only 50% to 60% of that necessary to maintain their original IQ scores. The above finding gives hope to the notion that the rate of learning could be accelerated in affected patients. In addition to IQ declines, specific problems with school achievement, dyslexia, and memory functions are reported among children surviving temporal lobe gliomas (Mulhern *et al.* 1988, Carpentieri and Mulhern 1993).

Risks for Neuropsychological Deficits

The analysis of risk factors for neurocognitive impairments is more complex among patients treated for brain tumors than among those treated for ALL because of the increased number and variety of putative sources of brain damage. In general, a young age at diagnosis, more aggressive CNS therapy, and tumor-associated factors such as location, seizures, and hydrocephalus are the most frequently cited risk factors.

Very young children treated for brain tumors, especially those below age 4 years, are exposed to potentially neurotoxic agents during a time of accelerated neuroanatomic as well as psychological development. Some of these neurotoxic events may be focal in nature, such as the tumor and associated mass effect as well as local RT; others may have a diffuse impact, such as full CRT or chemotherapy. The prevailing opinion is that very young children are at greater risk as the CNS is yet developing anatomically and functionally. Particularly in the young, diffuse insults may result in greater relative functional deficit as those exposed to focal insults have greater adaptive capacity to shift developing functions to unimpaired areas of the brain. Recent independent reviews of the pediatric brain tumor literature and the radiotherapy literature are in agreement that young age plays a preeminent role with regard to risks for treatment-related neurocognitive impairments (Roman and Sperduto 1995, Ris and Noll 1994).

Hydrocephalus, defined here as ventricular dilatation with increased intracranial pressure, is common as a presenting feature in newly diagnosed patients, especially those with obstruction of CSF flow through the fourth ventricle. This phenomenon is more common among children than adults with intracranial tumors, largely because of the greater prevalence of posterior fossa tumors in the younger age group (Klein 1984). Suprasellar tumors in both children and adults are often associated with hydrocephalus. If untreated, brain edema, periventricular white matter and vascular damage result. The association of chronic hydrocephalus with learning disability and mental retardation among children in settings other than that of brain tumors is well documented (Willis 1994). However, the effects of episodic and temporary increases in intracranial pressure are not well understood. Hydrocephalus has been variably reported as a risk factor for cognitive deficits in the setting of brain tumors. In the Ellenberg *et al.* (1987) mixed series of patients, 28 of 43 children presented with hydrocephalus at diagnosis. IQ deficits were documented at 1 and 4 months following tumor excision whether or not a shunt was required. All children showed gains, but those receiving a shunt showed the greatest gains, suggesting that their initial IQ scores in part reflected the effects of excess intracranial pressure. Hydrocephalus at diagnosis had no significant effect on IQ measured 1–4 years later. In a later series of a heterogeneous group of children, 40 presenting with hydrocephalus at diagnosis were compared to 22 with normal ventricles and no differences were found between the two groups with regard to mean IQ at follow-up; however, children presenting with hydrocephalus were twice as likely to be functioning in the intellectually deficient range with IQ scores less than 70 (Jannoun and Bloom 1990). In children with medulloblastoma, insertion of a VP shunt was associated with less pronounced intellectual and academic deficits at follow-up (Johnson *et al.* 1994).

Infiltrative tumors invade and destroy normal brain structures, whereas noninvasive or encapsulated tumors displace and compress normal brain structures. Subsequent alterations of brain function related to the area of insult may be transient, durable, or progressive. The manner in which tumor effects are manifested neuropsychologically may depend upon the developmental stage of the child. Two studies that investigated tumor location as a risk factor had positive findings (Mulhern *et al.* 1992b, Ellenberg *et al.* 1987). In each instance, patients surviving tumors of the cerebral hemispheres had lower IQ and/or quality of life than those with non-cerebral tumors. In two independent studies of children treated for temporal lobe tumors with surgery with or without RT, memory deficits and other cognitive changes have been associated with whether the tumor arose in the language dominant or non-dominant cerebral hemisphere (Carpentieri and Mulhern 1993, Cavazzuti *et al.* 1980).

Investigators from France have reported a cohort of 42 consecutively diagnosed children with low-grade cerebral hemispheric gliomas (Hirsch *et al.* 1989). Children were treated with surgery alone, comprising an important 'standard' for evaluating the late effects of other forms of treatment. Long-term follow-up revealed that 29% of children had IQ levels below 80, often with major problems in school. Although the authors did not associate a 20% incidence of poorly controlled postoperative seizures with low IQ or school problems, this additional influence cannot be ruled out. In contrast, Riva *et al.* (1989) reported normal IQ among children with posterior fossa (largely cerebellar) astrocytoma similarly managed with surgery alone, implying that tumor location is important among non-irradiated children. In contrast, cognitive decline has been documented in children with low-grade tumors of the brain stem following often limited surgery with or without local CRT (Mulhern *et al.* 1994).

The goal of CRT is the selective destruction of neoplastic cells. CT and MRI demonstrate white matter changes following irradiation that vary directly with the radiation dose (Corn *et al.* 1994). Changes are often limited to the high-dose radiation volume, but may progress from focal to diffuse 'encephalo-pathy' including significant volumes of one or both cerebral hemispheres. The late deleterious effects of RT for brain tumors in children and adults have been demonstrated using a variety of designs, primarily comparing the effect of the presence versus absence of RT as a treatment component or comparing local RT to full CRT. Given the previous discussion of mechanisms of action, studies relating total dose and fraction size to cognitive function would be important.

Although one study failed to detect an effect of RT volume (Jannoun and Bloom, 1990), another has found that the IQ values of children given CRT were significantly lower than those given local RT or no RT; the latter groups did not differ from each other (Ellenberg *et al.* 1987). Mostow *et al.*'s (1991) very long-term follow-up of adults who had been treated as children found the use of RT as part of the patient's treatment regimen was associated with an almost threefold increase in the risk of chronic unemployment. In general, the findings indicate that patients requiring CRT attain a lower level of cognitive function and quality of life than those treated with local CRT or no CRT. However, at least two qualifications to this statement must be made. Two studies from our group illustrate the potential for unexpected cognitive changes among children treated with local RT for brain stem gliomas and gliomas of the temporal lobes apparently related to the impact on normal temporal lobe areas (Carpentieri and Mulhern 1993, Mulhern *et al.* 1988).

Neurotoxicity has been related to several chemotherapeutic agents. Effects are generally acute and often self-limited for the central nervous system, typified by encephalopathies attributed to electrolyte disturbance (e.g., with cisplatinum) or direct drug effects (e.g., methotrexate or ifosfamide). Reduction of CRT-induced brain damage has been used to justify the use of primary chemotherapy, especially for very young children, with malignant or low-grade brain tumors. Neurotoxicities of chemotherapy in this clinical setting may relate to later functional change as in dose-related sensorineural hearing loss associated with cisplatin. Hearing loss extending into the speech frequencies can limit normal cognitive development and academic progress in children. In one study of infants and very young children treated for brain tumors with pre-irradiation chemotherapy, physical and psychological growth was abnormal in the majority of children and showed no 'catch up' effect during the time that CRT was delayed (Horowitz *et al.* 1988). In the series of mixed intracranial tumors of children receiving neuraxis RT by Jannoun and Bloom (1990), 8 of the 13 patients also received chemotherapy. The chemotherapy was not specified, and patient function was not analyzed using chemotherapy exposure as a potential risk factor. Interpretation of the effects of whole brain irradiation in this series is complicated by the high proportion of these patients who also received chemotherapy.

Other factors which may affect cognitive performance following treatment for brain tumors are only sporadically mentioned in the literature. These include family socioeconomic resources, premorbid levels of function, chronic sensory and motor deficits, and seizures. For example, in children without brain tumors poorly controlled seizures are associated with abnormal intellectual and academic development (Rankin, Adams and Jones 1996). Poorly controlled seizures among children surviving temporal lobe astro-cytomas are associated with psychopathology and poor academic achievement (Carpentieri and Mulhern 1993).

Surveys have found that a significant proportion of surviving patients have clinically significant visual (optic atrophy, hemianopsia), auditory, and motor disabilities (hemiparesis, ataxia) or seizures which grossly affect performance of age-appropriate activities of daily living such as self-care and socialization (Ris and Noll 1994). The precise etiology of these complications is often unknown, but chronic increased intracranial pressure, operative complications, and cisplatin-induced hearing loss are not uncommon. These deficits indirectly affect patient functional status because of the limitations placed on input and performance of tasks rather than on cognitive processing itself.

Sources of Neuropsychological Deficits

Unlike patients treated for ALL, those treated for brain tumors are exposed to the mechanical trauma of an invasive, space-occupying lesion of the CNS as well as the trauma associated with surgical resection and secondary effects (e.g., visual field cuts, seizures, hemiplegia, etc.) of both of these processes. It has been demonstrated that secondary, perioperative deficits adversely affect neuropsychological performance after controlling for the effects of treatment (Ris and Noll 1994).

Similar to studies of patients with ALL, the shared neurobiological substrate for neuropsychological deficits attributed to CRT is thought to be loss of normal white matter or the failure to develop normal white matter at an age-appropriate rate (Mulhern *et al.* 1999). For patients treated for malignant brain tumors, the adverse effects of ionizing irradiation on the cerebral micro-vasculature is thought to be the pathway leading to white matter loss as opposed to the direct effects of irradiation on glial cells or their precursors

(Hopewell and van der Kogel 1999). Although studies using qualitative methods of characterizing the type and frequency of brain abnormalities have sometimes resulted in ambiguous findings with respect to correlation with neuropsychological deficits, greater success has recently been achieved using quantitative methods of measuring brain morphology. For example, recent work from our institution has demonstrated that patients treated for medulloblastoma with craniospinal irradiation with or without chemotherapy following surgery exhibit smaller volumes of normal white matter than age-matched controls with low-grade posterior fossa tumors treated with surgery alone (Reddick *et al.* 1998). In addition, the patients had lower IQ scores as survivors than those treated for low-grade tumors, and increased volume of normal-appearing white matter was significantly correlated with higher IQ scores among the patients treated for medulloblastoma but not those treated for low-grade tumors (Mulhern *et al.* 1999), implying that there is a threshold for normal white matter impacting on IQ.

One provocative hypothesis is that the development of normal white matter may explain the well-documented adverse effects of a young at treatment for malignant brain tumors. A longitudinal study of patients treated for medulloblastoma with craniospinal irradiation and chemotherapy after surgical resection has demonstrated a progressive loss of normal white matter in contradistinction to the normally expected increase of normal white matter in persons under the age of 20 (Reddick *et al.* 2000). Recently, the clinical significance of this finding was tested in a cross-sectional study of 42 survivors of medulloblastoma. IQ was positively correlated with white matter volume and inversely correlated with age at CRT, and white matter volume and age at CRT were inversely correlated. After statistically controlling for the impact of normal white matter on IQ, the effects of age at CRT were no longer significant, implying that normal white matter mediated the relationship between age and IQ (Mulhern *et al.* 2001).

Young age at treatment, perioperative complications, more aggressive treatment (e.g., greater doses and volumes of radiation therapy), and more adverse impact on future brain development are risk factors previously discussed in this chapter that are probably not independent. Unlike research results with patients treated for ALL, patients treated for malignant brain tumors tend to have a greater number of potential sources of brain insult, more severe overall impairment as measured by IQ loss, and a greater number of specific neuropsychological deficits identified.

INTERVENTIONS FOR NEUROPSYCHOLOGICAL DEFICITS

Although research on the patterns and risks for neuropsychological and educational deficits among survivors of childhood cancer has been progressing for the past three decades, the development of empirically validated interventions for these deficits has not been as rapid. Broadly speaking, interventions can be divided into two approaches: those intended to avoid or reduce the neuropsychological toxicity of therapy directed toward the CNS, and those intended to minimize or rehabilitate deficits that cannot be avoided.

A formal plan of prospective surveillance of neuropsychological status should be set forth for each patient based upon known or suspected risk for problems. This assumes that a qualified psychologist has been identified as a consultant to the institution. For example, a middle-aged adult with a supratentorial low-grade glioma treated with surgery alone may require formal assessment only once or twice during the 2-year period following diagnosis with the focus being whether there is evidence of loss of abilities. On the other hand, a young child with the same tumor and treatment should have a neuropsychological evaluation scheduled at the completion of therapy and 3–5 years later, whereas an infant with a brain tumor should probably be evaluated every 6 months until the age of 3 or 4 years and then yearly until 5 years post-therapy. Such plans should not depend upon the presentation of symptoms because presymptomatic assessments oftentimes allow for early educational interventions that may minimize deficits.

Contemporary treatment protocols for children treated for cancer generally show an enlightened concern for the potential neurotoxicity of therapy, especially among very young patients. The elimination of CRT, delay of CRT until the patient is older, or CRT dose/volume reduction to spare more normal brain is one of the most frequently considered approaches. Several studies have documented benefit of CRT dose reduction in terms of IQ and achievement functioning in survivors of ALL and brain tumors. The benefits of more recent technological improvements, such as the use of three-dimensional conformal CRT, are not yet known. However, with ever-increasing cure rates, this approach to toxicity reduction is likely to continue to be very active.

If neuropsychological impairments are unavoidable, one may attempt to minimize their impact by direct intervention with cognitive rehabilitation or pharmacotherapy, and/or through more indirect approaches involving manipulations of the patient's environment. Cognitive rehabilitation is a term used to describe interventions intended to restore lost cognitive functions or to teach the patient skills to compensate for cognitive losses that cannot be restored. Although some evidence for efficacy is available from the child closed head injury literature, we are aware of only one program in the USA that is attempting to validate a standardized, 20-session program of cognitive rehabilitation for survivors of ALL and brain tumors in a seven-institution consortium funded by the National Cancer Institute (Butler and Copeland 2002).

Pharmacotherapy, especially the use of psychostimulants such as methyl-phenidate (Ritalin), has recently received interest. Impressive gains in activity level and quality of life were shown in one study of adult glioma patients treated with methylphenidate at the University of Texas/M.D. Anderson Cancer Center (Meyers, Weitzner and Valentine 1998). A subsequent study at our institution investigated the acute effects of methylphenidate on the cognitive functioning of pediatric patients treated for cancer (Thompson *et al.* 2001). In this double-blind, placebo-controlled study, patients given 0.6 mg/kg methylphenidate showed significant improvement on measures of attention when compared to those receiving placebo. Our current study, funded by the National Cancer Institute, expands upon these findings by conducting a 3-week crossover trial of two doses of methylphenidate and placebo in the home and school environments to establish the potential for efficacy prior to 12 months of treatment. Parent and teacher ratings of behavior as well as objective testing of the patients will allow the evaluation of effects on academic achievement and social relations.

Finally, one should not minimize the potential positive impact of optimal communication and education of the patient's caregivers (Armstrong, Blumberg and Toledano, 1999). Routine communication between the cancer treatment center and the patient's school should be the standard of care, especially in cases in which neurological (e.g., hearing loss in the speech frequencies, visual field cuts) or neuropsychological deficits (e.g., problems with attention, memory, or processing speed) can obviously impair the patient's ability to function in a normal classroom environment. Because all of the deficits listed above are unobservable to teachers, there may be a tendency to misinterpret the patient's behavior in the absence of knowledge of the deficits. For example, we have experience with children labeled as having attitude problems, or as being daydreamers or unmotivated to learn when, in fact, the patient had neurological and neuropsychological disabilities that were unknown to the teacher. Although parents can have an important role in facilitating communication between the cancer center and the school, we have found that a telephone call or visit from a representative from the cancer center teacher or social worker can have a profound impact on the adaptation of the classroom environment to meet the patient's needs.

SUMMARY AND CONCLUSIONS

Survivors of stem cell transplant in childhood represent a rapidly growing population who are at risk for adverse CNS outcomes and neurocognitive impairment. To date, studies of neurocognitive outcomes in specifically pediatric populations are few in number and suffer from a number of methodological limitations. Nevertheless, integration of the available literature leads to a reasonably coherent interpretation of the findings, with age at SCT a crucial determinant of outcome. For children age $\geqslant 6$ years at the time of transplant, SCT, even with TBI, poses low to minimal risks for late cognitive and academic deficits. However, for children less than 6 years, and particularly for those $\leqslant 3$ years, the risk of cognitive impairment is increased, regardless of whether or not TBI is used in conditioning.

The incidence and severity of neuropsychological impairments among children previously treated for ALL is variable, and depends upon the aggressiveness of CNS therapy, host factors such as age of the patient at the time of treatment and possibly gender, time elapsed from completion of treatment, and methods of assessment. Clearly, the contemporary focus is on the assessment of executive functions, such as working memory, and other cognitive processes that affect learning for ALL survivors, but are not apparent until later captured by declining IQ and academic achievement test scores.

The incidence of neurocognitive problems and resulting problems in attaining an adequate quality of life (e.g., employment, social relationships) is very high among persons treated for malignant brain tumors in childhood. Although neurocognitive problems are most often summarized by declining IQ values, one could use the ALL literature as a model for more in-depth studies of mental processing functions that may explain a lack of normal intellectual and academic development. Although demographic and clinical risk factors for neurocognitive deficits, such as young age at treatment and CRT, have been consistently identified, considerable work remains to be done regarding the biological substrates underlying these risks and methods of intervention.

This chapter has highlighted the most important issues relevant to neurocognitive late effects in childhood cancer, specifically those associated with ALL, malignant brain tumors, and stem cell transplantation. A summary of known risk factors for neuropsychological deficits in these patient groups is presented in Table 2.2.

Although neurocognitive problems have been traditionally defined by late IQ and achievement deficits, more recent studies, particularly with survivors of ALL, are defining the particular mental processing factors that antedate these late changes. However, clinical research in the area of late neuropsychological effects could be facilitated by several factors, including the removal of barriers to third-party payment for protocol-driven clinical neuropsychological evaluations of patients. Research goals should include improving methods of identifying the basis for declines in IQ and academic achievement, developing a better understanding of which children are at greatest risk for these changes, increasing our understanding of the biological substrates underlying neurocognitive deficits, and, most importantly, developing interventions at several levels to avoid or remediate deficits.

Table 2.2 Summary of risk factors for neuropsychological impairments from stem cell transplantation, acute lymphoblastic leukemia, and malignant brain tumors

Risk factor	Stem cell transplantation	Acute lymphoblastic leukemia	Malignant brain tumor
Disease process and associated problems	Graft vs. host disease may have a direct effect on the CNS but permanent association with NP deficits has not been demonstrated	Overt CNS leukemia is uncommon but usually requires more aggressive therapy and increased risk for NP deficits	Tumor volume, tumor location, seizures, hydrocephalus, and neurosurgical morbidities have all been associated with NP deficits
Radiation therapy	TBI is commonly used in SCT with variable association with NP deficits in the existing literature	CRT (18–24 Gy) is now avoided in the treatment of ALL except in the case of CNS leukemia	CRT is the only curative therapy for some tumors, although dose reductions with or without compensatory chemotherapy are now more common
Chemotherapy	Busulfan, cyclosporin, and corticosteroids are all potentially neurotoxic but their association with NP deficits in SCT is largely unproven	There is strong evidence for intrathecal and intravenous high dose methotrexate and some evidence for corticosteroids associated with NP deficits	Cisplatin chemotherapy is known to cause dose-related sensorineural hearing loss, beginning with the high frequencies
Age at treatment	There is some evidence that age moderates the effects of CNS treatment for SCT with younger children (<4 years) at greatest risk for NP deficits	There is strong evidence that age moderates the effects of CNS treatments for ALL with younger children (<4 years) at greatest risk for NP deficits	There is strong evidence that age moderates the effects of CNS treatments for brain tumors with younger children (<4 years) at greatest risk for NP deficits
Gender	None recognized	Female gender has been associated with increased risk for NP deficits in studies from several centers, although the biological mechanisms are not known	None recognized
Time from completion of treatment	Longitudinal studies have demonstrated a lag in the appearance of NP deficits for selected subgroups of patients	It is well recognized that NP deficits may take 2–5 years to manifest themselves by achievement and IQ loss, although more aggressive therapy may shorten the delay	As in ALL, cross-sectional and longitudinal studies have confirmed time-dependent changes that are not necessarily linear

Notes. CRT = cranial radiation therapy; RT = radiation therapy; TBI = total body irradiation; CNS = central nervous system; NP = neuropsychological; ALL = acute lymphoblastic leukemia.

ACKNOWLEDGEMENT

Preparation of this chapter was supported in part by the American Lebanese Syrian Associated Charities and grants CA 21765 and CA 20180 from the National Cancer Institute.

REFERENCES

Armstrong, F.D., Blumberg, M.J., Toledano, S.R. (1999) Neurobehavioral issues in childhood cancer. *School Psychology Review* **28**, 194–203.

Arvidson, J., Kihlgren, M., Hall, C., Lonnerholm, G. (1999) Neuropsychological functioning after treatment for hematological malignancies in childhood, including autologous bone marrow transplantation. *Ped. Hem. Oncol.* **16**, 9–21.

Baddeley, A.D. (1996) Exploring the central executive. *Quart. J. Exper. Psychol.* **49**, 5–28.

Baddeley, A.D., Logie, R.H. (1998) Working memory: The multiple-component model. In Miyake, A., Shah, P. (Eds) *Models of Working Memory: Mechanisms of Active Maintenance and Executive Control.* New York: Cambridge University Press.

Barkley, R.A. (1997) Attention-Deficit/Hyperactivity Disorder, self-regulation, and time: Toward a more comprehensive theory. *Developmental and Behavioral Pediatrics* **18**, 271–279.

Brouwers, P., Poplack, D. (1990) Memory and learning sequelae in long-term survivors of acute lymphoblastic leukemia: Association with attention deficits. *The American Journal of Pediatric Hematology/Oncology* **12**, 174–181.

Brouwers, P., Riccardi, R., Poplack, D., Fedio, P. (1984) Attentional deficits in long-term survivors of childhood acute lymphoblastic leukemia. *J. Clin. Neuropsychology* **6**, 325–336.

Brown, R.T., Madan-Swain, A. (1993) Cognitive, neuropsychological, and academic sequelae in children with leukemia. *J. Learning Disabilities* **26**, 74–90.

Brown, R.T., Madan-Swain, A., Pais, R. (1992) Cognitive status of children treated with central nervous system prophylactic chemotherapy for acute lymphocytic leukemia. *Arch. Clin. Neuropsychology* **7**, 481–497.

Brown, R.T., Madan-Swain, A., Walco, G.A., *et al.* (1998) Cognitive and academic late effects among children previously treated for acute lymphocytic leukemia receiving chemotherapy as CNS prophylaxis. *J. Pediat. Psychol.* **23**, 333–340.

Burger, P.C., Boyko, O.B. (1991) The pathology of central nervous system radiation injury. In Gutin, P.H., Leibel, S.A., Sheline, G.E. (Eds) *Radiation Injury to the Nervous System.* New York: Raven Press, pp. 3–15.

Butler, R., Copeland, D.R. (2002) Attentional processes and their remediation in children treated for cancer: A literature review and the development of a therapeutic approach. *J. Int. Neuropsychol. Soc.* **89**, 115–124.

Carpentieri, S., Mulhern, R.K. (1993) Patterns of memory dysfunction among children surviving temporal lobe tumors. *Arch. Clin. Neuropsychol.* **8**, 345–357.

Cavazzuti, V., Winston, K., Baket, R., Welch, K. (1980) Psychological changes following surgery for tumors in the temporal lobe. *J. Neurosurg.* **53**, 618–626.

Cetingul, N., Aydmok, Y., Kantar, M., *et al.* (1999) Neuropsychologic sequelae in the long-term survivors of childhood acute lymphoblastic leukemia. *Pediat. Hematol. Oncol.* **16**, 213–220.

Chou, R.H., Wong, G.B., Kramer, J.H., *et al.* (1996) Toxicities of total-body irradiation for pediatric bone marrow transplantation. *Int. J. Rad. Onc.* **34**, 843–851.

Cohen, R.A. (1993) *The Neuropsychology of Attention.* New York: Plenum Press.

Coley, S.C., Jager, H.R., Szydlo, R.M., Goldman, J.M. (1999) CT and MRI manifestations of central nervous system infection following allogeneic bone marrow transplantation. *Clin. Radiol.* **54**, 390–397.

Coley, S.C., Porter, D.A., Calamante, F., Chong, W.K., Connelly, A. (1999) Quantitative MR diffusion mapping and cyclosporin-induced neurotoxicity. *Am. J. Neuroradiol.* **20**, 1507–1510.

Connors, C.K. (1995) *Connors' Continuous Performance Test.* Toronto: Multi-Health Systems, Inc.

Cool, V.A. (1996) Long-term neuropsychological risks in pediatric bone marrow transplant: what do we know? *Bone Marrow Transpl.* **18**, Suppl. 3, S45–49.

Copeland, D.R., Moore, B.D., Francis, D.J., Jaffe, N., Culbert, S.J. (1996) Neuropsychologic effects of chemotherapy on children with cancer: a longitudinal study. *J. Clin. Oncol.* **14**, 2826–2835.

Corn, B.W., Yousem, D.M., Scott, C.B., *et al.* (1994) White matter changes are correlated significantly with radiation dose. *Cancer* **74**, 2828–2835.

Cousens, P., Waters, B., Said, J., Stevens, M. (1988) Cognitive effects of cranial irradiation in leukaemia: A survey and meta-analysis. *J. Child Clin. Psychiatry* **29**, 839–852.

Cousens, P., Ungerer, J.A., Crawford, J.A., Stevens, M.M. (1991) Cognitive effects of childhood leukemia therapy: A case for four specific deficits. *J. Pediat. Psychol.* **16**, 475–488.

Daneman, M., Carpenter, P.A. (1980) Individual differences in working memory and reading. *Journal of Verbal Learning and Verbal Behavior* **19**, 450–466.

Daniel Llach, M., Perez Campdepadros, M., Baza Ceballos, N., *et al.* Secuelas neuropsicologicas a medio y largo plazo del trasplante de medula osea en pacientes con enfermedades hematologicas. *Anales Pediatria* **54**, 463–467.

de Groot, J.C., de Leeuw, F.E., Oudkerk, M., *et al.* (2000) Cerebral white matter lesions and cognitive function: The Rotterdam scan study. *Annals of Neurology* **47**, 145–151.

Ellenberg, L., McComb, J.G., Siegel, S.E., Stowe, S. (1987) Factors affecting intellectual outcome in pediatric brain tumor patients. *Neurosurgery* **21**, 638.

Engle, R.W., Kane, M.J., Tulholski, S.W. (1999) Individual differences in working memory capacity and what they tell us about controlled attention, general fluid intelligence, and functions of the prefrontal cortex. In Miyake, A., Shah, P. (Eds) *Models of Working Memory: Mechanisms of Active Maintenance and Executive Control.* New York: Cambridge University Press.

Espy, K.A., Moore, I.M., Kaufmann, P.M., Kramer, J.H., Matthay, K., Hutter, J.J. (2001) Chemotherapeutic CNS prophylaxis and neuropsychologic change in children with acute lymphoblastic leukemia: a prospective study. *J. Pediat. Psychol.* **26**, 1–9.

Filley, C.M. (1998) The behavioral neurology of cerebral white matter. *Neurology* **50**, 1535–1540.

Garrick, R. (2000) Neurologic complications. In Atkinson, K. (Ed.) *Clinical Bone Marrow and Blood Stem Cell Transplantation* (2nd edn). New York: Cambridge University Press, pp. 958–979.

Golden, C.J. (1978) *Stroop Color and Word Test.* Wood Dale, IL: Stoelting Co.

Graus, F., Saiz, A., Sierra, J., *et al.* (1996) Neurologic complications of autologous and allogeneic bone marrow transplantation in patients with leukemia: a comparative study. *Neurology* **46**, 1004–1009.

Heideman, R.L., Packer, R.J., Albright, L.A., Freeman, C.R., Rorke, L.B. (1997) Tumors of the central nervous system. In Pizzo, P.A., Poplack, D.G. (Eds) *Principles and Practice of Pediatric Oncology* (2nd edn). Philadelphia, PA: Lippincott, pp. 633–681.

Hill, D.E., Ciesielski, K.T., Sethre-Hofstad, L., Duncan, M.H., Lorenzi, M. (1997) Visual and verbal short-term memory deficits in childhood leukemia survivors after intrathecal chemotherapy. *J. Pediat. Psychol.* **22**, 861–870.

Hirsch, J.F., Rose, C.S., Pierre-Kahn, A., Pfister, A., Hoppe-Hirsch, E. (1989) Benign astrocytic and oligodendrocytic tumors of the cerebral hemispheres in children. *J. Neurosurg.* **70**, 568.

Hopewell, J.W., van der Kogel, A.J. (1999) Pathophysiological mechanisms leading to the development of late radiation-induced damage to the central nervous system. In Wiegel, T., Hinkelbein, W., Brock, M., Hoell, T. (Eds) *Controversies in Neuro-Oncology: Frontiers of Radiation Therapy and Oncology*. Basle: Karger.

Horowitz, M.E., Mulhern, R.K., Kun, L.E., Kovnar, E.K., Sanford, R.A., Simmons, J., Hayes, A., Jenkins, J.J. (1998) Brain tumor in the very young child: Postoperative chemotherapy in combined-modality treatment. *Cancer* **61**, 428–434.

Hudson, M. (1999) Late complications after leukemia therapy. In Pui, C.H. (Ed.) *Childhood Leukemias*. Cambridge: Cambridge University Press, pp. 463–481.

Jannoun, L., Bloom, H.J.G. (1990) Long-term psychological effects in children treated for intracranial tumors. *Int. J. Radiat. Oncol. Biol. Phys.* **18**, 747.

Johnson, D.L., McCabe, M.A., Nicholson, H.S., *et al.* (1994) Quality of long-term survival in young children with medulloblastoma. *J. Neurosurg.* **80**, 1004–1010.

Jonides, J., Smith, E.E. (1997) The architecture of working memory. In Rugg, M.D. (Ed.) *Cognitive Neuroscience*. Cambridge, MA: MIT Press, pp. 243–276.

Jonides, J., Schumacher, E.A., Smith, E.E., Lauber, E.J., Awh, E., Minoshima, S., Koeppe, R.A. (1997) Verbal working memory load affects regional brain activation as measured by PET. *Journal of Cognitive Neuroscience* **9**, 462–476.

Kaleita, T.A., Shields, W.D., Tesler, A., Feig, S. (1989) Normal neurodevelopment in four young children treated for acute leukemia or aplastic anemia. *Pediatrics* **83**, 753–757.

Kaleita, T.A., Reaman, G.H., MacLean, W.E., Sather, H.N., Whitt, J.K. (1999) Neurodevelopmental outcome of infants with acute lymphoblastic leukemia: A children's cancer group report. *Cancer* **85**, 1859–1865.

Klein, D.M. (1984) Principles of neurosurgery. In Cohen, M., Duffner, P. (Eds) *Brain Tumors in Children*. New York: Raven Press, p. 92.

Kramer, J.H., Crittenden, M.R., Halberg, F.E., Wara, W.M., Cowan, M.J. (1992) A prospective study of cognitive function following low-dose cranial radiation for bone marrow transplantation. *Pediatrics* **90**, 447–450.

Kramer, J.H., Crittenden, M.R., DeSantes, K., Cowan, M.J. (1997) Cognitive and adaptive behavior 1 and 3 years following bone marrow transplantation. *Bone Marrow Transpl.* **19**, 607–613.

Lee, Y.Y., Nauert, C., Glass, P. (1986) Treatment-related white matter changes in cancer patients. *Cancer* **57**, 1473–1482.

Lockwood, K.A., Bell, T.S., Colegrove, R.W. (1999) Long-term effects of cranial radiation therapy on attention functioning in survivors of childhood leukemia. *J. Pediat. Psychol.* **24**, 55–66.

Margolin, J.F., Poplack, D.G. (1997) Acute lymphoblastic leukemia. In Pizzo, P.A., Poplack, D.G. (Eds) *Principles and Practice of Pediatric Oncology* (3rd edn). Philadelphia, PA: Lippincott-Raven, pp. 409–462.

Marks, P.V. (1998) Neurological aspects of stem-cell transplantation. In Barrett, J., Treleaven, J. (Eds) *The Clinical Practice of Stem-Cell Transplantation*, Vol. 1. Oxford: ISIS, pp. 787–794.

Mehta, J., Powles, R. (2000) The future of blood and marrow transplantation In Atkinson, K. (Ed.) *Clinical Bone Marrow and Blood Stem Cell Transplantation* (2nd edn). New York: Cambridge University Press, pp. 1457–1465.

Meyers, C.A., Weitzner, M.A., Valentine, A.D. (1998) Methylphenidate therapy improves cognition, mood, and function of brain tumor patients. *J. Clin. Oncol.* **16**, 2522–2527.

Meyers, C.A., Weitzner, M., Byrne, K., *et al.* Evaluation of the neurobehavioral functioning of patients before, during and after bone marrow transplantation. *J Clin. Oncol.* **12**, 820–826.

Meller, S., Pinkerton, R. (1998) Solid tumors in children. In Barrett, J., Treleaven, J. (Eds) *The Clinical Practice of Stem-Cell Transplantation*, Vol. 1. Oxford: ISIS, pp. 173–190.

Miale, T.D., Sirithorn, S., Ahmed, S. (1995) Efficacy and toxicity of radiation in preparative regimens for pediatric stem cell transplantation. I: Clinical applications and therapeutic effects. *Medical Oncology* **12**, 231–249.

Mildenberger, M., Beach, T.G., McGeer, E.G., Ludgate, C.M. (1990) An animal model of prophylactic cranial irradiation: Histological effects at acute, early, and delayed stages. *International Journal of Oncology, Biology, and Physics* **18**, 1051–1060.

Mirsky, A.F., Anthony, B.J., Duncan, C.C., Ahearn, M., Kellam, S.G. (1991) Analysis of the element of attention: A neuropsychological approach. *Neuropsychology Review* **2**, 109–145.

Miyake, A., Shah, P. (1999) Toward unified theories of working memory: Emerging general consensus, unresolved theoretical issues, and future research directions. In Miyake, A., Shah, P. (Eds) *Models of Working Memory: Mechanisms of Active Maintenance and Executive Control*. New York: Cambridge University Press.

Moleski, M. (2000) Neuropsychological, neuroanatomical, and neurophysiological consequences of CNS chemotherapy for acute lymphoblastic leukemia. *Arch. Clin. Neuropsychology* **15**, 603–630.

Monsell, S. (1996) Control of mental processes. In Bruce, V. (Ed.) *Unsolved Mysteries of the Mind: Tutorial Essays in Cognition*. Hove, UK: Erlbaum, pp. 93–148.

Mostow, E.N., Byrne, J., Connelly, R.R., Mulvihill, J.J. (1991) Quality of life in long-term survivors of CNS tumors of childhood and adolescence. *J. Clin. Oncol.* **9**, 592.

Mulhern, R.K., Fairclough, D., Ochs, J. (1991) A prospective comparison of neuropsychologic performance of children surviving leukemia who received 18-Gy, 24-Gy, or no cranial irradiation. *J. Clin. Oncol.* **9**, 1348–1356.

Mulhern, R.K., Phipps, S., Tyc, V.L. (1999) Psychosocial issues. In Pui, C.H. (Ed.) *Childhood Leukemias*. Cambridge: Cambridge University Press, pp. 520–541.

Mulhern, R.K., Kovnar, E.K., Kun, L.E., Crisco, J.J., Williams, J.M. (1988) Psychologic and neurologic function following treatment for childhood temporal lobe astrocytoma. *J. Child Neurol.* **3**, 47.

Mulhern, R.K., Kovnar, E., Langston, J., Carter, M., Fairclough, D., Leigh, L., Kun, L. (1992a) Long-term survivors of leukemia treated in infancy: Factors associated with neuropsychological status. *J. Clin. Oncol.* **10**, 1095–1102.

Mulhern, R.K., Hancock, J., Fairclough, D., Kun, L.E. (1992b) Neuropsychological status of children treated for brain tumors: a critical review and integrative analysis. *Med. Pediatr. Oncol.* **20**, 181.

Mulhern, R.K., Heideman, R.L., Khatib, Z.A., Kovnar, E.H., Sanford, R.A., Kun, L.E. (1994) Quality of survival among children treated for brain stem glioma. *Pediatr. Neurosurg.* **20**, 226–232.

Mulhern, R.K., Kepner, J.L., Thomas, P.R., *et al.* (1998) Neuropsychologic functioning of survivors of childhood medulloblastoma randomized to receive conventional or reduced-dose craniospinal irradiation: A pediatric oncology group study. *J. Clin. Oncol.* **16**, 1723–1728.

Mulhern, R.K., Reddick, W.E., Palmer, S.L., *et al.* (1999) Neurocognitive deficits in medulloblastoma survivors and white matter loss. *Annals of Neurology* **46**, 834–841.

Mulhern, R.K., Palmer, S.L., Reddick, W.E., *et al.* (2001) Risks of young age for selected neurocognitive deficits in medulloblastoma are associated with white matter loss. *Journal of Clinical Oncology* **19**, 472–479.

Pace, M.T., Slovis, T.L., Kelly, J.K., Abella, S.D. (1995) Cyclosporin A toxicity: MRI appearance of the brain. *Pediatr. Radiol.* **25**, 180–183.

Padovan, C.S., Tarek, Y.A., Schleuning, M., Holler, E., Kolb, H.J., Straube, A. (1998) Neurological and neuroradiological findings in long-term survivors of allogeneic bone marrow transplantation. *Ann. Neurol.* **43**, 627–633.

Padovan, C.S., Gerbitz, A., Sostak, P., *et al.* (2001) Cerebral involvement in graft-versus-host disease after murine bone marrow transplantation. *Neurology* **56**, 1106–1108.

Palmer, S.L., Goloubeva, O., Reddick, W.E., *et al.* (2001) Patterns of intellectual development among survivors of pediatric medulloblastoma: a longitudinal analysis. *Journal of Clinical Oncology* **19**, 2302–2308.

Patchell, R.A., White, C.L., Clark, A.W., Beschorner, W.E., Santos, G.W. (1985) Neurologic complications of bone marrow transplantation. *Neurology* **35**, 300–306.

Peper, M., Schraube, P., Kimming, C., Wagensommer, C., Wannenmacher, M., Haas, R. (1993) Long-term cerebral side-effects of total body irradiation and quality of life. *Recent Results in Cancer Research* **130**, 219–230.

Phipps, S., Barclay, D. (1996) Psychosocial consequences of pediatric bone marrow transplantation. *International Journal of Pediatric Hematology/Oncology* **3**, 171–182.

Phipps, S., Brenner, M., Heslop, H., Krance, R., Jayawardene, D., Mulhern, R. (1995) Psychological effects of bone marrow transplant on children: Preliminary report of a longitudinal study. *Bone Marrow Transpl.* **16**, 829–835.

Phipps, S., Dunavant, M., Srivastava, D.K., Bowman, L., Mulhern, R.K. (2000) Cognitive and academic functioning in survivors of pediatric bone marrow transplantation. *J. Clin. Onc.* **18**, 1004–1011.

Posner, M.I., Peterson, S.E. (1990) The attention system of the human brain. *Annual Review of Neuroscience* **13**, 25–42.

Pot-Mees, C.C. (1989) *The Psychological Aspects of Bone Marrow Transplantation in Children.* The Netherlands: Eburon Delft.

Rankin, E.J., Adams, R.L., Jones, H.E. (1996) Epilepsy and nonepileptic attack disorder. In Adams, R.L., Parsons, O.A., Culbertson, J.L., Nixon, S.J. (Eds) *Neuropsychology for Clinical Practice: Etiology, Assessment, and Treatment of Common Neurological Disorders.* Washington, DC: Amercian Psychological Association, pp. 131–173.

Raymond-Speden, E., Tripp, G., Lawrence, B., Holdaway, D. (2000) Intellectual, neuropsychological and academic functioning in long-term survivors of leukemia. *J. Pediat. Psychol.* **25**, 59–68.

Reddick, W.E., Mulhern, R.K., Elkin, T.D., *et al.* (1998) A hybrid neural network analysis of subtle brain volume differences in children surviving brain tumors. *Magnetic Resonance Imaging* **16**, 413–421.

Reddick, W.E., Russell, J.M., Glass, J.O., Xiong, X., Mulhern, R.K., Langston, J.W., Merchant, T.E., Kun, L.E., Gajjar, A. (2000) Subtle white matter volume differences in children treated for medulloblastoma with conventional or reduced dose craniospinal irradiation. *Mag. Res. Imag.* **18**, 787–793.

Reece, D.E., Frei-Lahr, D.A., Shepherd, J.D., *et al.* (1991) Neurologic complications in allogeneic bone marrow transplant patients receiving cyclosporin. *Bone Marrow Transplantation* **8**, 393–401.

Ris, M.D., Noll, R.B. (1994) Long-term neurobehavioral outcome in pediatric brain-tumor patients: Review and methodological critique. *J. Clin. Exper. Neuropsychology* **16**, 21–42.

Ris, M.D., Packer, R., Goldwein, J., Jones-Wallace, D., Boyett, J. (2001) Intellectual outcome after reduced-dose radiation therapy plus adjuvant chemotherapy for medulloblastoma: a Children's Cancer Group Study. *J. Clin. Oncol.* **19**, 3470–3476.

Riva, D., Pantaleone, C., Milani, N., Belani, F.F. (1989) Impairment of neuropsychological functions in children with medulloblastomas and astrocytomas in the posterior fossa. *Childs Nerv. Sys.* **5**, 107.

Rodgers, J., Horrocks, J., Britton, P.G., Kernahan, J. (1999) Attentional ability among survivors of leukaemia. *Archives of Disease in Childhood* **80**, 318–323.

Rogers, R.D., Monsell, S. (1995) Costs of a predictable switch between simple cognitive tasks. *Journal of Experimental Psychology: General* **124**, 207–231.

Roman, D.D., Sperduto, P.W. (1995) Neuropsychological effects of cranial irradiation: current knowledge and future directions. *Int. J. Radiat. Oncol. Biol. Phys.* **31**, 983–998.

Rouah, E., Gruber, R., Shearer, W., Armstrong, D., Hawkins, E.P. (1988) Graft-versus-host disease in the central nervous system. A real entity? *Am. J. Clin. Pathol.* **89**, 543–546.

Rubenstein, C.L., Varni, J.W., Katz, E.R. (1990) Cognitive functioning in long-term survivors of childhood leukemia: a prospective analysis. *Dev. Behavi. Pediat.* **11**, 301–305.

Sanders, J.E. (1997) Bone marrow transplantation in pediatric oncology. In Pizzo, P.A., Poplack, D.G. (Eds) *Principles and Practices of Pediatric Oncology* (3rd edn). New York: Lippincott-Raven, pp. 357–373.

Santos, G.W. (2000) Historical background to hematopoetic stem cell transplantation. In Atkinson, K. (Ed.) *Clinical Bone Marrow and Blood Stem Cell Transplantation* (2nd edn). New York: Cambridge University Press, pp. 1–12.

Schatz, J., Kramer, J.H., Ablin, A., Matthay, K.K. (2000) Processing speed, working memory, and IQ: A developmental model of cognitive deficits following cranial radiation therapy. *Neuropsychology* **14**, 189–200.

Shah, P., Miyake, A. (1999) Models of working memory: An introduction. In Miyake, A., Shah, P. (Eds) *Models of Working Memory: Mechanisms of Active Maintenance and Executive Control.* New York: Cambridge University Press.

Simms, S., Kazak, A.E., Golumb, V.A., Goldwein, J., Bunin, N. (1999) Cognitive and psychological outcome in 2 year survivors of childhood bone marrow transplantation. Paper presented at the University of Pennsylvania Cancer Center Annual Symposium, March.

Simms, S., Kazak, A.E., Gannon, T., Goldwein, J., Bunin, N. (1998) Neuropsychological outcome of children undergoing bone marrow transplantation. *Bone Marrow Transplantation* **22**, 181–184.

Smedler, A.C., Bolme, P. (1995) Neuropsychological deficits in very young bone marrow transplant recipients. *Acta Pediatr.* **84**, 429–433.

Smedler, A.C., Nilsson, C., Bolme, P. (1995) Total body irradiation: a neuropsychological risk factor in pediatric bone marrow transplant recipients. *Acta Pediatr.* **84**, 325–330.

Smedler, A.C., Ringden, K., Bergman, H., Bolme, P. (1990) Sensory-motor and cognitive functioning in children who have undergone bone marrow transplantation. *Acta Paediatr. Scand.* **79**, 613–621.

Sowell, E.R., Thompson, P.M., Holmes, C.J., Jernigan, T.L., Toga, A.W. (1999) In vivo evidence for post-adolescent brain maturation in frontal and striatal regions. *Nature Neuroscience* **2**, 859–861.

Steen, G., Mirro, J. (2000) *Childhood cancer: A Handbook from St. Jude Children's Research Hospital.* Cambridge, MA: Perseus Publishing.

Thompson, C.B., Sanders, J.E., Flournoy, N., *et al.* (1986) The risks of central nervous system relapse and leukoencephalopathy in patients receiving marrow transplants for acute leukemia. *Blood* **67**, 195–199.

Thompson, S., Leigh, L., Christensen, R., *et al.* (2001) Immediate neurocognitive effects of methylphenidate on learning-impaired survivors of childhood cancer. *J. Clin. Oncol.* **19**, 1802–1808.

Treleaven, J., Barrett, J. (1998) Introduction. In Barrett, J., Treleaven, J. (Eds) *The Clinical Practice of Stem-Cell Transplantation*, Vol. 1. Oxford: ISIS, pp. 2–16.

Tsuruda, J.S., Kortman, K.E., Bradley, W.G., *et al.* (1987) Radiation effects on white matter: MR evaluation. *Am. J. Roentgenology* **149**, 165–171.

Waber, D.P., Urion, D.K., Tarbell, N.J., *et al.* (1990) Late effects of central nervous system treatment of acute lymphoblastic leukemia in childhood are sex-dependent. *Developmental Medicine and Child Neurology* **32**, 238–248.

Waber, D.P., Tarbell, N.J., Kahn, C.M., Gelber, R.D., Sallan, S.E. (1992) The relationship of sex and treatment modality to neuropsychologic outcome in childhood acute lymphoblastic leukemia. *Journal of Clinical Oncology* **10**, 810–817.

Waber, D.P., Carpentieri, S.C., Klar, N., *et al.* (2000) Cognitive sequelae in children treated for acute lymphoblastic leukemia with dexamethasone or prednisone. *J. Pediat. Hematol./Oncol.* **22**, 206–213.

Willis, K.E. (1994) Neuropsychological functioning in children with spina bifida and/or hydrocephalus. *J. Clin. Child Psychol.* **22**, 247.

Wingard, J.R. (1997) Bone marrow to blood stem cells: past, present, future. In Whedon, M.B., Wujcik, D. (Eds) *Blood and Marrow Stem Cell Transplantation: Principles, Practice, and Nursing Insights* (2nd edn). Boston: Jones and Bartlett, pp. 3–24.

Wiznitzer, M., Packer, R., August, C., *et al.* (1984) Neurological complications of bone marrow transplantation. *Ann. Neurol.* **16**, 569–576.

3

Palliative Care for Children with Advanced Cancer

JOANNE WOLFE

Children's Hospital Boston, Dana-Farber Cancer Institute, Harvard Medical School, Boston, MA, USA

ANNE TOURNAY

Division of Pediatric Neurology, University of California at Irvine, CA, USA

LONNIE R. ZELTZER

David Geffen School of Medicine at University of California at Los Angeles, CA, USA

INTRODUCTION

Definition of Palliative Care

This chapter will present a philosophy of cancer care that promotes communication between providers, patients (regardless of age), and parents *throughout the illness* with the goal of achieving the best possible quality of life for the child and family. Palliative care can be defined as the active total care of patients and families, including control of pain, other symptoms, and psychological, social and spiritual concerns (Frager 1996). Our emphasis will be on including communication as a primary tenet of palliative care, and on integrating palliative care along the entire disease trajectory, whether the anticipated outcome is cure, chronic disease or death.

Psychosocial Aspects of Pediatric Oncology. Edited by S. Kreitler and M. Weyl Ben Arush
© 2004 John Wiley & Sons Ltd: ISBN 0 471 49939 0

History of Palliative Care

The origin of palliative care lies in the hospices of Europe in the Middle Ages. These provided care to people on pilgrim routes. The Latin word *hospes* initially meant 'stranger', but with time evolved to *hospitium*, which at first described the warmth between guest and host, and later the building where this was experienced (Saunders 1993). The modern era of hospice and palliative care stems from the dedication and enthusiasm of an English physician, Dame Cicely Saunders. She had previously trained as a nurse, and before entering medical school, worked as a voluntary nurse at St Luke's Home for the Dying Poor in London. After qualifying from medical school, Saunders worked at St Joseph's Hospital in Hackney, London, where she explored the use of opioids to achieve pain control in dying patients. She discovered that regular doses of opiates in higher doses than were then standard practice could relieve patients' pain and allow them to talk openly about their illness. Saunders wrote and taught about her experiences, and by 1967 had persuaded the National Health Service to support the building of St Christopher's Hospice in Sydenham, England.

In the North America, nurses and physicians became interested in the ethos of palliative care at St Christopher's. In 1974, funded by the National Cancer Institute, the Connecticut Hospice began offering home-based care. The same year, in New York, a team of specialists in care of the dying started a consulting service at St Luke's Hospital. In 1975, Mount established the Palliative Care Service at The Royal Victoria Hospital, Montreal. Hospice and palliative care were thus demonstrated to be concepts that could be practiced in very varied settings (Saunders 1993).

As palliative care for adults became better established, Chapman and Goodall (1979) drew attention to the need for symptom control in dying children. In 1978, Edmarc Hospice for Children was founded in Virginia by a couple whose son, Marcus, was dying. Edward, the pastor of their church (himself terminally ill), was very supportive of their efforts. The hospice was named in honor of both Edward and Marcus, hence Edmarc. It was a volunteer agency providing home-based nursing support. Later, ancillary services including bereavement counseling were offered by the program (Armstrong-Dailey and Zarbock 2001). The Hospice of Northern Virginia became the first adult home-based care group to provide services for children, in 1979 (Armstrong-Dailey and Zarbock 2001). The first inpatient pediatric palliative care unit was opened at St Mary's Hospital for Children in Bayside, New York in 1985 (Armstrong-Dailey and Zarbock 2001). Initially the majority of admissions were children with chronic disorders, but as AIDS became common amongst inner city children, the program started to care for affected families, as well as children with cancer and other forms of terminal illness.

In 1983, Children's Hospice International (CHI), a US non-profit organization, was founded by Ann Armstrong-Dailey (2001). It provides information and support to families with children who have life-threatening conditions. The group has also been instrumental in offering advice to health care professionals looking after dying children. According to CHI, there are currently 250 hospice programs throughout the USA which provide specialist palliative care to terminally ill children (Armstrong-Dailey and Zarbock 2001).

In the UK, there is a network of over 20 freestanding, charitably funded children's hospices that provide respite and palliative care for children with life-limiting conditions. The first such hospice to be established was Helen House, in Oxford. It was built in response to the realization for the need for such services by the parents of Helen, a child left severely neurologically impaired after brain tumor surgery, and a nun, Mother Frances Dominica, who became friends with the family (Worswick, 1993). Similar children's hospices have been set up in Canada (Davies 1998) and Australia (Stevens and Pollard 1998).

Martinson (1996) has written an overview of international pediatric palliative care. Home-based programs exist in several eastern European countries (such as Poland, Belarus and Russia), while efforts are under way to expand care to dying children in Africa and Asia.

Extent of Need for Pediatric Palliative Care for Children with Cancer

Although the prognosis for children with cancer has improved considerably over the past three decades, the disease remains the leading cause of non-accidental death in childhood. In 1999, 2500 children died of cancer or treatment complications in the USA. Sadly, advances in the control of symptoms in children dying of cancer have not kept pace with treatment directed at curing the underlying disease. In a survey of 103 parents of children who had died of cancer, Wolfe (2000) reported that 89% of the children had suffered 'a great deal' or 'a lot' from at least one symptom during their last month of life. The most common symptoms were pain, fatigue and dyspnea. Attempts at relief of suffering were frequently regarded as unsuccessful by parents; only 27% of children with pain, and 16% with dyspnea were felt to have had adequate control of their symptoms.

Barriers to the Provision of Pediatric Palliative Care

The traditional model of palliative care has represented the relief of symptoms to be the major goal of treatment only when aggressive therapy directed at a cure has been unsuccessful. The overall improvement in prognosis in childhood cancer, and the enormous emotional issues involved in trying to save a child's life can prevent both caregivers and parents from abandoning cancer-directed therapy. Pursuit of intensive cancer-directed therapy can overshadow attention to quality of life and symptom control, which can result in substantial suffering during the last phase of a child's life. However, it is often not possible for parents and/or the child to forgo further cancer-directed therapy, and this should not be required in order to achieve optimal palliative care. The need to ensure that everything possible has been done may be the only way that some parents can live and cope with their child's death (Vickers and Carlisle 2000).

Hospice care for adults dying of cancer is now quite accessible. Unfortunately, children are not 'little adults', either emotionally or physiologically, and relatively few adult hospice care providers receive adequate training in the care of children to feel comfortable looking after them. Since childhood death is uncommon, many primary care pediatricians and pediatric oncologists may even lack training in care of the dying child. In 2000 the American Academy of Pediatrics (2000a) published guidelines on palliative care for children which outlined recommendations for training and minimum standards of care. The lack of an evidence base poses another challenge. As one example, there are very few developmentally appropriate tools to use for symptom and quality-of-life assessments in children (Wong and Baker 1998).

Numerous financial barriers impede early integration of palliative care. The communication required on the part of physicians, nurses, social workers, child life workers, and others, is very time-consuming as we guide families from diagnosis to death. Lack of reimbursement for communication time, typical of pediatrics, is a much larger problem in this setting. More significantly, many state Medicaid hospice programs are based on the federal Medicare model, which was designed for adult patients with cancer. Admission is restricted to patients with a life expectancy of 6 months or less. This stipulation makes it difficult to provide hospice services to many pediatric patients, whose providers, and parents may find it difficult to recognize when a child meets this criterion.

Furthermore, hospice benefits may not cover treatments intended to improve the quality of a child's remaining life, such as transfusions, ventilator support for neuromuscular disorders, or palliative surgery. The total daily reimbursement for hospice services is around $100. At present only 1% of dying children are receiving hospice care. In the USA there are about 2500 adult hospice programs, while only a tenth of that number offer care for children.

Finally, caring for a dying child is emotionally very difficult. It may be particularly difficult for physicians and other caregivers to consider the integration of palliative care because this may be perceived as 'giving up'. More importantly, parental loss of a child is certainly considered to be the most difficult type of loss (Saunders 1979–1980, Whittam 1993). As a result, the emotional cost of recognizing that a child may die impedes planning for optimal care and support.

COMMUNICATION AND DECISION MAKING

Optimal palliation requires the establishment of open and ongoing communication between all careteam members, the child and the family. Wolfe and colleagues (2000) have shown that parents first recognize that the child has no realistic chance for cure more than three months after the primary oncologist realizes this likelihood. Involvement of a child psychologist or social worker was associated with parents and physicians coming to understand the child's terminal prognosis closer together in time. The study also showed that earlier recognition by the physician and parent that the child had no realistic chance for cure was associated with better integration of palliative care. Thus, early and ongoing interdisciplinary discussions aimed at informing parents of the possibility of a child's death might be critical to easing suffering during the end of a child's life.

Introducing Palliative Care

Many have suggested strategies for 'breaking bad news' (Buckman 1992, Suchman *et al.* 1997, Girgis and Sanson-Fisher 1995); however, it remains less clear how to discuss palliative care with families. Billings (1998) suggests the following introduction of palliative care to families: 'Palliative care is a special service, a team approach to providing comfort and support for persons living with life-threatening illness and for their families', leaving out reference to the terminal prognosis. Often the most effective communication begins with open-ended questions such as, 'What concerns you most about you/your child's illness?', 'How is treatment going for you/your child and your family?', 'As you think about your/your child's illness, what is the best and worst that might happen?', 'What are your/your child's hopes (expectations, fears) for the future?' (Lo, Quill and Tulsky 1999). These open-ended questions provide a means to explore the possibility of a child's dying.

Discussing Palliative Care with Children

Very little is known regarding communication about palliative care with children with advanced cancer; however, knowledge of the developmental understanding of death should help guide this generally unexplored area (Table 3.1). Most children learn to recognize when something is 'dead' before they reach 3 years of age, but at this early age death, separation, and sleep are almost synonymous in the child's mind. As children become preschool age, they can recognize that a dead person cannot function, but may believe that death is temporary. Their egocentric reasoning can lead them to believe they can cause death with their thoughts or actions.

Table 3.1 Overview of children's concepts of death

Age range, years	Concept
Birth to 2	Death is perceived as separation or abandonment Protest and despair from disruption in caretaking No cognitive understanding of death
2 to 6	Death is reversible or temporary Death is personified and often seen as punishment Magical thinking that wishes can come true
6 to 11	Gradual awareness of irreversibility and finality Specific death of self or loved one difficult to understand Concrete reasoning with ability to see cause-and-effect relationships
Older than 11	Death is irreversible, universal, and inevitable All people and self must die, although latter is far off Abstract and philosophical reasoning

From American Academy of Pediatrics, Committee on Psychosocial Aspects of Child and Family Health, The pediatrician and childhood bereavement. Reproduced with permission from *Pediatrics*, Vol. 105, pages 445–447, Table 1, Copyright 2000.

School-age children begin to have logical thought and during these years they normally acquire a much more complete understanding of death. By the age of 7, most children understand that death is irreversible, universal, that the dead do not function, and that people die from both internal and external causes. They can be interested in the specific details of death, and in the latter part of this phase they are able to envision their own deaths.

As children become adolescents, their thinking about death is usually consistent with reality. They can begin to also appreciate the effect death has on other people and on society as a whole. However, their future orientation makes it difficult for them to recognize their own deaths as a present possibility, although they can conceive this occurring at some point in the future.

Children with chronic, advanced illness appear to have a precocious understanding of the concepts of death and their personal mortality (Schonfeld 1993, Spinetta, Rigler and Karon 1973, Spinetta 1974, Greenham and Lohmann 1982). Yet, for each individual child, prior experience, social and cultural factors will impact greatly on their understanding of death. Importantly, studies have indicated that children with cancer want to know about their prognosis. In a survey of 50 children with cancer, ages 8–17, 95% of patients wanted to be told if they were dying (Ellis and Leventhal 1993). Although most of the children felt that treatment decisions were up to the physicians, 63% of the adolescents and 28% of the younger children wanted to make their own decisions about palliative therapy. Nitschke *et al.* (1982) reported on their experience of including children between 6 and 20 years in a 'final stage conference' in which progression of disease, minimal chance of cure, imminence of death, and therapeutic options were discussed. These children appeared capable of making rational decisions about further therapy. Others have suggested that children under 11 years of age may not be able to grasp these concepts (Leikin and Connell 1983, Shumway, Grossman and Sarles 1983). The approach should be tailored to the individual child and family.

In order to preserve a relationship that is built on trust and caring the caregiver should always be honest with the child. Children will often know when they are dying and may feel tremendous isolation if they are not given permission to talk openly about their illness and impending death (Hilden, Watterson and Chrastek 2000). Furthermore, it is now generally accepted that children give their assent in medical decision making (Bartholome 1995). In talking to children it is important to stay open and receptive when the child initiates a conversation. 'Teachable moments' may be fleeting, and an immediate response is necessary to capitalize on them. Alternatively, many children communicate best through nonverbal means such as artwork or music. For example, they may be more willing to 'talk things over' with puppets or stuffed animals rather than real people. Finally, euphemistic expressions about death can be very confusing or even frightening for children (for instance, equating death with sleep may result in the child being afraid of going to bed), and should always be avoided.

Resuscitation Status

It can be very difficult to initiate discussions about the appropriateness of cardiopulmonary resuscitation efforts for children with advanced cancer (Goold, Williams and Arnold 2000). As a result, medical caregivers may avoid these conversations until respiratory or cardiac collapse appears imminent or may not initiate them at all (SUPPORT 1995). This may account for why 45% of children with advanced cancer who die in the hospital die in the intensive care unit (Wolfe *et al.* 2000). Clearly, parents would be better able to consider this decision if they were not in the midst of a crisis. Thus advanced discussion about resuscitation status may be very beneficial to the child and family.

Wolfe and Grier suggest approaching this sensitive topic by framing it as 'in the worst case scenario, we would like you to consider whether your child should undergo cardiopulmonary resuscitation (CPR) efforts if we believe s/he has an irreversible problem' (Pizzo and Poplack 2002). This approach, along with reassurance that a life-threatening event is not imminent, may allow parents to maintain hope while facing this decision. It may also be helpful to reassure parents that should the child's condition improve, this status would be reconsidered. At the same time, if parents are unable to make a decision about resuscitation status, caregivers should not labor the point, and recognize that for some parents this is an impossible decision to make. Ideally, optimal palliative care should be delivered wherever the child is residing, even in the intensive care unit.

Careful thought should be placed on the exact words used during a discussion about resuscitation status. Parents often think that agreeing to 'do not resuscitate' (DNR) status is choosing death over life for their children. It is helpful to explain that it is the uncontrolled cancer that would be the cause of death. More concretely, using the phrase 'do not resuscitate' may imply that, when attempted, resuscitation is always successful. However, among children with far-advanced cancer, the likelihood of being extubated once on a ventilator and surviving is extremely low. Thus, when approaching families about this issue, it is recommended to use the phrase: 'do not *attempt* resuscitation' (DNAR) (Foex 2000).

Location of Care

Over half of children with progressive cancer die at home (Wolfe *et al.* 2000, Sirkia *et al.* 1997). Some have suggested that a home death may promote better family adjustment and healing (Lauer *et al.* 1983, 1989). This may be related to fewer feelings of helplessness and greater opportunity for family intimacy offered by being at home. Others have found family relationships to be better when the child died in the hospital (Birnbaum and Robinson 1991). While many have suggested that most children prefer to die at home, this too has not been systematically evaluated.

Regardless, it is critically important to discuss preferences regarding the primary location of care as early as possible. Options include inpatient care or home care with or without the support of a home care team. Presently, more and more hospitals are developing palliative care services, the impact of which has yet to be evaluated (Hockley 1999, Adam 1999, Liben and Goldman 1998, Weissman and Griffie 1994). Home care teams might include a visiting nurse association, bridge programs or hospice. There are very few inpatient pediatric hospice units in the USA. A parental decision to care for their terminally ill child at home involves consideration of medical, psychological, social and cultural factors together with such practical considerations as the availability of respite care, physician access, and financial resources (Liben and Goldman 1998). Whatever the decision is regarding the primary location of care, families should be reassured that they can change from one option to another and that the primary team will remain closely involved (Collins, Stevens and Cousens 1998).

CANCER-DIRECTED THERAPY

Parents will most often opt for continued treatment of the underlying cancer even when there is no realistic hope for cure (Wolfe *et al.* 2000, Goldman and Heller 2000). This is often motivated either by hope for a miracle, a desire to extend life, or a desire to palliate symptoms related to progressive disease. In discussions of treatment options with families, Wolfe and Grier suggest the following statement, 'The very nature of miracles is that they are rare. However, we have seen miracles, and they have occurred both on and off treatment' (Pizzo and Poplack 2002). In other words, a child does not have to continue on cancer-directed therapy in order to preserve hope, especially when the therapy significantly impacts the child's remaining quality of life. Regardless, decisions regarding continued cancer-directed therapy need to be carefully considered, weighing the potential for life extension and impact on quality of life.

Chemotherapy

Chemotherapy can both prolong life and lessen suffering. However, administration of treatments may also lead to increased numbers of physician–patient interactions, visits to clinic, admissions to the hospital and most importantly treatment-related complications requiring increased supportive care. Among adult patients, a number of studies show improved quality of life in patients receiving chemotherapy compared to those who were not (Cassileth *et al.* 1991, Coates *et al.* 1987, Ellis *et al.* 1995, Poon *et al.* 1999, Geels *et al.* 2000). Possible reasons for this include placebo effect, provision of hope, and/or increased medical attention associated with being on treatment. The impact of chemotherapy in children with advanced cancer has not been studied and may depend on the developmental stage of the child and awareness of disease state. For example, increased interactions with medical personnel may outweigh any improvements in quality of life for the child. Parents may also have differing views on the role of continued cancer-directed therapy. Wolfe and colleagues (2000) found that only 13% of parents reported that the primary goal of cancer-directed therapy for their child during the end-of-life care period was to lessen suffering. The majority of parents maintained a primary goal of extending life. Communication around this issue must be very clear and tailored to the individual family.

Several agents have been shown to be well tolerated in children and to have some anti-tumor effect. For example, oral etoposide has anti-tumor effect with limited toxicity in children with refractory neuroblastoma, germ cell tumors, brain tumors, rhabdomyosarcoma and other solid tumors (Kushner, Kramer and Cheung 1999, Porcu *et al.* 2000, Davidson *et al.* 1997, Chamberlain 1997, Chamberlain and Kormanik 1997, Needle 1997, Ashley *et al.* 1996, Mathew *et al.* 1994). Relapsed acute lymphoblastic leukemia may be temporarily controlled with regimens including vincristine, methotrexate, prednisone and 6-mercaptopurine. The decision about whether or not to continue cancer-directed therapy must carefully balance considerations of efficacy, potential treatment-related complications and psychological impact.

Phase I Trials

The goal of phase I research is to determine the toxicities and maximum-tolerated dose of an investigational drug or drugs. However, only one-third of adults enrolled in a phase I trial were able to state the purpose of the trial (Daugherty *et al.* 1995). Most cancer patients who participate in phase I trials are strongly motivated by the hope of therapeutic benefit and not altruistic feelings. Yet overall, the chance of tumor response in phase I trials is low, ranging from 4% to 6% (Daugherty *et al.* 1995, Decoster, Stein and Holdener 1990). In children the response rate is similar (Shah *et al.* 1998). At the same time the chance of fatal toxicity is also low at approximately 0.5% (Decoster, Stein and Holdener 1990, Shah *et al.* 1998). Physicians also tend to assume more positive potential benefit from experimental chemotherapy than statistics would warrant (Daugherty *et al.* 1995). Although these biases are not presented to the family with any intention of doing harm, they may make the informed consent process exceedingly difficult and potentially raise serious ethical questions (Emanuel 1995).

Similar to discussions around chemotherapy, it is critical to ensure effective communication when discussing phase I therapy for children with advanced cancer. Furthermore, it is strongly recommended that children give their assent to participation in clinical trials (American Academy of Pediatrics 1995).

Radiation Therapy

Approximately half of all courses of radiation therapy are delivered with palliative intent with the goal of relieving symptoms, and complete elimination of the tumor is not necessary (Kirkbride 1995). Larger fraction sizes over shorter timeframes can be used in most cases, as late-arising complications are not of major concern (Gaze 1997). Munro and Sebag-Montefiore (1992) have devised the concept of 'opportunity cost', i.e. what the time spent on the treatment of a dying patient costs in terms of lost opportunities in his or her remaining lifespan. Common indications for palliative radiation include (Kirkbride 1995):

- Pain relief from bone metastases or pulmonary metastases, and tumors causing nerve root and soft tissue infiltration.
- Control of bleeding.
- Control of fungation and ulceration.
- Relief of impeding or actual obstruction – for example of the large airways.
- Shrinkage of tumor masses causing symptoms – such as brain metastases, skin lesions, and other sites.
- Oncological emergencies – such as spinal cord compression, superior vena-caval obstruction.

In the absence of symptoms to palliate, there is probably little value in giving treatment unless it is apparent that significant problems are incipient.

SYMPTOM MANAGEMENT

Children with advanced cancer experience a high prevalence of symptoms during the last month of life and parents report limited success in alleviating symptom distress (Wolfe *et al.* 2000, Collins *et al.* 2000). Any distress should be considered a medical emergency requiring direct evaluation of the patient and immediate implementation of interventions.

The constellation of symptoms that a child dying of cancer may experience is determined by the site of the tumor and any metastatic disease, and the side effects or complications of treatment. In children, many tumors spread widely and aggressively, so that the terminal stage of illness may be short when compared to an adult with cancer (Goldman 1998). Pain management forms a major part of the care of a child dying of cancer, but other symptoms may also need to be addressed. The extent to which the precise underlying cause of a symptom needs to be established should be tempered by the child's ability to tolerate investigations; it may be more appropriate to just try to alleviate the suffering.

Fatigue

Fatigue is the most common symptom experienced by children with terminal cancer in the last month of life yet little is known about the pathogenesis or treatment of this patient population.

- Causes
  - Progressive disease
  - Anemia
  - Malnutrition
  - Intercurrent illness such as infection
  - Respiratory compromise
  - Cardiac, renal, hepatic compromise
  - Sleep disturbance
  - Medication side-effect
  - Psychological factors such as depression
- Evaluation
  - Thorough history and physical exam
  - Laboratory tests can be helpful such as hemoglobin level
- Treatment
  - If related directly to advanced disease, expectations for reversal are limited and should be explained to the patient and parents

– Dextroamphetamine can be helpful to counteract opioid-related somno-
lence and depression
– Transfusions
– Amitriptyline can help with sleep disturbance

Pain

More than 80% of children with advanced cancer experience pain, regardless of
the underlying diagnosis and this symptom is often inadequately controlled
(Wolfe *et al.* 2000, Sirkia 1998). For a complete discussion of pain, see Chapter 4.
Undertreatment of pain may be related to several critical barriers to effective pain
management. These include, a general deficit in knowledge and experience
(Ingham and Foley 1998, Buchanan and Tolle 1995), the unsubstantiated fear of
inducing addiction (Porter and Hick 1980, Levin, Cleeland and Dar 1985, Fife,
Irick and Painter 1993, Elliott *et al.* 1995), the symbolic implication that
beginning a morphine drip is equivalent to 'giving up on a patient' (Field and
Cassel 1997), and importantly the inappropriate fear of hastening death through
respiratory depression, excess sedation, or both (Solomon *et al.* 1993). Open
communication regarding these issues among medical caregivers and the
family may be an important means to overcoming these barriers.

- Causes
  - Progressive disease
  - Procedural pain
- Evaluation
  - Thorough history and physical exam
  - Radiological tests can be helpful depending on the goals of the patient
    and family
- Treatment
  - Important to take a multimodal approach using medications, cognitive
    interventions, and local anesthetics when appropriate
  - Stepwise approach from weak analgesics (e.g., acetaminophen or non-
    steroidal anti-inflammatory drugs (NSAIDS)) to strong ones (e.g.
    morphine, fentanyl, or hydromorphone) (WHO 1998)
  - Adjuvant drug therapies can be very helpful such as anticonvulsants or
    tricyclic antidepressants for neuropathic pain (Billings 1994)
  - Non-pharmacological strategies, including guided imagery, hypnosis,
    meditation, acupuncture, and acupressure, can also be helpful (Rusy and
    Weisman 2000)

Neurological Symptoms

Seizures

Seizures are frightening for family members to witness. They may have a
variety of underlying etiologies.

- Causes
  - Primary or metastatic tumor in the brain
  - Metabolic derangement (hypo- or hyper-natremia, hypomagnesemia, hypoglycemia, uremia)
  - Vascular (stroke, bleed)
  - Medication effects (neoplastic agents such as intrathecal methotrexate, vincristine, cisplatin, L-asparaginase. Some antibiotics, such as imipenem, can also lower seizure threshold, as can psychotropic medications such as buproprion)
- Evaluation
  - Make sure that the airway is clear, check vital signs, response to stimulus, examine for new neurological abnormalities. Check for papilledema (evidence of raised intracranial pressure)
  - Check blood glucose, electrolytes, renal, hepatic function and a disseminated intravascular coagulation (DIC) panel
  - MRI may show lesions not seen on CT scan, especially in early stages of stroke, or brain injury secondary to treatment (the radiologist may be helpful in recommending particular MRI sequences)
  - EEG can help to clarify the seizure type, and guide medication use
- Management
  - Reassure the family. The vast majority of seizures stop spontaneously within seconds or minutes. Short seizures do not cause brain damage, and death during a seizure is extremely rare
  - Do not put anything in the child's mouth. This may result in damage to the tongue or teeth. If possible, turn the child on their side to allow saliva or vomit to drain out
  - Move away any objects on which the child may injure themselves
  - Administer lorazepam 0.1 mg/kg intravenously (maximum 2 mg as a single dose, may repeat once) or rectal diazepam. If this is unsuccessful in stopping the seizure, an intravenous load of either phenobarbital or phenytoin may be necessary. The dose for each medication is 20 mg/kg. Phenytoin needs to be given at no greater than 1–3 mg/kg/min (maximum 50 mg/min) as it is potentially cardiotoxic and a vein irritant

Spinal cord compression

Although not life-threatening, spinal cord compression may cause severe and irreversible neurological impairment including paralysis, and loss of bowel and bladder control, which can be very distressing. Back pain occurs in 80% of children with cord compression (Lewis *et al.* 1986).

- Causes
  - Solid tumors (such as sarcoma, neuroblastoma)

  - Leukemia (initial presentation or relapse)
  - Osteoporosis or vertebral collapse
- Evaluation
  - Detailed neurological examination including motor and sensory testing
  - Percuss spine
  - Assess sphincter tone
  - MRI of the spine is essential. Plain X-ray films are rarely adequate
- Management
  - Emergency evaluation addressing underlying problem. Consider radiation, chemotherapy, decompression laminectomy
  - Dexamethasone 1–2 mg/kg as loading dose followed by 1.5 mg/kg divided Q6 hours (maximum dose 4 mg) to decrease edema.

Respiratory Symptoms

Dyspnea

Many children dying of cancer have respiratory symptoms, the commonest of which is dyspnea. This is an unpleasant, often frightening sensation of shortness of breath. It is a subjective feeling – hypoxia or hypercarbia do not need to be present.

- Causes
  - Metastatic cancer
  - Pneumonia
  - Pleural effusion
  - Congestive heart failure
- Evaluation
  - Detailed evaluation of chest including auscultation and percussion
  - Chest radiography or CT scans may be helpful
- Management
  - Reassurance, and, if necessary, anxiolytics
  - Open a window, use a fan near the bedside
  - Blow-by air is often as effective as oxygen
  - Nebulized opioids can produce good relief of dyspnea. They have been associated with bronchospasm in patients with underlying reactive airways disease. Fentanyl has less histamine effect. The usual starting dose is 4 hours' worth of the patient's total IV opioid dose

Cough

- Causes
  - Lung or pleura involvement by primary or metastatic tumor
  - Pleural effusion
  - Underlying asthma
  - Infection

- Gastro-esophageal reflux
- Heart failure
- Post-nasal drip/sinusitis
- Medications
- Evaluation
  - Usually not indicated. Consider chest X-ray if concern regarding pleural effusion that may require drainage for symptom relief
- Management
  - Address underlying cause if possible
  - *Dry cough:* Simple linctus, linctus containing codeine if not on opioids. If on opioids, morphine sulfate and dexamethasone
  - *Wet cough (patient able to produce sputum):* Humidify air, albuterol nebulizers and chest physical therapy to loosen secretions
  - *Wet cough (patient unable to raise sputum):* Scopolamine patch (use a quarter of a patch at first, increasing in increments of a quarter patch as needed). Medication can rarely provoke seizures, especially if a whole patch is used initially. Glycopyrrolate (does not have a central effect), opioids, anxiolytics

Hemoptysis

Fortunately, this is rare, but is terrifying for the child and family.

- Causes
  - Bleeding from an extra-pulmonary source (nose, mouth)
  - Bleeding from a vessel into a bronchus
  - Pneumonia
  - Pulmonary embolism
- Evaluation
  - Inspect locally
  - Chest X-ray
- Management
  - *Small amount of blood (specks or streaks):* Cough suppressants, reassurance, anxiolytics
  - *Massive hemoptysis:* Morphine sulfate, Trendelenburg position to decrease the symptoms of suffocation. Lie child with affected side (if known) down to decrease bleeding into good lung, anxiolytics. Use dark-colored towels or blankets to clear away blood

Gastro-intestinal Symptoms

Mucositis

This is a common and painful complication of chemotherapy, bone marrow transplantation, and radiation. It is due to an inflammatory necrosis of the upper and lower gastro-intestinal tract.

- Causes
  - *Chemotherapy related:* Peaks by the end of the first week following treatment
  - *Radiation therapy related:* Presents by the second week of treatment, and may increase in severity between 2 and 3 weeks after the end of the therapy
- Management
  - Mucositis is self-limiting, recovery taking place when the neutrophil count rises above 500–1000
  - Ice chips orally at the time of infusion of fluorouracil and adriamycin may decrease mucositis
  - Mouth care every 4 hours. A 'star and rewards' chart is helpful
  - Topical analgesics, e.g., Benadryl/viscous lidocaine/Maalox 1:1:1 mixture
  - Avoid heavily seasoned and acidic foods
  - Moisten food with gravy or sauces
  - Frozen yoghurt may be soothing

Anorexia and dehydration

Poor nutrition and dehydration in the terminal child are complex issues evoking intense emotional response in medical caregivers and families. When present, anorexia is usually more distressing to the parents than the dying child. Reassurance that decreasing appetite is a normal part of the dying process is necessary, and aggressive measures to provide nutrition should be avoided, as they may not improve wellbeing. The goal of nutrition and fluid management should be to alleviate any hunger and thirst, to reduce anxiety and to preserve the social aspects of meal time.

- Evaluation
  - Find out the child's food likes and dislikes, and accommodate them
  - Look for mucositis
  - Check for problems with taste or sense of smell
  - Ask about nausea and vomiting
  - Make sure that the child is not having problems with bowel movements
  - Consider malabsorption
  - Laboratory investigations if indicated
- Management
  - To improve quality of life
  - Reassure the parents to let the child eat what they want
  - Serve small portions of attractively presented food
  - Dexamethasone, cannabinoids or megestrol acetate can improve appetite if anorexia is distressing to the child

– Nasogastric and total parenteral nutrition should be considered depending on the patient and families' values and needs

Hiccups

These are infrequent, but can cause irritation. They are probably generated by the interference in a complex neurologically mediated loop connecting the brain stem, midbrain and respiratory center. Their frequency is usually between 4 and 60 hiccups per minute. Hiccups are usually self-limiting.
- Causes
  - Gastric distension (decreased motility, 'squashed stomach')
  - Central nervous system disturbance (release of higher center inhibition of the hiccup reflex)
  - Irritation of the vagus or phrenic nerve
  - Metabolic derangements – uremia, hypocalcemia, hyponatremia, sepsis
  - Drugs – IV corticosteroids, barbiturates, benzodiazepines
- Evaluation
  - Establish the severity and duration of hiccups
  - Determine the relationship to sleep (if hiccups stop during sleep, likely to be psychogenic)
  - Review medications
  - Check electrolytes
  - Consider chest X-ray
- Management
  - *Non-pharmacologic:* (1) Nasopharyngeal stimulation (e.g., lifting uvula with a cotton tip swab, swallowing a spoonful of dry sugar, forced traction of the tongue to provoke a gag response, sipping ice water). (2) Vagal afferent stimulation (e.g., valsalva maneuver, breath-holding, rebreathing. This increases the pCO_2, decreasing hiccup frequency.)
  - *Pharmacologic:* (1) Metaclopramide (increases gastric emptying, has a central antidopaminergic action). (2) Antacids with simethicone (useful if gastric distension is part of the problem). (3) Peppermint water (opposes the action of metaclopramide, relaxing lower esophageal sphincter). (4) Haloperidol (central effect). (5) Anticonvulsants (phenytoin, carbamazepine, valproate). (6) Baclofen

Constipation

Constipation is distressing to both the child and the family.
- Cause
  - Inactivity
  - Opioids

- Poor oral intake
- Direct compression of the bowel by tumor
- Neurological impairment due to tumor invasion of spinal cord or sacral nerve roots
- Evaluation
  - When did the child last have a bowel movement?
  - Consistency of stool
  - Any pain with stooling?
  - Any incontinence?
  - Blood or mucus in stool?
  - Use of laxatives/suppositories/enemas
  - Examine for abdominal distension, hard impacted feces, empty rectum (?proximal fecal impaction), hemorrhoids, fissures, perineal mucositis
- Management
  - Start a stool softener (e.g., docussate sodium) and a bowel stimulant (senna) in appropriate doses at the same time as starting an opioid
  - Add a stool lubricant (e.g. mineral oil) if necessary
  - Suppositories (rarely, enemas) may help in severe constipation
  - In neurological impairment, use stool softeners together with gentle disimpaction and evacuation if necessary
  - Irradiation to shrink an impinging tumor may not significantly benefit the dying child

Bowel obstruction

Bowel obstruction may cause severe pain and vomiting.

- Causes
  - *Cancer related:* Tumor mass pressing on the outside of the bowel, within the bowel lumen, intussusception with tumor as the focal point, or invasion of the neural plexus supplying the gut
  - *Treatment related:* Adhesions following surgery, fecal impaction, drug-induced (opioids, neurotoxicity from vinca alkaloids, tricyclics), small bowel damage due to radiation, paralytic ileus (due to electrolyte abnormalities, pneumonia)
- Evaluation
  - Attempt to identify clinically the cause of the obstruction, whether high in the gut (duodenum), low (colon) or due to paralytic ileus
  - X-ray examination may be indicated if the child is not imminently dying, and may be a candidate for palliative surgery
  - *High intestinal obstruction:* Pain is severe, colicky, often epigastric, vomiting occurs early, contains bile and mucus, and is copious.

Abdomen is not greatly distended, bowel sounds may be normal, succussion splash may be present
- *Lower intestine obstruction:* Pain often suprapubic, less intense, vomiting occurs late, may be feculent, abdomen is distended, hyperactive bowel sounds
- *X-ray findings in bowel obstruction:* Bowel is distended proximal to obstruction, empty distally. Air-fluid levels present on upright film in a 'step-ladder pattern'. Differentiate from severe constipation, where the colon has a ground-glass appearance throughout due to feces
- *Paralytic ileus:* Pain is not colicky, may be present due to abdominal distension. Vomiting is frequent but not usually copious but contains bile. Hiccups are common. X-ray shows widespread gas and fluid distension of both small and large bowel. Upright film shows balanced air-fluid levels in long loops
- Management
  - Try to avoid nasogastric suction, which is uncomfortable, interferes with coughing, and can lead to aspiration. If other medical management is ineffective in relief of symptoms, especially vomiting, nasogastric suction may be indicated
  - *Colicky abdominal pain:* Stop irritant laxatives (e.g., senna) and medications which increase gastric motility (e.g., metaclopramide). Antispasmodics, such as scopolamine patch, may be helpful
  - *Constant abdominal pain:* Use morphine sulfate orally or in a syringe pump
  - *Nausea and vomiting:* Droperidol or haloperidol may be useful.

MEANINGFULNESS AND QUALITY OF LIFE AT THE END OF LIFE

Adequate pain and symptom management, strengthening relationships with loved ones, and avoiding inappropriate prolongation of dying are among a set of priorities elicited from adult patients with terminal illness (Singer, Martin and Kelner 1999). Similar research has not been conducted in children or their parents. However, experience teaches us that these are critical considerations. Furthermore, families must have the opportunity to carry out important family, religious, and/or cultural rituals during the child's end-of-life care period (Levetown 1998). The families' sense of spirituality or engagement in a religious community may provide a structure for positive coping strategies for both parent and child (Barnes *et al.* 2000). 'The goal is to add life to the child's years, not simply years to the child's life' (American Academy of Pediatrics 2000a). Facilitating memory building during this period can be the greatest gift to the child and family.

Table 3.2 Life cycle stories for children

Book	Notes
Al-Chokhachy, E. *The Angel with the Golden Glow*. Marblehead, MA: The Penny Bear Co., 1998.	A story about a special little boy and his family and how they savored every moment they shared.
Branderburg, A. *The Two of Them*. New York: Mulberry Books, 1979.	The story of the special relationship between a girl and her grandfather.
Breebart, J. and Breebart, P. *When I Die, Will I Get Better?* Belgium: Peter Bedrick Books, 1993.	A story about rabbit brothers written by a 6-year-old boy as he tries to come to terms with the death of his younger brother.
Brown, L. and Brown, M. *When Dinosaurs Die*. Boston: Little, Brown & Co., 1996.	A guide for understanding death, using dinosaurs as the characters.
Buscaglia, L. *The Fall of Freddie the Leaf: A Story of Life for All Ages*. Thorofare, NJ: Slack, Inc., 1982.	Freddie and his companion leaves change with the passing seasons, finally falling to the ground with winter's snow.
Carlstrom, N. *Blow Me a Kiss, Miss Lilly*. New York: HarperCollins, 1990.	The relationship between a young girl and her elderly neighbor during her illness.
Coerr, E. and Young, E. *Sadako and the Thousand Paper Cranes*. New York: G.P. Putnam & Sons, 1993.	Sadako's journey through illness and death, illustrating her courage and strength.
Coleman, W. *When Someone You Love Dies*. Minneapolis, MN: Augsburg, 1994.	Advice and support for children ages 8–12 and their parents on fears and questions they have when someone they love dies.
Fahy, M. *The Tree that Survived the Winter*. New York: Paulist Press, 1989.	For survivors who find joy and compassion on the other side of suffering.
Gootman, M. *When a Friend Dies: A Book for Teens about Grieving and Healing*. Minneapolis, MN: Free Spirit Publishing Inc., 1994.	A book of wisdom and compassion for grieving teens, their parents and educators.
Grollman, E. *Straight Talk about Death for Teenagers*. Boston: Beacon Press, 1993.	For teenagers who have lost a friend or relative to death. Includes a journal section to record memories, feelings, and hopes.
Holden, D. *Gran-Gran's Best Trick: A Story for Children Who Have Lost Someone They Love*. Washington, DC: Magination Press, 1989.	A young girl whose beloved grandfather battles cancer learns that those we love never leave our hearts and that this is 'love's best trick'.
Johnson, J. and Johnson, M. *Where's Jess?* Omaha, NE: Centering Corp., 1982.	When a brother or sister dies, a child may have these questions and feelings.

(Continued)

Table 3.2 (*Continued*)

Book	Notes
Levy, J. *The Spirit of Tío Fernando: A Day of the Dead Story*. Morton Grove, IL: Albert Whitman & Company, 1995.	This bilingual story describes a young boy's understanding of death through the Mexican Day of the Dead celebration.
London, J. and Long, S. *Liplap's Wish*. San Francisco: Chronicle Books, 1994.	Little bunny Liplap wrestles with his grandmother's death and finds solace in his mother's tale about the First Rabbits becoming 'stars in the sky'.
Mills, J.C. *Gentle Willow*. New York: Magination Press, 1993.	How friends help a willow tree face a terminal illness.
Mundy, M. *Sad Isn't Bad*. St. Meinrad, IN: Abbey Press, 1998.	A good grief guidebook for children dealing with loss.
Romain, T. *What on Earth Do You Do When Someone Dies?* Minneapolis, MN: Free Spirit Publishing, 1999.	Children's questions about death.
Sasso, S. E. *For Heaven's Sake, What is Heaven? Where do we find it?* Woodstock, VT: Jewish Lights Publishing, 1999.	Isaiah goes on a search for heaven after his grandfather dies and finds it where he least expects it.
Stickney, D. *Water Bugs and Dragonflies*. Cleveland, OH: The Pilgrim Press, 1982.	A beautiful life cycle story.
Varley, S. *Badger's Parting Gifts*. New York: A Mulberry Paperback Book, 1984.	An aging badger prepares for his death.
Viorst, J. *The Tenth Good Thing about Barney*. New York: Atheneum Books, 1971.	Plans for a funeral for pet cat Barney.
Wigand, M. *Heavenly Ways to Heal from Grief and Loss*. St. Meinrad, IN: Abbey Press, 1998.	Let the angel in you lend strength and comfort as you journey from grief to grace.
Wild, M. *Old Pig*. New York: Penguin Books, 1995.	Old Pig and her grand-daughter say 'good-bye' in the best way they know.

For many children, the social context of school and friendship is most important. The care team should encourage the child's continued participation in a school setting, even if attendance is limited by the child's physical deterioration to 'social' visits. Whether the child is based at home or in an institution, regular social contact with other children and adults should be strongly encouraged. This may involve a shift of attitude in families that have been very protective about visitors for fear of introducing infection to the child on chemotherapy.

Intense support of siblings during the final phase of a child's life is critical to ensuring healing. Siblings of a dying child often hold misconceptions and misunderstandings about the child's illness. Specific, concrete information about the dying child's illness as well as the siblings' own health, may do much to allay fears (American Academy of Pediatrics 2000b). Many children's books on dying, death, and bereavement are available for families to use in helping siblings mourn (Table 3.2).

SUMMARY

High-quality care for children with advanced cancer is now an expected standard (American Academy of Pediatrics 2000a, Field and Behrman 2002). However, there remain significant barriers to achieving optimal care related to lack of formal education, reimbursement issues and the emotional impact of caring for a dying child. Whenever possible, treatment should focus on continued efforts to control the underlying illness. At the same time, children and their families should have access to interdisciplinary care aimed at promoting optimal physical, psychological and spiritual wellbeing. Open and compassionate communication can best facilitate meeting the goals of these children and families. Future research efforts should focus on ways to enhance communication, symptom management and quality of life for children with advanced cancer and their families. Being present with children with advanced cancer and their families is at the same time a great gift and intensely rewarding on a personal level.

REFERENCES

Adam, J. (1999) Palliative care service in an acute teaching hospital – the first three years. *Oncol. Nurs. Forum* **26**(8), 1281–1282.

American Academy of Pediatrics (1995) Informed consent, parental permission, and assent in pediatric practice. Committee on Bioethics, American Academy of Pediatrics [see comments]. *Pediatrics* **95**(2), 314–317.

American Academy of Pediatrics (2000a) Committee on Bioethics and Committee on Hospital Care. Palliative care for children. *Pediatrics* **106**(2 Pt 1), 351–357.

American Academy of Pediatrics (2000b) The pediatrician and childhood bereavement. American Academy of Pediatrics. Committee on Psychosocial Aspects of Child and Family Health. *Pediatrics* **105**(2), 445–447.

Armstrong-Dailey, A. (2001) Preface. In Armstrong-Dailey, A., Zarbock, S. (Eds) *Hospice Care for Children*. Oxford: Oxford University Press.

Armstrong-Dailey, A., Zarbock, S. (2001) Introduction. In Armstrong-Dailey, A., Zarbock, S. (Eds) *Hospice Care for Children*. Oxford: Oxford University Press.

Ashley, D.M., *et al.* (1996) Response of recurrent medulloblastoma to low-dose oral etoposide. *J. Clin. Oncol.* **14**(6), 1922–1927.

Barnes, L.J., *et al.* (2000) Spirituality, religion, and pediatrics: Intersecting worlds of healing. *Pediatrics* **104**(6), 899–908.

Bartholome, W.G. (1995) Informed consent, parental permission, and assent in pediatric practice [letter; comment]. *Pediatrics* **96**(5 Pt 1), 981–982.

Billings, J.A. (1994) Neuropathic pain. *J. Palliat. Care* **10**(4), 40–43.

Billings, J.A. (1998) What is palliative care? *Journal of Palliative Medicine* **1**, 73–82.

Birenbaum, L.K., Robinson, M.A. (1991) Family relationships in two types of terminal care. *Soc. Sci. Med.* **32**(1), 95–102.

Buchan, M.L., Tolle, S.W. (1995) Pain relief for dying persons: dealing with physicians' fears and concerns. *J. Clin. Ethics* **6**(1), 53–61.

Buckman, R. (1992) *How to break bad news.* Baltimore: Johns Hopkins University Press.

Cassileth, B.R., *et al.* (1991) Survival and quality of life among patients receiving unproven as compared with conventional cancer therapy [see comments]. *N. Engl. J. Med.* **324**(17), 1180–1185.

Chamberlain, M.C. (1997) Recurrent supratentorial malignant gliomas in children. Long-term salvage therapy with oral etoposide. *Arch. Neurol.* **54**(5), 554–558.

Chamberlain, M.C., Kormanik, P.A. (1997) Chronic oral VP-16 for recurrent medulloblastoma. *Pediatr. Neurol.* **17**(3), 230–234.

Chapman, J., Goodall, J. (1979) Dying children need help too. *Brit. Med. J.* **1**, 593–594.

Coates, A., *et al.* (1987) Improving the quality of life during chemotherapy for advanced breast cancer. A comparison of intermittent and continuous treatment strategies. *N. Engl. J. Med.* **317**(24), 1490–1495.

Collins, J.J., Stevens, M.M., Cousens, P. (1998) Home care for the dying child. A parent's perception. *Aust. Fam. Physician* **27**(7), 610–614.

Collins, J.J., *et al.* (2000) The measurement of symptoms in children with cancer. *J. Pain Symptom Manage.* **19**(5), 363–377.

Daugherty, C., *et al.* (1995) Perceptions of cancer patients and their physicians involved in phase I trials [see comments] [published erratum appears in *J. Clin. Oncol.* 1995 Sep. **13**(9), 2476]. *J. Clin. Oncol.* **13**(5), 1062–1072.

Davidson, A., *et al.* (1997) Phase II study of 21 day schedule oral etoposide in children. New Agents Group of the United Kingdom Children's Cancer Study Group (UKCCSG). *Eur. J. Cancer* **33**(11), 1816–1822.

Davies, B. (1998) Paediatric palliative care – development in Canada. In Doyle, D., Hanks, G., MacDonald, N. (Eds) *Oxford Textbook of Palliative Medicine.* Oxford: Oxford University Press.

Decoster, G., Stein, G., Holdener, E.E. (1990) Responses and toxic deaths in phase I clinical trials. *Ann. Oncol.* **1**(3), 175–181.

Elliott, T.E., *et al.* (1995) Physician knowledge and attitudes about cancer pain management: a survey from the Minnesota cancer pain project. *J. Pain Symptom Manage.* **10**(7), 494–504.

Ellis, P.A., *et al.* (1995) Symptom relief with MVP (mitomycin C, vinblastine and cisplatin) chemotherapy in advanced non-small-cell lung cancer. *Br. J. Cancer* **71**(2), 366–370.

Ellis, R., Leventhal, B. (1993) Information needs and decision-making preferences of children with cancer. *Psycho-Oncology* **2**, 277–284.

Emanuel, E.J. (1995) A phase I trial on the ethics of phase I trials [editorial; comment]. *J. Clin. Oncol.* **13**(5), 1049–1051.

Field, M.J., Cassel, C.K., Institute of Medicine (U.S.) (1997) Committee on Care at the End of Life, *Approaching Death: Improving Care at the End of Life.* Washington, DC: National Academy Press, pp. xvii, 437.

Field, M.J., Behrman, R.E. (Eds) (2002) *When Children Die: Improving Palliative and End-of-Life Care for Children and their Families.* Washington, DC: National Academy Press.

Fife, B.L., Irick, N., Painter, J.D. (1993) A comparative study of the attitudes of physicians and nurses toward the management of cancer pain. *J. Pain Symptom Manage.* **8**(3), 132–139.

Foex, B.A. (2000) The do-not-attempt resuscitation ('DNAR') order [letter; comment]. *Anaesthesia* **55**(3), 292.

Frager, G. (1996) Pediatric palliative care: building the model, bridging the gaps. *J. Palliat. Care* **12**(3), 9–12.

Gaze, M.N., *et al.* (1997) Pain relief and quality of life following radiotherapy for bone metastases: a randomised trial of two fractionation schedules. *Radiother. Oncol.* **45**(2), 109–116.

Geels, P., *et al.* (2000) Palliative effect of chemotherapy: objective tumor response is associated with symptom improvement in patients with metastatic breast cancer. *J. Clin. Oncol.* **18**(12), 2395–2405.

Girgis, A., Sanson-Fisher, R.W. (1995) Breaking bad news: consensus guidelines for medical practitioners. *J. Clin. Oncol.* **13**(9), 2449–2456.

Goldman, A. (1998) Life threatening illnesses and symptom control. In Doyle, D., Hanks, G., MacDonald, N. (Eds) *Oxford Textbook of Palliative Medicine.* Oxford: Oxford University Press.

Goldman, A., Heller, K.S. (2000) Integrating palliative and curative approaches in the care of children with life-threatening illnesses. *Journal of Palliative Medicine* **3**(3), 353–359.

Goold, S.D., Williams, B., Arnold, R.M. (2000) Conflicts regarding decisions to limit treatment: a differential diagnosis [see comments]. *JAMA*, **283**(7), 909–914.

Greenham, D.E., Lohmann, R.A. (1982) Children facing death: recurring patterns of adaptation. *Health Soc. Work* **7**(2), 89–94.

Hilden, J.M., Watterson, J., Chrastek, J. (2000) Tell the children [In Process Citation]. *J. Clin. Oncol.* **18**(17), 3193–3195.

Hockley, J. (1999) Specialist palliative care within the acute hospital setting [see comments]. *Acta Oncol.* **38**(4), 491–494.

Ingham, J.M., Foley, K.M. (1998) Pain and the barriers to its relief at the end of life: a lesson for improving end of life health care. *Hosp. J.* **13**(1–2), 89–100.

Kirkbride, P. (1995) The role of radiation therapy in palliative care. *J. Palliat. Care* **11**(1), 19–26.

Kushner, B.H., Kramer, K., Cheung, N.K. (1999) Oral etoposide for refractory and relapsed neuroblastoma. *J. Clin. Oncol.* **17**(10), 3221–3225.

Lauer, M.E., *et al.* (1983) A comparison study of parental adaptation following a child's death at home or in the hospital. *Pediatrics* **71**(1), 107–112.

Lauer, M.E., *et al.* (1989) Long-term follow-up of parental adjustment following a child's death at home or hospital. *Cancer* **63**(5), 988–994.

Leikin, S.L., Connell, K. (1983) Theraputic choices by children with cancer. *Pediatrics* **103**(1), 167.

Levetown, M. (1998) Palliative care in the intensive care unit. *New Horizons* **6**, 383–397.

Levin, D.N., Cleeland, C.S., Dar, R. (1985) Public attitudes toward cancer pain. *Cancer* **56**(9), 2337–2339.

Lewis, D.W., Packer, R.J., Raney, B., Rak, I.W., Belasco, J., Lange, B. (1986) Incidence, presentation and outcome of spinal cord disease in children with systemic cancer. *Pediatrics* **78**(3), 438–443.

Liben, S., Goldman, A. (1998) Home care for children with life-threatening illness. *J. Palliat. Care* **14**(3), 33–38.

Lo, B., Quill, T., Tulsky, J. (1999) Discussing palliative care with patients. ACP-ASIM End-of-Life Care Consensus Panel. American College of Physicians – American Society of Internal Medicine. *Ann. Intern. Med.* **130**(9), 744–749.

Martinson, I. (1996) An international perspective on palliative care for children. *J. Pall. Care* **12**, 13–15.

Mathew, P., *et al.* (1994) Phase I study of oral etoposide in children with refractory solid tumors. *J. Clin. Oncol.* **12**(7), 1452–1457.

Munro, A.J., Sebag-Montefiore, D. (1992) Opportunity cost – a neglected aspect of cancer treatment [editorial]. *Br. J. Cancer* **65**(3), 309–310.

Needle, M.N., *et al.* (1997) Phase II study of daily oral etoposide in children with recurrent brain tumors and other solid tumors. *Med. Pediatr. Oncol.* **29**(1), 28–32.

Nitschke, R., *et al.* (1982) Therapeutic choices made by patients with end-stage cancer. *J. Pediatr.* **101**(3), 471–476.

Pizzo, P.A., Poplack, D.G. (Eds) (2002) *Principles and Practice of Pediatric Oncology* (4th edn). Philadelphia, PA: Lippincott Williams & Wilkins.

Poon, M.A., *et al.* (1989) Biochemical modulation of fluorouracil: evidence of significant improvement of survival and quality of life in patients with advanced colorectal carcinoma. *J. Clin. Oncol.* **7**(10), 1407–1418.

Porcu, P., *et al.* (2000) Results of treatment after relapse from high-dose chemotherapy in germ cell tumors. *J. Clin. Oncol.* **18**(6), 1181–1186.

Porter, J., Jick, H. (1980) Addiction rare in patients treated with narcotics [letter]. *N. Engl. J. Med.* **302**(2), 123.

Rusy, L.M., Weisman, S.J. (2000) Complementary therapies for acute pediatric pain management. *Pediatr. Clin. North Am.* **47**(3), 589–599.

Saunders, C.M. (1979–1980) A comparison of adult bereavement in the death of a spouse, child, and parent. *Omega* **10**, 302–322.

Saunders, C. (1993) Foreword – The early hospices. In Doyle, D., Hanks, G., MacDonald, N. (Eds) *Oxford Textbook of Palliative Medicine*. Oxford: Oxford University Press, pp. v–ix.

Schonfeld, D.J. (1993) Talking with children about death. *Journal of Pediatric Health Care* **7**, 269–274.

Shah, S., *et al.* (1998) Phase I therapy trials in children with cancer. *J. Pediatr. Hematol. Oncol.* **20**(5), 431–438.

Shumway, C.N., Grossman, L.S., Sarles, R.M. (1983) Theraputic choices by children with cancer. *Pediatrics* **103**(1), 168.

Singer, P.A., Martin, D.K., Kelner, M. (1999) Quality end-of-life care: patients' perspectives [see comments]. *JAMA* **281**(2), 163–168.

Sirkia, K., *et al.* (1997) Terminal care of the child with cancer at home [see comments]. *Acta Paediatr.* **86**(10), 1125–1130.

Sirkia, K., *et al.* (1998) Pain medication during terminal care of children with cancer. *J. Pain Symptom Manage.* **15**(4), 220–226.

Solomon, M.Z., *et al.* (1993) Decisions near the end of life: professional views on life-sustaining treatments [see comments]. *Am. J. Public Health* **83**(1), 14–23.

Spinetta, J. (1974) The dying child's awareness of death: A review. *Psychological Bulletin* **81**, 256–260.

Spinetta, J., Rigler, D., Karon, M. (1973) Anxiety in the dying child. *Pediatrics* **52**, 841–845.

Stevens, M., Pollard, B. (1998) Paediatric pallliative care – development in Australia. In Doyle, D., Hanks, G., MacDonald, N. (Eds) *Oxford Textbook of Palliative Medicine*. Oxford: Oxford University Press.

Suchman, A.L., *et al*. (1997) A model of empathic communication in the medical interview [see comments]. *JAMA* **277**(8), 678–682.

SUPPORT (1995) A controlled trial to improve care for seriously ill hospitalized patients. The study to understand prognoses and preferences for outcomes and risks of treatments (SUPPORT). The SUPPORT Principal Investigators [see comments] [published erratum appears in *JAMA* 1996 Apr. 24; **275**(16), 1232] *JAMA* **274**(20), 1591–1598.

Vickers, J.L., Carlisle, C. (2000) Choices and control: parental experiences in pediatric terminal home care. *J. Pediatr. Oncol. Nurs.* **17**(1), 12–21.

Weissman, D.E., Griffie, J. (1994) The Palliative Care Consultation Service of the Medical College of Wisconsin. *J. Pain Symptom Manage.* **9**(7), 474–479.

Whittam, E.H. (1993) Terminal care of the dying child. Psychosocial implications of care. *Cancer* **71**(10 Suppl.), 3450–3462.

WHO (1998) *Cancer Pain and Relief and Palliative Care in Children*. Geneva: World Health Organization.

Wolfe, J. (2000) Symptoms and suffering at the end of life in children with cancer (see comments). *N. Engl. J. Med.* **342**(5), 326–333.

Wolfe, J., *et al*. (2000) Understanding of prognosis among parents of children who died of cancer: Impact on treatment goals and integration of palliative care. *Journal of American Medical Association* **284**(19), 2469–2475.

Wong, D., Baker, C. (1998) Pain in children: a comparison of assessment scales. *Pediatric Nursing* **14**, 9–17.

Worswick, J. (1993) *A House Called Helen. The development of hospice care for children*. Oxford: Oxford University Press.

4

Pain in Children with Cancer

RICHARD D. W. HAIN

Department of Child Health, University of Wales College of Medicine, Llandough Hospital, Cardiff, Wales, UK

INTRODUCTION

Ultimately the aim of all medical intervention is to improve the quality of life. The net value of any intervention must be considered by balancing its benefit against the burden it imposes on the patient. When there is the prospect of cure, it is often justifiable to impose measures that significantly impair the quality of life in the short term for the sake of long-term benefit. Chemotherapy is a good example.

If curative treatment is one way to improve a patient's quality of life, good symptom control is another. A curative and a palliative approach are not in any way mutually exclusive. Rather, the judgement of burden versus benefit is different depending on the stage of treatment. With this in mind, it is clear that there is no point in an illness at which good symptom control has no part to play.

As physicians, we often find it difficult to address problems that have no clear-cut solution. If cure of the disease is the only goal of our involvement with a patient, it is difficult to address issues of symptom control in which the possibility of cure, if any, is only incidental. On the other hand, for the child him- or herself, the immediacy of severe pain may eclipse any consideration of long-term survival.

The purpose of these guidelines is to demonstrate that good symptom control is an active adjunct to curative therapy. It demands the same rigorous and rational approach to assessment and treatment as all other medical

Psychosocial Aspects of Pediatric Oncology. Edited by S. Kreitler and M. Weyl Ben Arush
© 2004 John Wiley & Sons Ltd: ISBN 0 471 49939 0

interventions. This approach is familiar to doctors and should give them confidence dealing with children when there is little or no chance of cure and the goal of the doctor's involvement has become rather different.

PAIN

One rational and commonsense approach to pain in a child has been summarised in the letters 'QUEST' (Baker and Wong 1987), that is: Question the child, Use pain rating tools, Evaluate behaviour, Sensitise parents and Take action (or Treat). This is not very different from the approach we are taught at medical school for the rational diagnosis and management of other medical problems: history, examination, special tests and treatment.

HISTORY

Points to note in the history of pain have been conveniently grouped under the headings 'PQRST':

(1) Precipitating factors
(2) Quality of pain
(3) Radiation of pain
(4) Severity
(5) Timing

(1) *Precipitating factors* can give an indication of cause of pain as well as for management. For example, pain that is experienced only during movement (incident pain) will need a specific management strategy and should lead one to consider the possibility of a pathological fracture.
(2) *Quality.* The quality of pain is perhaps the most important in making a differential diagnosis. It is usually possible to classify pain as one of the following:
   (a) *Bone pain.* Bone is characterised by a pain that is very intense and well circumscribed. Typically the patient points to the area with one finger. The pain may be described as 'like toothache'. Children can be very imaginative in their descriptions and will often use a far wider range of adjectives than their adult counterparts. It is important to consider the context in which the pain is occurring. For example, bony metastasis is common in osteosarcoma but very rare in brain tumours.
   (b) *Neuropathic pain.* This is characterised by altered sensation, i.e. hyperaesthesia (increased sensitivity, including to pain), paraesthesia (pins and needles) and numbness. Patients will describe burning, pins

and needles, electric shock or lightning pains. Patients will often use a whole hand in sweeping movement to illustrate that the pain is not localised but occurs in a distribution which is often recognisably dermatomal. The context is often tumours pressing on the spinal cord or those that cause bony metastasis in the spinal column itself. Neuropathic pain is also encountered in the soft tissue components of Ewing's and neuroblastoma (these being of neural origin).

(c) *Colicky pain*. As its name suggests, colicky pain is characterised by intense but intermittent pain separated by periods when the patient is absolutely or relatively pain-free. As with incident pain, the danger is that analgesia that is adequate for the pain at its maximum is too toxic for pain at its minimum. Colicky pain typically characterises intestinal obstruction and can therefore occur in the context of some lymphomas and in the late stages of other abdominal solid tumours such as neuroblastoma.

(d) *Soft tissue pain*. Pain that arises directly from the local effects of the tumour itself may not fit easily into any of the above categories, or have elements of all of them. Soft tissue pain is often diffuse and difficult to describe even for older children and adolescents. A child may not volunteer that he or she is in pain. It is important to recognise subtle evidence of pain such as a loss of interest in social interaction or play.

(3) *Radiation*. Neuropathic pain is classically characterised by its radiation in a recognisable distribution. If the distribution is dermatomal this may be easy to recognise but neuropathic pain may be in a less familiar distribution. For example, tumours that impinge on the coeliac plexus, such as advanced Wilms' or neuroblastoma, can cause a 'boring'-type pain which radiates from the epigastrium to the back or vice versa. Neuropathic pain may also follow the distribution of the sympathetic nerves, that is to say in a vascular rather than obviously nerve distribution. Bone pain is typically characterised by its very well circumscribed nature with little or no radiation. However, it is common for many bony pains to occur simultaneously in different locations and this may masquerade as radiation. Children are adept at distinguishing between the same pain occurring in two places, and two different pains. Colicky pain is typically localised to the abdomen, but painful muscle spasms can occur elsewhere and are particularly common in non-malignant pain.

(4) *Severity*. It is important to make some assessment of the severity of pain in order to judge the effectiveness of an intervention. This is not always easy as children may lack the necessary abstract and verbal skills to rate pain effectively. Two recent reviews (Franck, Greenberg and Stevens 2000, Hain 1997) reveal that there are a large number of scales available for children, most of which are based on a visual analogue scale (VAS). The VAS has

been well validated in an adult population (Huskisson 1983, Price *et al.* 1983) and many of its modifications seem to be effective, at least in acute pain for children (Beyer and Wells 1989, Beyer 1986, 1988, Beyer, Villarruel and Denyes 1988, Hester, Foster and Krestenzen 1990, Kuttner and LePage 1989, Bieri *et al.* 1990). Such scales simply ask the patient to select the severity of pain between two extremes, usually 0–10 or 0–100. In order for there to be some kind of fixed anchor point at either end, it is essential to explain beforehand that '0 means no pain at all and 10 represents the worst pain you can imagine'.

Children who are too young to express pain may demonstrate it by behaviour changes. The child may, for example, adopt a posture that minimises pain or over time appear to become resigned to it. This syndrome, termed 'psychomotor atonia', has been likened to adult depression (Gauvain-Piquard, Rodary and Lemerle 1988), and measuring it is the basis of an observational pain scale developed in France that is well suited to the management of a child's cancer pain (Gauvain-Piquard *et al.* 1991, 1999).

It is always important to ask those who are with the child all the time – usually the parents – for their opinion. This should only allow you to revise your estimate of pain severity upwards. It is not usually appropriate to conclude that a child is overstating the severity of pain, only that he or she is understating it. Ideally, pain scales should be in routine use for all children receiving analgesia of any kind. Realistically, such scales are not yet always practical.

(5) *Timing*. The timing of pain can give valuable clues as to the cause. For example, abdominal pain that is relieved by defaecation is likely to be due to constipation while pain that is at its most severe immediately before attending hospital is likely to have a large psychological component. This in no way argues, of course, that the pain is any less 'real' – only that the strategy used to treat it needs to be considered accordingly.

EXAMINATION

As always, the examination should be guided by the history. At the end of the history it should be possible to make a reasonable clinical diagnosis of the nature of the pain and to have a differential diagnosis of the causes. The aims of the examination are:

(1) to distinguish between the differential diagnoses
(2) to exclude related pain problems (for example, other painful metastases that have not been reported)
(3) identify factors that might complicate treatment

The examination itself is no different from other paediatric examinations. It should start with a global assessment of the child. The site of pain may be immediately obvious if the child adopts an antalgic posture or is simply able to indicate the area of pain. However, the signs may be more subtle. It has been said that a normal child is always sleeping, eating or playing. If the child is doing none of these things, pain may be the explanation. It is rarely possible to distinguish definitively between signs of anxiety and pain. Where pain is likely (either because the child has reported it or simply because your knowledge of the clinical context leads you to expect it) it is usually better to assume it than to diagnose anxiety alone. Pain and anxiety are only definitively distinguished by a response to pure analgesics such as opioids. If it later becomes clear that prescribing adequate doses of analgesia has made no difference to the child's clinical state, it is reasonable to assume that pain was not the cause and to review the need for analgesia.

The rest of the examination is guided by the history. If neuropathic pain is considered it is important to delineate the distribution. This will not only help establish the underlying cause of the pain but may also be important in managing it, for example if a local nerve block is to be considered. Where the history suggests bone pain, it is particularly important to exclude the possibility of pathological fracture as these require a different therapeutic approach from other causes of bone pain. Colicky pain should prompt careful examination to exclude intestinal obstruction. This is not because surgical intervention will necessarily be appropriate, but because the management of other symptoms, particularly nausea and vomiting, is quite different if it is present. Soft tissue pain should prompt careful examination of the area. Soft tissue pain is common around the site of the tumour itself but may also occur at sites of metastasis, particularly the liver. Again, this is important as the management of pain due to stretching of the capsule around the liver or a tumour is different from other forms of pain.

Lastly, the examination should identify factors that might complicate the management of symptoms. For example, demonstrating severe epigastric pain would suggest that caution will be necessary in prescribing non-steroidal anti-inflammatory drugs.

INVESTIGATIONS

Investigations are often considered inappropriate when there is no longer any prospect of cure. Certainly it is true that the benefit of an investigation in terms of how it will help improve the patient's symptoms has to be weighed very carefully against the need for the child to come to the hospital and perhaps to undergo venepuncture. However, this is only a special case of something that is always true of medical interventions: that is that they should only be undertaken when the benefit outweighs the burden. This balance should be carefully considered before undertaking any investigations, but the balance will sometimes mean that they are justified even where palliation is the only aim.

Plain X-ray

Plain X-rays are usually painless but require the child to attend hospital. During the period of treatment when a cure is still possible, this may be very appropriate but at other times children may choose to avoid all contact with the hospital. In practice, the potential value of a plain X-ray is usually relatively small. Metastases that are symptomatic do not need to be demonstrated; those that cause no symptoms do not need to be treated. The main clinical situation in which a plain X-ray can be very helpful is in distinguishing the pain of a metastasis from that of a pathological fracture; this will have an impact on management and is therefore a real benefit.

Bone Scan

The bone scan is of considerable diagnostic value in demonstrating for the first time that there has been disease progression or metastasis. Once this has been established, however, there is usually little benefit in repeating the procedure. It is uncomfortable and demands a hospital visit. It is not usually necessary to demonstrate the presence of a metastasis if there are clinical signs and symptoms to suggest one. Once again, bony lesions that are symptomatic do not need to be demonstrated radiologically and those that are not require no treatment. Palliative radiation of bone metastases does not usually require them to be demonstrated radiologically.

MRI or CT Scan

These tests are often surprisingly frightening and uncomfortable for children and should be avoided unless there is a good reason. Such good reasons include excluding imminent cord compression or to localise a tumour prior to neurolytic procedure such as coeliac access block. Missing a cord compression can mean a child's being paraplegic for the last weeks or even months of his or her life so that despite being uncomfortable these can be very valuable investigations. MRI and CT can also be required in preparation for palliative radiotherapy.

Blood Tests

Generally speaking, blood tests should be avoided even in patients who have indwelling central lines. For the child, accessing these lines can often be an unpleasant reminder of uncomfortable treatment that has ultimately failed. At the very least, it runs the risk of further medicalising the child. However, once again there are circumstances under which blood tests can be of value. For example, anaemia that is symptomatic may benefit from palliative transfusion and sudden onset of opioid toxicity can be caused by an acute deterioration in renal function which should be demonstrated.

Other Investigations

The exact judgement as to when an investigation becomes justifiable will depend not only on the individual situation but on the individual patient. Many continue to see the hospital as a lifeline and welcome evidence that palliative care is an active plan of management. Others prefer to forget they were ever ill and to cut themselves off from the hospital. The important thing is not whether investigations are ordered more or less often for the purposes of symptom control but that they continue to be ordered appropriately after considering the balance of burden and benefit.

MANAGEMENT

Before the 1980s, management of pain tended to be chaotic and ill-thought-through. The World Health Organization sought to improve the delivery of analgesia by clarifying and simplifying it (Ventafridda et al. 1989, World Health Organization 1984, 1998). They did this by means of the concept of the 'pain ladder' (Figure 4.1). While this was developed and validated in adults, the principles on which it was based can be extrapolated to children. They are:

(1) That, as pain increases in severity, more powerful analgesia should be offered.
(2) There is no advantage in exchanging one analgesia for another of similar type and potency. If a previously analgesic drug becomes inadequate, either the dose should be reviewed or a more powerful drug substituted.
(3) The simplest medication and the oral route should be selected wherever possible.
(4) Adjuvant therapy (that is, medications that are not usually considered to be analgesics but which become analgesic in certain situations) should be used as soon as a specific diagnosis of pain is made. This means, for example, that NSAID therapy should be instituted as soon as a diagnosis of bone pain is made, rather than waiting until other measures have failed.
(5) Opioid medication should be given regularly and never only 'as needed'.
(6) Breakthrough medication should remain a fixed proportion of the regular medication and always be prescribed simultaneously.

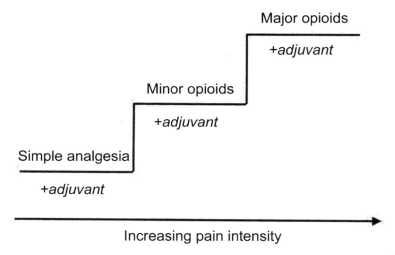

Figure 4.1 WHO pain ladder

WHO Pain Ladder

Step 1 (simple analgesia)

In paediatrics, the only simple analgesia widely available is paracetamol. In palliative situations, it may sometimes be appropriate to consider using aspirin which is a powerful anti-inflammatory, antipyretic and analgesic.

Step 2 (minor opioid)

Minor opioids include codeine, dihydrocodeine and dextropropoxyphene. These are often conveniently combined with paracetamol. This may improve compliance but imposes a ceiling dose as there is a maximum safe daily dose of paracetamol.

In practice, the middle step (minor opioid) is probably unnecessary in children. There is no difference in effect between a large dose of a minor opioid and a small dose of a major opioid. Even in adults there is considerable overlap; in children who are resistant to the effects of opioids and who clear them very quickly, it is often justifiable to go straight from simple analgesia (step 1) to a small dose of a major opioid (step 3).

Step 3 (major opioid)

It is the third step in which there is most variety. Morphine is the archetype major opioid and is both effective and relatively non-toxic. Unlike many opioids, the pharmacology of morphine has been studied in children (Esmail *et al.* 1999, McRorie *et al.* 1992, Collins 1996, Hunt *et al.* 1999, Hain *et al.* 1999, Lynn *et al.* 1998, Hartley *et al.* 1993). There have been numerous commercial attempts to develop superior major opioids to morphine, most of which have failed. However, a small number of synthetic or semi-synthetic opioids such as fentanyl (Collins *et al.* 1996, Ahmedzai and Brooks 1997, Hunt *et al.* 2001), do offer genuine advantages over morphine and these are listed in Table 4.1. As a rule of thumb, the best approach is to use morphine orally unless there is a good reason not to.

Other opioids

A number of opioids are intermediate between major and minor. These include tramadol and pethidine. They probably offer no advantage over more major opioids and are relatively toxic compared with morphine (Silvasti *et al.* 1999, Naguib *et al.* 1998, Moore *et al.* 1998, Pokela *et al.* 1992, Hamunen *et al.* 1993, Kussman and Sethna 1998, Pryle *et al.* 1992, Kyff and Rice 1990, Waterhouse 1967). They have no proven place in the management of paediatric pain.

Practical Application

There are essentially three phases in managing a child's pain:

(1) Choosing a starting dose
(2) Finding the right dose (titration)
(3) Maintenance of analgesia

Table 4.1 Conversion of common major opioids in children

Opioid	Advantage over morphine	Relative potency compared with oral morphine (approx.)
Morphine		
Diamorphine (po)	More soluble	1.5
Fentanyl (patch)	Patch formulation Less constipation Less itch (?) Less retention (?)	100
Methadone (po)	Possible anti-neuropathic activity	Variable
Hydromorphone (po)	None	5
Pethidine	None	0.125
Tramadol	None	0.25
Oxycodone	None	1

Choosing a starting dose

The starting point on the WHO pain ladder must depend on a clinical assessment as outlined above. Starting doses for drugs at steps 1 and 2 are given in various paediatric formularies including *Medicines for Children* (Hull *et al.* 1999).

In selecting a starting dose for a major opioid, one of two approaches can be taken. Either an empiric starting point can be selected (equivalent of 2 mg/kg/day of oral morphine) or a conversion can be made from existing opioid requirements using conversions in Table 4.1. The most appropriate approach is usually the one that will result in the higher dose of opioid.

A prescription of both *regular* and *breakthrough* dose must be made.

Regular medication

Having established the dose, the starting opioid should usually be immediate-release morphine 4-hourly by mouth. Rarely, it may be preferable to commence immediately on parenteral opioids (usually subcutaneous diamorphine or transdermal fentanyl, see Table 4.1).

Breakthrough medication

The dose of breakthrough medication is calculated simply by prescribing the regular 4-hourly dose of immediate-release morphine and prescribing the same dose PRN. Children appear to clear morphine more quickly than adults and it is often my practice to prescribe half the 4-hourly dose but increase the frequency to 2-hourly PRN. Usually medication for breakthrough pain should be the same as that for regular pain. However, there is sometimes an advantage in using two different formulations. For example, children having a fentanyl patch for regular analgesia will prefer to have oral morphine for breakthrough than fentanyl which is currently only available as an injection.

Finding the right dose (titration)

The primary purpose of breakthrough medication is to ensure adequate analgesia during the period of assessment of the correct dose of opioids. A secondary purpose, however, is to provide an indirect measure of the child's experience of pain. It is therefore very important to encourage the child and/or parents to administer breakthrough medication as soon as there is any sign of pain. Unless this is clearly articulated to the child's family, his or her requirements for analgesia will almost always be underestimated.

The requirements for breakthrough pain should ideally be reviewed after 48 hours. If there have been two or more requirements for breakthrough pain in each 24-hour period, the regular dose should be increased by the amount of breakthrough that has been required. To do these calculations, all doses should be converted to milligram equivalents of oral morphine (Table 4.1).

It is sometimes necessary to titrate more quickly. Where possible, this should be avoided as it typically takes 48 hours for the full effect of any modification of the regular dose to become apparent. Too rapid an escalation of opioid dose can cause intolerable adverse effects which can jeopardise future symptom management by causing the patient to lose confidence in the medications.

Adverse Effects

Morphine is a well tried and trusted medication. The adverse effects are few and well-recognised. Fortunately, the body develops tolerance to many of these effects well before the analgesic effectiveness of morphine is lost.

(1) *Drowsiness*. During the first 48 hours of opioid therapy, or following an increase in opioid dose, drowsiness is universal. This will resolve spontaneously with no modification of the dose and it is important to warn the patient and family that it will occur. It is caused partly by the direct central effect of morphine but also by the relief of pain which can sometimes allow sleep for the first time in many weeks.

(2) *Constipation*. Constipation is one of the adverse effects for which no tolerance develops. A stimulant laxative should always be prescribed. Lactulose is not appropriate for this purpose as it is mainly osmotic. Instead, a combination of senna and magnesium hydroxide, or else co-danthrusate in the palliative phase should be considered. Alternatively, constipation may be an indication to change to fentanyl which may cause less of the problem (Ahmedzai and Brooks 1997).

(3) *Urinary hesitancy*. Urinary retention and hesitancy appear anecdotally to be more common in children than in adults. It is still relatively unusual, but if it occurs is an indication for considering an alternative opioid, particularly fentanyl which is a synthetic opioid and appears much less likely to cause the problem.

(4) *Pruritus*. Again, skin itching as a result of histamine release from mast cells that have been directly activated by the morphine molecule, is much more common in children than in adults. It is still rare. Antihistamines and topical preparations such as calamine can be very helpful but once again this is probably an indication for selecting an alternative from a different class, such as fentanyl.

(5) *Nausea and vomiting*. Nausea and vomiting due to opioids in children are distinctly unusual. There is certainly no need to prescribe prophylactic anti-emetics. If they do occur, the most effective anti-emetics are haloperidol, ondansetron and Nozinan (or other dopamine and $5HT_3$ antagonists).

(6) *Dysphoria*. Dysphoria is relatively uncommon in children but may simply be under-reported. It is often transient and self-limiting but, again, fentanyl may be a suitable alternative if it is difficult to treat.

Maintaining Analgesia

The result of titration should be a clear idea of what the patient's immediate analgesia needs are. Clearly, as the disease progresses it may be necessary to increase the dose of opioids. However, this is not universal and the complex and multidimensional nature of pain means that despite disease progression opioid requirements sometimes even decrease. The process of reviewing 48-hourly requirements for breakthrough should therefore continue. This relies on good record keeping so that the healthcare professional (usually doctor or nurse) advising on prescription can see exactly how much has been required. It is unlikely that regular medication will be able to provide complete pain relief and it is acceptable for a patient to require breakthrough medication once every day, or even occasionally twice. Again, it is often helpful to make the child and family aware of this before embarking on therapy.

Once the dose of opioid has become clear, the next stage is to simplify its prescription. Morphine is conveniently available as slow-release (MST). In adults, the dosage interval is 12-hourly and the starting dose interval in children should be the same. However, a large proportion of children require a smaller interval than this (Hunt and Kaiko 1991) and it is often necessary to change the dosing interval to 8-hourly. Once-daily preparations of slow-release morphine are also available, though not licensed in children.

Fentanyl patches offer numerous potential advantages over morphine for some children (see Table 4.1). The patches are designed to last for 72 hours but, again, the more rapid clearance of opioids in children means that this not uncommonly needs to be reduced to 48-hourly. The conversion from morphine dose to fentanyl patch is given in the product monologue. Calculating the conversion without this is complex. The 'size' of the patch that is usually quoted refers not to the total amount of drug in the patch but to the hourly rate of fentanyl delivered by it.

An oral 'lollipop' delivery system has been developed for fentanyl with equivocal results (Sharar 1998). It appears to be effective but the taste is not altogether pleasant and in some children the lollipop causes uncomfortable numbness of the oral mucosa.

Non-opioid and Adjuvant Therapy

Introduction

It has already been seen that a rational and analytical approach to the history and examination of a child in pain should mean that some attempt can be made to categorise it.

An alternative and very practical way to categorise pain is into opioid sensitive, opioid partially sensitive, and opioid resistant. These three categories obviously represent points on a spectrum. The clinician should consider pain under these headings at the same time as considering the diagnostic category of the pain. The two systems are linked but are not the same. For example, neuropathic pain is typically relatively resistant to treatment with opioids but the individual child with neuropathic pain may nevertheless experience great relief from opioid therapy.

The WHO Guidelines suggest that once diagnosis of pain is made, an appropriate adjuvant therapy should be used (Ventafridda *et al.* 1989, World Health Organization 1984, 1998). The use of such adjuvants does not replace the rest of the pain ladder – simple analgesia, minor opioid, major opioid – but proceeds in parallel with it. For example, as soon as a diagnosis of bone pain is made, non-steroidals should be considered even if the severity of the pain warrants only simple analgesia. In other words, the selection of an adjuvant is on the basis of the nature of the pain rather than the severity of it (Tables 4.2 and 4.3). It is worth emphasising that even in pain that is only partially sensitive to opioids, few adjuvants can offer the chance of good analgesia provided by morphine.

Adjuvants

A drug that is not usually considered to be an analgesic, but can provide pain relief in certain situations, is termed an 'adjuvant' medication. Many of the drugs in this category have, in fact, been shown to have analgesic properties in their own right.

Bone pain

The classical adjuvant for bone pain are the non-steroidal anti-inflammatory drugs (Thomsen, Crawford and Sjogren 1997, Johnson and Miller 1994, Portenoy 1993, 1995, Payne 1997). Their side effect profile in children appears to be very good (Levick 1988). Most children experience no adverse effects. Others experience mild gastrointestinal upset which resolves spontaneously without a need for a change in dose. Where adverse effects are more persistent and mean that the child is unable to tolerate them, enteric-coated preparations or Cox-2 selective non-steroidal anti-inflammatory drugs are available (Shah *et al.* 2001, Mandell 1999, Miyamoto *et al.* 2000). Proton blockers such as

Table 4.2 Principles of symptom management in children

1	All pain is multidimensional, having physical, psychosocial and existential (spiritual) aspects.
2	Pain is subjective: 'it is what the child says it is'.
3	Management of pain should be rational, based on an understanding of the pathophysiology of pain and of the underlying condition after systematic history, examination and investigation. However, it should also be empirical; if something works, use it and if it doesn't, reconsider.
4	Like all medical interventions, palliative manoeuvres should be undertaken only when the benefit outweighs the burden in the individual child. Appropriate weight needs to be given to non-physical aspects, both of burden and benefit, in making this judgement, particularly in the palliative phase.

Table 4.3 Adjuvant therapies in management of pain in children. (N.B. most pains are at least partially opioid responsive. Adjuvants should accompany rather than replace appropriate opioid therapy)

Physical pain	Characteristic	Suggested adjuvants
Neuropathic pain	Altered sensation (numbness, dysaesthesia, hyperaesthesia, paraesthesia), weakness, characteristic distribution	Tricyclic antidepressants Anticonvulsants Steroids in first 48 hours Radiotherapy Neurolytic procedures
Bone pain	Severe, well-circumscribed 'like toothache', in context of metastatic cancer	Radiotherapy (local) Non-steroidal anti-inflammatory drugs
Colicky pain	Constipation Malignant obstruction	Anticholinergics
Incident pain	Worse on movement	Reduce movement (e.g. immobilise pathological fracture) Parenteral opioids 20 mins before procedure Entonox

omeprazole should probably be prescribed prophylactically if non-steroidals are co-prescribed with steroids for more than a few days (Piper *et al.* 1991). The gastric mucosal protectant misoprostol is also effective in adults; both are more effective than H_2 blockers (Yeomans *et al.* 1998, Hawkey *et al.* 1998, Yeomans 1998). All non-steroidal anti-inflammatory drugs inhibit platelet aggregation through their effect on the cyclo-oxygenase system and should be used with caution in children with a low platelet count or defective coagulation. H_2 blockers such as ranitidine may be useful in managing established gastrointestinal irritation but appear to be of little or no help in prophylaxis.

All children with bone pain due to proven or probable metastatic disease should be assessed for radiotherapy. A small, localised dose of radiation as a single fraction can often provide lasting relief of symptoms with little or no side effects. It is therefore worth considering even in relatively radio-resistant tumours such as osteosarcoma.

Neuropathic pain

Neuropathic pain is usually at least partially opioid responsive. The pain is typically caused by compression or outright damage of a peripheral nerve, for example by tumour at the spinal cord. Within the first 48 hours of the onset of neuropathic pain compression can be relieved with the use of steroids (dexamethasone is the most widely used in palliative care – see under 'liver capsule pain' below). This may be enough to convert an opioid resistant to an opioid sensitive pain. For pain of longer duration, it is likely that actual nerve damage has occurred and that steroids will be ineffective. Tricyclic antidepressants are very effective in management of neuropathic pain (McQuay *et al.* 1996). Amitriptyline has more side effects than nortriptyline but both are well tolerated by most children despite their potential for anticholinergic side effects. Carbamazepine is a good second line (McQuay *et al.* 1995) and, because of the long history of its safe use in children, is often chosen in preference to the tricyclics.

Drugs that interfere with the N-methyl-D-aspartate system are also effective in relieving neuropathic pain. They have a particular role in managing phantom limb pain and the 'wind up phenomenon' in which chronic exposure to repeated painful procedures leads to ever-increasing sensation of pain on each occasion. Of these, ketamine is the one most often used in children. Methadone is unusual among opioids in possessing additional NMDA blocking activity (Stringer *et al.* 2000) which would *in theory* (Carpenter *et al.* 2000) make it ideal for managing neuropathic pain. There are reports of the use of methadone in children (Shir *et al.* 1998, Miser 1986) but more research is required.

It has been implied (Watson and Babul 1998) that other opioids such as oxycodone and tramadol have specific activity in neuropathic pain, both major. There is no evidence that any of them are more effective than existing treatments. It is likely that other anti-convulsants will have some impact on neuropathic pain but, again, this has not yet been definitively shown in children.

Episodic pain

The difficulty in managing episodic pain is that a dose of analgesic that is adequate for pain at its worst is likely to be too toxic for pain at its least.

Breakthrough morphine is often ineffective for severe episodic pain, since the time taken for it to reach its effective serum levels means that the pain has subsided before the medication can work.

Pain may be episodic for three reasons. The dose of regular medication may be too small, resulting in intermittent breakthrough pain for which the solution is to review the regular medication. The cause of the pain may be episodic: for example, pain from a pathological fracture or from some bone metastases can be provoked by movement ('incident pain'). Management of the underlying lesion (for example using radiotherapy), and identifying and avoiding the provoking factors (for example by immobilisation of a fracture) may be practical. Anticipating the need for breakthrough medications before painful procedures can be helpful if it is impossible to avoid them. Rapidly acting analgesics such as parenteral opioids, Palfium or Entonox can moderate but rarely abolish procedure-related pain (Pal, Cortiella and Herndon 1997, Michaud et al. 1999, Martin et al. 2000). Arranging for the child or parent to be able to administer the analgesia, rather than having to wait for a healthcare professional to do so, allows a sense of control as well as minimising the lag period between experiencing pain and experiencing relief.

Finally, the pain may simply be of an episodic nature, for example intestinal colic or muscle spasm. The pain from intestinal colic can be excruciating but is typically short-lived. Where possible, the frequency of colic spasms should be reduced. This is often possible using anticholinergics such as buscopan. Octreotide, a synthetic analogue of somatostatin may reduce the frequency of spasms but increase their force (Fallon 1994, Khoo 1994).

Pain caused by muscle spasm is relatively unusual in the context of cancer, though it is a common problem among other life-limiting diseases such as cerebral palsy. It may respond to benzodiazepines or antispasmodics such as baclofen.

Psychological components to pain

Properly speaking, the syndrome of 'total pain' describes all pain. It embodies the concept that the physical, nociceptive aspect is only one factor among many in determining the degree of discomfort caused by the pain. Thus, the pain of an ankle injury acquired during a game of football is very different from the pain of the same intensity when relapsed osteosarcoma is the proven or even the suspected cause.

However, total pain is often used to describe those pains in which the psychological, emotional and existential elements of the pain are such that analgesics alone are unlikely to provide adequate analgesia. Ideally, these aspects should be dealt with by discussion, exploration and where necessary support from pastoral or psychology services. In practice, it is often necessary to supplement these with medications that have some influence on the psyche.

Depression is typically under-diagnosed in childhood but much more common is anxiety. This can be moderated with careful use of benzodiazepines such as medazolam or phenothiazines such as levopromazine. Levopromazine is a particularly useful drug since it combines its sedative effects with excellent anti-emesis and even a degree of analgesia. See later chapters for more details about these and other drugs useful in the management of anxiety.

Liver capsule pain

Liver capsular pain is characterised by severe pain in the right upper quadrant of the abdomen. It occurs in the context of metastatic disease, particularly neuroblastoma, Wilms' or osteosarcoma, where spread to the liver is relatively common, and is often accompanied by nausea and vomiting.

Like most pains, it is usually at least partially sensitive to opioids but adjuvant therapy using steroids (dexamethasone orally: anecdotally, it is best given in two divided doses, one at 6.00 amd and one at 12.00 md to minimise mood and sleep disturbance). The adverse effects of long-term steroids mean that for most indications their use in children should be restricted to five-day courses. The course can if necessary be repeated if symptoms recur.

Neurolytic procedures

Some forms of neuropathic pain can respond well to carefully performed infusion of local anaesthetic or even permanent blockade using phenol. This requires great expertise and the services of a specialised paediatric anaesthetist. Since the procedure involves both needles and general anaesthetic, it is less often used in treating pain in children than in adults. Epidurals are much more readily available in children and can be very helpful in the management of pain in the lower limbs unresponsive to other modalities, particularly where mobility is not an issue.

SUMMARY

The clinical evidence is accumulating that major opioids can be used safely and effectively in children with moderate to severe pain. They should be used as part of a rational approach to the diagnosis, assessment and management of pain. The WHO pain ladder gives a straightforward structure to such an approach and is recommended to all those who wish to approach the management of a child with pain.

The evolution of clinical expertise and experience has been paralleled and supported by an expansion of the research evidence base. This seems to show that, where children differ from adults in their handling of morphine, the result is that they are more resilient rather than more sensitive to its effects.

Good symptom control should be seen as an active intervention which at different stages in the progress of a disease will complement or replace potentially curative interventions. Like them, interventions for symptom control should be a judicious mix of the empirical and the evidence-based but should always be rigorously rational.

REFERENCES

Ahmedzai, S., Brooks, D. (1997) Transdermal fentanyl versus sustained-release oral morphine in cancer pain: preference, efficacy, and quality of life. The TTS-Fentanyl Comparative Trial Group. *J. Pain Symptom Manage.* **13**(5), 254–261.

Baker, C.M., Wong, D.L. (1987) QUEST: a process of pain assessment in children. *Orthopaedic Nursing* **6**(1), 11–21.

Beyer, A. (1986) Content validity of an instrument to measure young children's perception of the intensity of their pain. *Journal of Pediatric Nursing* **1**(6), 386–395.

Beyer, A. (1988) Convergent and discriminant validity of a self-report measure of pain intensity for children. *Children's Health Care* **16**(4), 274–282.

Beyer, J.E., Villarruel, A.M., Denyes, M. (1993) *The Oucher: The new user's manual and technical report.* Dept Paeds, University of Colorado Health Center.

Beyer, J.E., Wells, N. (1989) The assessment of pain in children. *Pediatric Clinics of North America* **36**(4), 837–854.

Bieri, D., Reeve, R.A., Champion, G.D., Addicoat, L., Ziegler, J.B. (1990) The faces pain scale for the self-assessment of the severity of pain experienced by children: development, initial validation, and preliminary investigation for ratio scale properties. *Pain* **41**, 139–150.

Carpenter, K.J., Chapman, V., Dickenson, A.H. (2000) Neuronal inhibitory effects of methadone are predominantly opioid receptor mediated in the rat spinal cord *in vivo*. *European Journal of Pain* **4**, 19–26.

Collins, J.J., Geake, J., Grier, H.E., Houck, C.S., Thaler, H.T., Weinstein, H.J. *et al.* (1996) Patient-controlled analgesia for mucositis pain in children: a three-period crossover study comparing morphine and hydromorphone. *J. Pediatr.* **129**(5), 722–728.

Esmail, Z., Montgomery, C., Courtrn, C., Hamilton, D., Kestle, J. (1999) Efficacy and complications of morphine infusions in postoperative paediatric patients. *Paediatr. Anaesth.* **9**(4), 321–327.

Fallon, M.T. (1994) The physiology of somatostatin and its synthetic analogue, octreotide. *European Journal of Palliative Care* **1**(1), 20–25.

Franck, L.S., Greenberg, C.S., Stevens, B. (2000) Pain assessment in infants and children. *Pediatr. Clin. North Am.* **47**(3), 487–512.

Gauvain-Piquard, A., Rodary, C., Lemerle, J. (1988) L'atonie psychomotrice: signe majeur de douleur chez l'enfant de moins de 6 ans. *Journées Parisiennes de Pédiatrie*, 249–252.

Gauvain-Piquard, A., Rodary, C., Francois, P., Rezvani, A., Kalifa, C., Lecuyer, N., *et al.* (1991) Validity assessment of DEGR scale for observational rating of 2–6-year-old child pain. *J. Pain Symp. Manage.* **6**(3), 171.

Gauvain-Piquard, A., Rodary, C., Rezvani, A., Serbouti, S. (1999) The development of the DEGR(R): A scale to assess pain in young children with cancer. *Eur. J. Pain* **3**(2), 165–176.

Hain, R.D.W. (1997) Pain scales in children: a review. *Palliative Medicine* **11**, 341–350.

Hain, R.D., Hardcastle, A., Pinkerton, C.R., Aherne, G.W. (1999) Morphine and morphine-6-glucuronide in the plasma and cerebrospinal fluid of children. *Br. J. Clin. Pharmacol.* **48**(1), 37–42.

Hamunen, K., Maunuksela, E.L., Seppala, T., Olkkola, K.T. (1993) Pharmacokinetics of i.v. and rectal pethidine in children undergoing ophthalmic surgery. *Br. J. Anaesth.* **71**(6), 823–826.

Hartley, R., Green, M., Quinn, M., Levene, M.I. (1993) Pharmacokinetics of morphine infusion in premature neonates. *Arch. Dis. Child.* **69**(1 Spec. No.), 55–58.

Hawkey, C.J., Karrasch, J.A., Szczepanski, L., Walker, D.G., Barkun, A., Swannell, A.J. *et al.* (1998) Omeprazole compared with misoprostol for ulcers associated with nonsteroidal antiinflammatory drugs. Omeprazole versus Misoprostol for NSAID-induced Ulcer Management (OMNIUM) Study Group. *N. Engl. J. Med.* **338**(11), 727–734.

Hester, N.K.O., Foster, R., Kristensen, K. (1990) Measurement of pain in children: generalizability and validity of the pain ladder and the poker chip tool. In Tyler DC, Krane EJ. (Ed.) *Advances in Pain Research Therapy*. New York: Raven Press Ltd, pp. 79–84.

Hull, D., Burns, A., Stephenson, T., Cockburn, F., Carson, D., Rylance, G. *et al.* (1999) *Medicines for Children* (1st edn). London: Royal College of Paediatrics and Child Health.

Hunt, A.M., Goldman, A., Devine, T., Phillips, M. (2001) Transdermal fentanyl for pain relief in a paediatric palliative care population. *Palliative Medicine* **15**, 405–412.

Hunt, A., Joel, S., Dick, G., Goldman, A. (1999) Population pharmacokinetics of oral morphine and its glucuronides in children receiving morphine as immediate-release liquid or sustained-release tablets for cancer pain. *J. Pediatr.* **135**(1), 47–55.

Hunt, T.L., Kaiko, R.F. (1991) Comparison of the pharmacokinetic profiles of two oral controlled-release morphine formulations in healthy young adults. *Clin. Ther.* **13**(4), 482–488.

Huskisson, E.C. (1983) Visual analogue scales. In: Melzack R. (Ed.) *Pain Management and Assessment*. New York: Raven Press, pp. 33–37.

Johnson, J.R., Miller, A.J. (1994) The efficacy of choline magnesium trisalicylate (CMT) in the management of metastatic bone pain: a pilot study. *Palliative Medicine* **8**(2), 129–135.

Khoo, D., Hall, E., Motson, R., Riley, J., Denman, K., Waxman, J. (1994) Palliation of malignant intestinal obstruction using octreotide. *European Journal of Cancer* **30A**(1), 28–30.

Kussman, B.D., Sethna, N.F. (1998) Pethidine-associated seizure in a healthy adolescent receiving pethidine for postoperative pain control. *Paediatr. Anaesth.* **8**(4), 349–352.

Kuttner, L., LePage, T. (1989) Face scales for the assessment of pediatric pain: a critical review. *Canadian Journal of Behavioural Sciences/Review of Canadian Science and Comp* **21**(2), 198–209.

Kyff, J.V., Rice, T.L. (1990) Meperidine-associated seizures in a child. *Clin. Pharm.* **9**(5), 337–338.

Levick, S., Jacobs, C., Loukas, D.F., Gordon, D.H., Meyskens, F.L., Uhm, K. (1988) Naproxen sodium in treatment of bone pain due to metastatic cancer. *Pain* **35**(3), 253–258.

Lynn, A., Nespeca, M.K., Bratton, S.L., Strauss, S.G., Shen, D.D. (1998) Clearance of morphine in postoperative infants during intravenous infusion: the influence of age and surgery. *Anesth. Analg.* **86**(5), 958–963.

Mandell, B.F. (1999) COX 2-selective NSAIDs: biology, promises, and concerns. *Cleve. Clin. J. Med.* **66**(5), 285–292.

Martin, J.P., Sexton, B.F., Saunders, B.P., Atkin, W.S. (2000) Inhaled patient-administered nitrous oxide/oxygen mixture does not impair driving ability when used as analgesia during screening flexible sigmoidoscopy. *Gastrointest. Endosc.* **51**(6), 701–703.

McQuay, H.J., Carroll, D., Jadad, A.R., P. W, Moore, A. (1995) Anticonvulsant drugs for management of pain: a systematic pain. *British Medical Journal* **311**, 1047–1052.

McQuay, H.J., Tramer, M., Nye, B.A., Carroll, D., Wiffen, P.J., Moore, R.A. (1996) A systematic review of antidepressants in neuropathic pain. *Pain* **68**, 217–227.

McRorie, T.I., Lynn, A.M., Nespeca, M.K., Opheim, K.E., Slattery, J.T. (1992) The maturation of morphine clearance and metabolism. *Am. J. Dis. Child* **146**(8), 972–976.

Michaud, L., Gottrand, F., Ganga-Zandzou, P.S., Ouali, M., Vetter-Laffargue, A., Lambilliotte, A. *et al.* (1999) Nitrous oxide sedation in pediatric patients undergoing gastrointestinal endoscopy. *J. Pediatr. Gastroenterol. Nutr.* **28**(3), 310–314.

Miser, A.W., Chayt, K.J., Sandlund, J.T., Cohen, P.S., Dothage, J.A., Miser, J.S. (1986) Narcotic withdrawal syndrome in young adults after the therapeutic use of opiates. *Am. J. Dis. Child* **140**(6), 603–604.

Miyamoto, H., Saura, R., Harada, T., Doita, M., Mizuno, K. (2000) The role of cyclooxygenase-2 and inflammatory cytokines in pain induction of herniated lumbar intervertebral disc. *Kobe J. Med. Sci.* **46**(1–2), 13–28.

Moore, P.A., Crout, R.J., Jackson, D.L., Schneider, L.G., Graves, R.W., Bakos, L. (1998) Tramadol hydrochloride: analgesic efficacy compared with codeine, aspirin with codeine, and placebo after dental extraction. *J. Clin. Pharmacol.* **3**8(6), 554–560.

Naguib, M., Seraj, M., Attia, M,, Samarkandi, A.H., Seet, M., Jaroudi, R. (1998) Perioperative antinociceptive effects of tramadol. A prospective, randomized, double-blind comparison with morphine. *Can. J. Anaesth.* **45**(12), 1168–1175.

Pal, S.K., Cortiella, J., Herndon, D. (1997) Adjunctive methods of pain control in burns. *Burns* **23**(5), 404–412.

Payne, R. (1997) Mechanisms and management of bone pain. *Cancer* **80** (suppl 8), 1608–1613.

Piper, J.M., Ray, W.A., Daugherty, J.R., Griffin, M.R. (1991) Corticosteroid use and peptic ulcer disease: role of nonsteroidal anti-inflammatory drugs. *Ann. Intern. Med.* **114**(9), 735–740.

Pokela, M.L., Olkkola, K.T., Koivisto, M., Ryhanen, P. (1992) Pharmacokinetics and pharmacodynamics of intravenous meperidine in neonates and infants. *Clin. Pharmacol. Ther.* **52**(4), 342–349.

Portenoy, R.K. (1993) Cancer pain management. [Review]. *Seminars in Oncology* **20** (2 suppl 1), 19–35.

Portenoy, R.K. (1995) Pharmacological management of cancer pain. [Review]. *Seminars in Oncology* **22** (2 suppl 3), 112–120.

Price, D.D., McGrath, P.A., Rafii, A., Buckingham, B. (1983) The validation of visual analogue scales as ratio scale measures for chronic and experimental pain. *Pain* **17**, 45–56.

Pryle, B.J., Grech, H., Stoddart, P.A., Carson, R., O'Mahoney, T., Reynolds, F. (1992) Toxicity of norpethidine in sickle cell crisis. *BMJ* **304**(6840), 1478–1479.

Shah, A.A., Thjodleifsson, B., Murray, F.E., Kay, E., Barry, M., Sigthorsson, G. *et al.* (2001) Selective inhibition of COX-2 in humans is associated with less gastrointestinal injury: a comparison of nimesulide and naproxen. *Gut* **48**(3), 339–346.

Sharar, S.R., Bratton, S.L., Carrougher, G.J., Edwards, W.T., Summer, G., Levy, F.H. *et al.* (1998) A comparison of oral transmucosal fentanyl citrate and oral hydromorphone for inpatient pediatric burn wound care analgesia. *J. Burn Care Rehabil.* **19**(6), 516–521.

Shir, Y., Shenkman, Z., Shavelson, V., Davidson, E.M., Rosen, G. (1998) Oral methadone for the treatment of severe pain in hospitalized children: a report of five cases. *Clin. J. Pain* **14**(4), 350–353.

Silvasti, M., Tarkkila, P., Tuominen, M., Svartling, N., Rosenberg, P.H. (1999) Efficacy and side effects of tramadol versus oxycodone for patient-controlled analgesia after maxillofacial surgery. *Eur. J. Anaesthesiol.* **16**(12), 834–839.

Stringer, M., Makin, M.K., Miles, J., Morley, J.S. (2000) *d*-morphine, but not *l*-morphine, has low micromolar affinity for the non-competitive *N*-methyl-D-aspartate site in rat forebrain. Possible clinical implications for the management of neuropathic pain. *Neurosci. Lett.* **295**(1–2), 21–24.

Thomsen, C.B., Crawford, M.E., Sjogren, P. (1997) Malignant bone pain. *Ugeskrift for Laeger* **159**(16), 2364–2369.

Ventafridda, V., Tamburini, M., Caraceni, C., De Conno, F., Naldi, F. (1987) A validation study of the WHO method for cancer pain relief. *Cancer* **59**, 850–856.

Waterhouse, R.G. (1967) Epileptiform convulsions in children following premedication with Pamergan SP100. *Br. J. Anaesth.* **39**(3), 268–270.

Watson, C.P.N., Babul, N. (1998) Efficacy of oxycodone in neuropathic pain. *Neurology* **50**, 1837–1841.

World Health Organization. (1984) *Cancer as a Global Problem.* Geneva: WHO.

World Health Organization. (1998) Guidelines for analgesic drug therapy. In *Cancer Pain Relief and Palliative Care in Children.* Geneva: WHO/IASP; pp. 24–28.

Yeomans, N.D. (1998) New data on healing of nonsteroidal anti-inflammatory drug-associated ulcers and erosions. Omeprazole NSAID Steering Committee. *Am. J. Med.* **104**(3A), 56S–61S; discussion 79S–80S.

Yeomans, N.D., Tulassay, Z., Juhasz, L., Racz, I., Howard, J.M., van Rensburg, C.J. *et al.* (1998) A comparison of omeprazole with ranitidine for ulcers associated with nonsteroidal antiinflammatory drugs. Acid Suppression Trial: Ranitidine versus Omeprazole for NSAID-associated Ulcer Treatment (ASTRONAUT) Study Group. *N. Engl. J. Med.* **338**(11), 719–726.

5

Care of a Child Dying of Cancer

SERGEY POSTOVSKY AND MYRIAM WEYL BEN ARUSH

Pediatric Hematology Oncology Department, Meyer Children's Hospital, Rambam Medical Center, Technion Faculty of Medicine, Haifa, Israel

In the case of a dying child, the goal of therapy is to maintain the child's comfort and provide support to the child and the family (Masera *et al.* 1999, McGrath 1996, Wolfe 2000). It is the responsibility of the healthcare team to provide the child in the last phase of his or her life adequate control of pain as well as of all other bothersome symptoms.

Despite significant success that has been achieved in the past two decades in the treatment of children with cancer, it is estimated that long-term survival may be achieved only in about 75–80% of patients (Gatta *et al.* 2002). This implies that every fourth child suffering from cancer will eventually die.

The life of a child lasts to its last second. Loss of a child's life is a tragic and illogical event for all those involved and especially for the child's parents who have come to believe, as so many people do, that it is the children who should witness their parents' death and not vice versa.

Last days, hours and minutes of a child's life will most probably remain engraved forever in the parents' mind. Moreover, the way their child dies may play a critical role in the future life of the parents and possibly of the other siblings too. Therefore, it is difficult to overestimate the importance of a competent, comprehensive and sensitive management of the terminal phase of child's life.

DNR AND DNAR ORDER

Parents are frequently reluctant to discuss the 'Do Not Resuscitate' (DNR) order regarding their children because they tend to equate such a decision with

Psychosocial Aspects of Pediatric Oncology. Edited by S. Kreitler and M. Weyl Ben Arush
© 2004 John Wiley & Sons Ltd: ISBN 0 471 49939 0

the abandonment of hope and capitulation in face of impending death. Parents may sometimes consider a decision of this kind as outright betrayal of their child.

The responsibility of a palliative team is to help parents to make a correct decision in the best interests of the child. It may be prudent to initiate conversations with parents about this topic long before a child suffering from progressive cancer approaches imminent death. This approach conforms also to the modern concept which promotes incorporating palliative care into the standard care of a child sick with cancer from the very initial stages of the child's disease (American Academy of Pediatrics 2000).

It is important to note that resuscitative measures may be successful in the 'technical' sense of the word, allowing the treating team to sustain the continued performance of the vital functions, but at the same time rendering the child unconscious and leaving him without any ability to communicate with his parents and other loved ones. Given the progressive nature of the child's cancer, and the mostly irreversible nature of the symptoms causing the present distress, the net result of resuscitation may often exert a devastating effect on both the sick child and his relatives. Hence, it is of vital importance to introduce to parents the concept of 'Do Not Attempt To Resuscitate' (DNAR) (Foex 2000). In certain instances avoiding unnecessary interventions may be more appropriate than to 'go ahead to the end' and thus to prolong suffering.

However it may be, it would be advisable to discuss all issues regarding possible interventions in the end of the child's life before the critical moment approaches, and to place in the patient's medical chart written notification to forgo or to initiate (and to what extent) resuscitation. Planned discussion of the DNAR order long before the patient's final deterioration, which may be rapid and not always anticipated, allows parents to ponder upon the possibility of their child's final phase of life without the enormous psychological and emotional strain, which usually accompanies witnessing of the dying process of their beloved child. Furthermore, it is likely to enable the parents to take a more considered and reasoned decision in the best interests of a child. In view of the above considerations, discussion of the DNAR order appears to be of paramount importance. It is very useful to clarify with parents all aspects of this order, for example, not to initiate intubation and indirect cardiac massage, without concurrently forgoing drug therapy such as anti-seizures drugs and oxygen supply.

While discussing various aspects of the treatment of a child during his last days and hours, it is always useful to remember that his parents are those who are the primary decision-makers for the child. This is true not only because of the legal aspects of this situation, but primarily because no-one else knows better what their child would have preferred if he had been able to decide for himself in a given situation. Hence, in most circumstances parents should be encouraged to clearly express their intention to initiate or forgo resuscitation during the terminal phase of child's cancer.

Unfortunately, all too often in clinical practice, a DNR order is written only close to the time of the child's death. McCallum, Byrne and Bruera (2000) noted that the median time intervening between DNR and death was less than 24 hours in the case of 77 pediatric patients with cancer and other life-threatening diseases; and in 8% of the cases, the DNR order was not given at all. Only in 13 cases did death occur in the pediatric or oncology ward or at home, while the majority of deaths were registered in the intensive care unit.

Wolfe *et al.* (2000) noted that there is a significant discrepancy in understanding of ultimate prognosis between physicians and parents of pediatric cancer patients. In general, physicians realized that there was no realistic chance for cure significantly earlier than parents of children with progressive cancer (mean 106 versus 206 days before child's death, $p = 0.01$). Earlier recognition of the incurability of a child's cancer and earlier initiation of discussion of all aspects of management of the terminal phase enabled both treating physician and the child's parents to come to terms with instituting the DNR order long before the approach of the final phase.

Possible problems may arise when clearly clarified written permission from the parents has not been procured in time while the child in the terminal phase of cancer is rapidly deteriorating and develops cardiopulmonary arrest. In a situation of this kind it may be advisable to initiate resuscitation using indirect cardiac massage and artificial ventilation with an Ambu bag. Concurrently, an emergency session with the parents may be organized, sometimes in the proximity of the patient's bed. It should be conducted in a sensitive and empathic manner, preferably by the treating pediatric oncologist who has been in close contact with the family all through the child's disease. The session could be decisive regarding continuation or withdrawal of resuscitative measures. But if the parents do not give their permission to abandon life-supporting therapy it should be continued in full range.

It is to be emphasized that, even if parents choose to proceed with resuscitation despite the apparent futility of this mode of action, they neither should nor can be blamed for this. Under no circumstances is it the parents' fault but rather a failure of the palliative team to come to terms with the parents when the possibility of withdrawing resuscitative measures was contemplated.

Despite the apparent 'finality' of a DNAR order, in clinical reality it sometimes is not so. It is not inconceivable that even a child with widespread multiform glioblastoma of the brain, resistant to treatment, who has lost consciousness and deteriorated hemodynamically and respiratorily, may sometimes regain his cognitive status and resume his cardio-respiratory functioning, provided all necessary supportive measures have been properly instituted. Given the current status of our medical knowledge, we are not always able to assess a clinical situation correctly. Thus, even a child with widespread brain tumor may deteriorate because of seizures or transient elevation of intracranial pressure – namely, causes, which are potentially treatable but may go unrecognized in a child with cancer, which might be referred to as 'terminal'. If such a child is treated promptly and correctly with anti-seizures drugs and Mannitol, he may be stabilized and even discharged home for quite a long period of time. The correct decision in this sort of situation is a matter of the art of medicine and clinical experience.

DEPRESSION DURING THE TERMINAL PHASE OF CANCER

The prevalence of depression in the population of children suffering from progressive cancer has not been evaluated with precision so far (Wolfe *et al.* 2000, Steif and Heiligenstein 1989). But it is well known that depression is highly prevalent among adult cancer patients (Angelino and Treisman 2001, Breitbrat *et al.* 2000, Barraclough 1997, Chochinov *et al.* 1997). There is no doubt that children of various ages may suffer from severe and diverse psychological problems including depression. Anyone dealing with children dying from cancer encounters these problems in their everyday practice. It is sufficient to look at the eyes of many such children in order to understand that. There are several possible sources of depression in children, both physical and existential (Stevens 1998, Bluebond-Langner 1978, Spinetta, Rigler and Karon 1973, Hilden, Watterson and Chrastek 2000). The most common physical cause of depression is unremitting and poorly controlled pain (Steif and Heiligenstein 1989). In young children suffering from neuroblastoma with bone metastases and neuropathic pain, the signs of depression may become evident not only on the verbal level but also on the nonverbal one. Such children often look sad; they cry even when they stay still without moving and usually demonstrate withdrawal from playing activities with their favorite toys – the kind of activity, which had been pleasurable for them prior to the disease. Other sources of pain in children may be adverse effects of antitumor treatment, such as mucositis resulting from palliative chemotherapy and radiotherapy in a child with locally advanced rhabdomyosarcoma of head. Thus, paradoxically, palliative treatment itself may become a source of further suffering.

Other physical causes of depression in children may be nausea and vomiting, increasing respiratory difficulties and other distressing symptoms.

There are many non-physical, psychological and existential causes of depression in children with advanced cancer. Younger children may suffer from fear (Bluebond-Langner 1978, Spinetta, Rigler and Karon 1973, Hilden, Watterson and Chrastek 2000). There are at least two non-physical sources of fear: (1) fear of abandonment: one can see it every time when a parent leaves the room where the child spends his last period of life; and (2) fear of separation: when a child is afraid of losing his loved ones due to approaching death. Basically, we know little about existential sources of suffering in young children (Wolfe 2000, Attig 1996).

Older patients may suffer from depression caused by many aspects of existential crisis (Attig 1996, Cassel 1982, 1999, Sullivan 2001). It is well-known that adolescence is a crucial period of life when understanding of the surrounding world is being formed and approaches the image that adults have. In addition, children's concept of death evolves with age and during adolescence children become able to fully comprehend the irreversibility and inevitability of death (Spinetta 1974). These developments may enhance the fears of an adolescent with cancer who ponders his imminent death so that the anxiety turns into an existential crisis leading to severe depression, sometimes with devastating outcome (Attig 1996).

Taking into account all the abovementioned considerations leads to the conclusion that a palliative team should initiate treatment of suspected depression as soon as any clinical concern is raised. Sometimes a brief therapeutic trial with antidepressants helps to clarify whether a given patient suffers from depression or not (Barraclough 1997, Block 2000). In the context of terminal cancer, when many such children have neuropathic pain, antidepressants may be helpful adjunct drugs, even if clinical suspicion of depression were not proven correct (Block 2000).

PALLIATIVE SEDATION IN PEDIATRIC CANCER PATIENTS

Most children with progressive cancer in the terminal phase of their life suffer from various symptoms, where pain is the most common one (McGrath 1996, American Academy of Pediatrics 2000, Wolfe *et al.* 2000, Stevens *et al.* 1994, Collins *et al.* 1995, Galloway and Yaster 2000). With modern treatment modalities an effective control of pain, vomiting and other symptoms of physical distress is attainable in more than 90% of pediatric cancer patients (Collins *et al.* 1995, Galloway and Yaster 2000).

Difficult symptoms are identified as those symptoms which, despite their severity, may be alleviated by standard, sometimes rather rigorous, therapy, without causing unbearable side effects. This therapy does not cause sedation and excessive side effects which outweigh the positive effects of the therapy itself. This therapy should be effective within an acceptable timeframe when it is applied to a dying patient (Cherny and Portenoy 1994).

Symptoms of suffering would be designated as *refractory symptoms* (Cherny and Portenoy 1994), when all our interventions are either:

(1) incapable of providing adequate relief, or
(2) associated with excessive and intolerable side effects, or

(3) unable to provide relief to the dying child within the relevant period of time.

When all interventions directed at alleviating the suffering of a child in the terminal phase of his cancer have proven to be ineffective, conducting a therapy which is accompanied by sedation may be the only and last mode of action we have in use. This therapy is frequently designated *terminal sedation*.

The definition of terminal sedation is rather elusive. First, we do not always actually know if the child has entered the terminal phase of his disease because our ability to predict survival in patients with advanced cancer is sometimes limited. Second, there is an often-stated belief that terminal sedation is aimed at terminating the patient's suffering by hastening death. According to this belief, terminal sedation is a form of slow euthanasia (Galloway and Yaster 2000, Cherny and Portenoy 1994, Meisel 1991). Morita *et al.* (2001) showed that palliative sedation does not affect survival of adult cancer patients. Actually, this therapy may even prolong life since alleviating suffering decreases the severe physiologic stress, which may exhaust the patient and accelerate death.

It is to be emphasized that alleviating pain in dying children enhances the children's quality of life and eases the distress of the grieving parents.

There is a major difference between palliative sedation and euthanasia. Palliative sedation is intended for alleviation of existing symptoms of physical and existential suffering, while euthanasia is primarily a course of action initiated by the physician and intended to hasten death (Chater *et al.* 1998, Quill, Lo and Brock 1997, Rushton 2001). The objective of palliative sedation is not to shorten the duration of the remaining life but to alleviate pain and other symptoms, although some risk of facilitating death exists (Cherny and Portenoy 1994, Chater *et al.* 1998). In order to minimize this risk, palliative sedation should be applied only by personnel who have special expertise and training in palliative care and under thorough monitoring with regular reassessment of the child's status.

As a result, several other terms for this mode of action have been proposed, such as:

(1) Palliative sedation (Yanov 2000)
(2) Sedation for intractable distress of a dying patient (Chater *et al.* 1998, Krakauer *et al.* 2000)
(3) Sedation in the imminently dying (Sulmasy *et al.* 2000)
(4) Heavy sedation (Krakauer *et al.* 2000)

We prefer the term 'palliative sedation' in order to avoid the possible negative connotations of termination of life.

Regardless of the term, it is sedation for intractable problems near the end of life. Therefore, it is justified to raise the question: what problems may be encountered that could serve as indications for initiation of palliative sedation? The following are the most frequent ones:

(1) Severe uncontrollable pain
(2) Refractory dyspnea
(3) Refractory seizures
(4) Various psychiatric disturbances, such as confusion, agitation, or restlessness
(5) Existential suffering (Morita *et al.* 2000, Rousseau 2001, Cherny 1998)

Palliative sedation is directed solely at alleviating otherwise uncontrollable suffering. This is the main and only aim that we pursue when initiating this treatment. There is no intent to shorten the life of suffering patient. Nevertheless, under certain circumstances, when we apply palliative sedation to a dying child we cannot exclude the potential for accelerating death. In order to provide a moral justification for applying palliative sedation, a certain moral code has been invented. It is called the principle of double effect (Cherny and Portenoy 1994, Rushton 2001, Quill, Dresser and Brock 1997, Sulmasy and Pellegrino 1999).

Palliative sedation in terms of the principle of double effect means that:

(1) Our primary and only aim is to help the patient
(2) Palliative sedation is undertaken with the intention to achieve the possible alleviation of suffering without intending to shorten life even though it may be foreseen
(3) We do not want to end suffering by termination of life
(4) Palliative sedation is undertaken in a dying child when all other interventions have been unsuccessful.

There exist various methods of palliative sedation. Usually it is a combination of administering an opioid drug with some other drug that has sedative properties (Collins *et al.* 1995, Galloway and Yaster 2000, Cherny and Portenoy 1994, Kenny and Frager 1996, Fainsinger *et al.* 2000). Because many dying children with cancer have severe pain, we advocate the use of an opioid as a part of sedation in most cases.

Ideally, a decision regarding conducting palliative sedation is a multistep process. First, a palliative team should perform a thorough clinical and laboratory re-evaluation of the patient and, if needed, restaging of the disease in a given child. The primary goal of this re-evaluation is to reassure that we deal with refractory symptoms in a child with terminal cancer. Second, revision of all therapies, including psychological intervention, directed toward the alleviation of suffering is performed. Further, on the consilium of all involved medical and psychosocial staff, including the treating senior physician, nurses, the psychologist and the social worker, the possibility of presenting the proposal of palliative sedation to the child's parents is discussed. If such a decision is made, the next step is the discussion of the issue with the patient's parents.

Not all parents are ready immediately to accept a proposal of this kind at this stage, because of the immense emotional significance carried by such a decision. Hence, sometimes performance of other additional medical tests, usually some kind of imaging scan, may be useful in order to help parents understand the real state of affairs and to accept reality. After their approval palliative sedation is commenced.

Because the majority of cancer patients at the end of life suffer from pain, one of the components of palliative sedation is usually morphine administered intravenously or subcutaneously. Usually the patient gets some opioid medication at the start of palliative sedation. Hence, all that is often necessary is merely to adjust the dose of the opioid drug to the extent that pain becomes absent or minimal and to switch to the parenteral route of administration, if this has not been done before.

If the patient has not been placed on opioids earlier and is in pain, at the beginning of palliative sedation one usually applies a loading dose of morphine in order to switch off the child's consciousness, while maintaining a subsequent continuous intravenous drip of morphine with the aim of keeping the patient unconscious without, however, causing respiratory depression. This is usually achieved with doses of morphine between 0.5 and 5 mg/hour with upward titration when needed. Sometimes significantly higher doses are used to achieve the desirable effect. Use of morphine is especially convenient when the patient suffers from cancer with lung metastases causing respiratory distress and the feeling of air hunger (Collins *et al.* 1995).

Use of Meperidine in the practice of clinical pediatric oncology is limited mainly to the treatment of chills, as a side effect resulting from transfusion of various blood products or infusion of Amphothericine B. In these situations Meperidine may be a rapidly effective drug. When Meperidine is administered in repeated doses or as a continuous infusion, its toxic metabolite, normeperidine, may accumulate in the plasma and exert its excitatory effect leading to convulsions. Therefore it is recommended to omit the use of Meperidine as an opioid in the context of palliative sedation (Kaiko *et al.* 1993, Marinella 1997).

In addition to its known sedative effects, Midazolam also has prominent anticonvulsive properties. Therefore, it is especially useful for patients with seizures at present or in the past and for those who have intracranial metastases or brain tumor as a primary cancer (Collins *et al.* 1995). After the loading dose of 0.2–0.3 mg/kg of Midazolam, it should be continued by intravenous drip.

It is to be emphasized, that initiating palliative sedation is not always dictated by unbearable and uncontrolled pain. Therefore, morphine or some other opioid are not always administered and hence must not necessarily be viewed as an integral component of this kind of treatment. For example, if palliative sedation is initiated in a child with a brain tumor because of intractable seizures, sedation only with Midazolam or other sedative agents may suffice.

It is important to try to avoid any temporal association between initiation or performance of palliative sedation and the occurrence of death because such an association, even if it is merely coincidental, may become of great negative symbolic significance in the minds of parents. It is still customary in clinical practice to conduct palliative sedation with the combination of morphine, chlorpromazine and phenergan. Chlorpromazine has adrenolitic properties and tends to decrease the level of arterial pressure. Hence, it may precipitate a cardiovascular collapse in a patient, and should not be used in the context of palliative sedation. Because of the possibility of ensuing death as a result of administering chlorpromazine, it is preferable to avoid as much as possible using this drug. For the same reason, increments in drug doses should be made gradually rather than by push.

ROLE OF NUTRITION AND HYDRATION DURING TERMINAL PHASE

Providing a sick person with fluids and food is a basic requirement of human and compassionate care (MacFie 1995, Morita et al. 1999, Nelson et al. 1995). Timely and correct nutritional support may significantly improve outcome in patients with cancer. More specifically, they have been shown to facilitate successful recovery after surgical interventions (Bozzetti et al. 2000) and recovery after high-dose chemotherapy with stem cell support (Weisdorf et al. 1987). Nutritional support represents a highly emotion-laden theme with serious ethical considerations in the practice of pediatric palliative care. It is widely assumed that forgoing nutrition and fluids to a terminally ill child contradicts the very essence of compassionate care. This point of view is frequently supported by parents and other lay persons who tend to think that withholding fluids and food may lead to the patient's accelerated demise. Given the fact that most pediatric cancer patients have a central line in place during their last phase of life, it might seem tempting to use it as a vehicle for providing nutrition and hydration to the dying child. Nevertheless, one has to keep in mind all possible and unfortunately not rare drawbacks of total parenteral nutrition (TPN), which may occur with even higher frequency in debilitated cancer patients (Wesley 1992). Since in most instances the projected life expectancy is very short, whereas TPN may be potentially useful when it is given for sufficiently long periods of time (say, weeks to months), it is evident that TPN cannot play a central role in the context of palliative medicine. Exceptions to this conclusion would be those rare instances when the terminal phase of cancer is expected to be prolonged in a child who cannot be fed in any other way (for example, cases in which a surgically uncorrectable intestinal obstruction or severe respiratory distress develop in a child with pulmonary metastases after insertion of a nasogastric tube).

It has been shown that most patients with progressive cancer do not feel hunger and thirst. McCann, Hall and Groth-Juncker (1994) in their study of 32 adult patients with a life expectancy of 3 months or less (31 patients suffered from cancer) found that 63% of patients never experienced any hunger and 34% additional patients complained of hunger only during the initial phase of starvation. Similarly, 62% of patients either experienced no thirst or experienced thirst only initially during their terminal illness. In those patients who had some complaints of either hunger or thirst, it was possible to achieve alleviation by very simple measures, such as providing small amounts of food, or water and by moistening of lips. In another study, Torelli, Campos and Meguid (1999) tried to determine whether providing TPN may actually improve the quality of life and alter the ultimate outcome of terminally ill adult cancer patients. The authors evaluated the possible influence of TPN provided either as an adjunct to in-hospital intensive therapy for cancer or for in-hospital supportive treatment and found that in both settings providing TPN was of no value either for quality of life or for the ultimate outcome of these cancer patients. Unfortunately, there are no similar studies performed with terminally ill pediatric cancer patients. But common sense and clinical experience suggest that the same holds true for pediatric oncology as well.

A lot has been written about the ethical aspects of forgoing nutritional support to terminally sick patients (MacFie 1995, Nelson et al. 1995, Sullivan 1993, Barber et al. 1998). A current concept prevailing in medicine is that nutrition and hydration are medical interventions as much as any other treatment modalities and, therefore, their administration should be subsumed under the same moral and ethical principles (Nelson et al. 1995, Bozzetti et al. 1996). It is ethically justified to withhold or even withdraw some medical interventions in patients suffering from progressive cancer in the terminal phase, in order to prevent unnecessary suffering by providing futile treatments (Nelson et al. 1995). According to this postulate, providing nutrition and hydration should be ruled only by medical indications. However, in the reality of pediatric palliative oncology, this apparently clear decision to forgo provision of nutrition to the child dying of cancer is not so easily accepted. Parents very often, and sometimes even the treating medical personnel, find it emotionally too difficult to agree not to give food or fluids to a dying child. In certain instances, when there is no consensus between the parents of a dying child and the treating physician, it may be prudent to provide the child with hydration through either a nasogastric tube (Boyd and Beeken 1994) or a central/peripheral line while forgoing nutritional support. Explaining to the parents that the fluids contain a certain amount of glucose necessary for providing energy may facilitate parental agreement to accept the physician's proposal.

PLACE OF DEATH

It is generally assumed that most people would prefer to die at their homes surrounded by close family members and friends. It is logically easy to assume that children do not constitute an exception to this general rule (Lauer and Camitta 1980, Mulhern, Lauer and Hoffmann 1983). As McCallum, Byrne and Bruera (2000) put it 'death in hospital is the default situation when support for death in the home is inadequate'. Unfortunately, it is only rarely that the child's death occurs at his or her home. There are several possible reasons for this. First, the progressive nature of cancer itself is often accompanied by multiple symptoms, sometimes difficult to control, which necessitate hospitalization of a dying child. Second, the intense psychological impact that imminent death of the child poses for other family members may preclude the child's staying at home in the last phase of sickness. Third, there are sometimes certain human, financial and other difficulties that limit or even completely preclude the possibility of managing the terminal phase of cancer in an ill child at home. This becomes all too evident when we consider that, in order to enable successful terminal care of the child with cancer at home, it is necessary to create a palliative care team specifically dedicated for the management of such children (Sirkia *et al*. 1997). Optimally, this multidisciplinary team should consist of a pediatric oncologist, a pediatric oncology nurse, a psychologist and a social worker. The presence of a chaplain or another spiritual personality may be very helpful as well.

If death at home is not an option, the dying child spends his or her last days in the hospital. But even in a hospital ward the medical personnel should make everything possible in order to create a sense of 'home' for the dying child and his relatives. It is insensitive and therefore unacceptable to ask parents to leave the room where their child is dying, even using the excuse that it is too stressful for parents to witness the last agony of their loved one. These last minutes spent together may be very precious for those who continue to live, indeed they are all too precious to be ignored or slighted. It is likely that they may even help the parents to undergo a normal bereavement process during this difficult time. The responsibility of the palliative team is to make everything possible in order to mask signs of agony by properly performed medical assistance to a dying child (by optimal dosing of opioids and sedatives). It may sometimes be very useful to explain tactfully to parents about physiologic changes their child is undergoing during the process of dying as soon as they occur, while constantly reassuring parents that all possible sources of suffering during this period are properly addressed and controlled.

It occurs only very rarely in clinical practice of pediatric oncology that parents do not want to be present at the bed of their dying child. In that case the parents' wishes should be respected and a quiet place should be provided for them to stay or wait not far from the child's ward. In these cases it is very helpful if a psychologist or another person familiar to the parents stay near the grieving parents.

CONCLUSION

For a parent witnessing the death of a child is a tragic event, which cannot be compared in its severity and intensity with anything else. The physician often is unable to prevent this death but is responsible for making it as peaceful and free of suffering as possible. The ultimate gratification of the physican in his work as a palliative care specialist is rendering it possible for the bereaved parents to detect meaning in the death of the child. This is achieved by vigorous control of all physical symptoms in a dying child and close attention to all existential, emotional and social demands of both the child and his or her relatives.

REFERENCES

American Academy of Pediatrics (2000) Committee on Bioethics and Committee on Hospital Care. Palliative care for children. *Pediatrics* **106**(2 Pt 1), 351–357.

Angelino, A.F., Treisman, G.J. (2001) Major depression and demoralization in cancer patients: diagnostic and treatment considerations. *Support Care Cancer* **9**, 344–349.

Attig, T. (1996) Beyond pain: The existential suffering of children. *J. Palliat. Care* **12**, 20–23.

Barber, M.D., Fearon, K.C.H., Delmore, G., Loprinzi, C.L. (1998) Should cancer patients with incurable disease receive parenteral or enteral nutritional support? *Eur. J. Cancer* **34**, 279–285.

Barraclough, J. (1997) ABC of palliative care. Depression, anxiety, and confusion. *BMJ* **315**, 1365–1368.

Block, S.D. (2000) Assessing and management depression in the terminally ill patient. ACP-ASIM End-of-life Care Consensus Panel. American College of Physicians: American Society of Internal Medicine. *Ann. Intern. Med.* **132**, 209–218.

Bluebond-Langner, M. (1978) *The Private Words of Dying Children*. Princeton, NJ: Princeton University Press.

Boyd, K.J., Beeken, L. (1994) Tube feeding in palliative care: benefits and problems. *Palliat. Med.* **8**, 156–158.

Bozzetti, F., Amadori, D., Bruera, E., Cozzaglio, L., Corli, O., Filiberti, A., Rapin, C.H., *et al.* (1996) Guidelines on artificial nutrition versus hydration in terminal cancer patients. European Association for Palliative Care. *Nutrition* **12**, 163–167.

Bozzetti, F., Gavazzi, C., Miceli, R., Rossi, N., Mariani, L., Cozzaglio, L., Bonfanti, G., Piacenza, S. (2000) Perioperative total parenteral nutrition in malnourished, gastrointestinal cancer patients: a randomized, clinical trial. *J. Parenter. Enter. Nutr.* **24**, 7–14.

Breitbrat, W., Rosenfeld, B., Pessin, H., Kaim, M., Funesti-Esch, J., Galietta, M., Nelson, C.J., Brescia, R. (2000) Depression, hopelessness, and desire for hastened death in terminally ill patients with cancer. *JAMA* **284**, 2907–2911.

Cassel, E.J. (1982) The nature of suffering and the goals of medicine. *N. Engl. J. Med.* **306**, 639–645.

Cassel, E.J. (1999) Diagnosing suffering: a perspective. *Ann. Intern. Med.* **131**, 531–534.

Chater, S., Viola, R., Paterson, J., Jarvis, V. (1998) Sedation for intractable distress in the dying – a survey of experts. *Palliat. Med.* **12**, 255–269.

Cherny, N.I. (1998) Sedation in response to refractory existentional distress: Walking the fine line. *J. Pain & Symptom Management* **16**, 404–406.

Cherny, N.I., Portenoy, R.K. (1994) Sedation in the management of refractory symptoms: guidelines for evaluation and treatment. *J. Palliat. Care* **10**, 31–38.

Chochinov, H.M., Wilson, K.G., Anns, M., Lander, S. (1997) 'Are you depressed?' Screening for depression in the terminally ill. *Am. J. Psychiatry* **154**, 674–676.

Collins, J.J., Grier, H.E., Kinney, H.C., Berde, C.B. (1995) Control of severe pain in children with terminal malignancy. *J. Pediatr.* **126**, 653–657.

Fainsinger, R.L., Waller, A., Bercovoci, M., Bengston, K., Landman, W., Hoskins, M., *et al.* (2000) A multicentre international study of sedation for uncontrolled symptoms in terminally ill patients. *Palliat. Med.* **14**, 257–265.

Foex, B.A. (2000) Do-not-attempt resuscitation ('DNAR') order. *Anaesthesia* **55**, 292.

Galloway, K.S., Yaster, M. (2000) Pain and symptom control in terminally ill children. *Pediatr. Clin. North America* **47**, 711–746.

Gatta, G., Capocaccia, R., Coleman, M.P., Ries, L.A., Berrino, F. (2002) Childhood cancer survival in Europe and the United States. *Cancer* **95**(8), 1767–1772.

Hilden, J.M., Watterson, J., Chrastek, J. (2000) Tell the children. *J. Clin. Oncol.* **18**, 3193–3195.

Kaiko, R.F., Foley, K.M., Grabinski, P.Y., Heindrich, G., Rogers, A.G., Inturrisi, C.E., Reidenberg, M.M. (1983) Central nervous system excitatory effects of Meperidine in cancer patients. *Ann. Neurol.* **13**, 180–185.

Kenny, N.P., Frager, G. (1996) Refractory symptoms and terminal sedation of children: Ethical issues and practical management. *J. Palliat. Care* **12**, 40–45.

Krakauer, E.L., Penson, R.T., Truog, R.D., King, L.A., Chabner, B.A., Lynch, T.J. Jr (2000) Sedation for intractable distress of a dying patient: acute palliative care and the principle of double effect. *Oncologist* **5**, 53–62.

Lauer, M.E., Camitta, B.M. (1980) Home care for dying children: A nursing model. *J. Pediatr.* **97**, 1032–1035.

MacFie, J. (1995) Ethics and nutritional support. *Nutrition* **11**, 213–216.

McCallum, D.E., Byrne, P., Bruera, E. (2000) How children die in hospital. *J. Pain & Symptom Management* **20**, 417–423.

McCann, R.M., Hall, W.J., Groth-Juncker, A. (1994) Comfort care for terminally ill patients. The appropriate use of nutrition and hydration. *JAMA* **272**, 1263–1266.

McGrath, P. (1996) Development of the World Health Organization guidelines on cancer pain relief and palliative care in children. *J. Pain & Symptom Management* **12**, 87–92.

Marinella, M.A. (1997) Meperidine-induced generalized seizures with normal renal function. *South. Med. J.* **90**, 556–558.

Masera, J., Spinetta, J.J., Jankovic, M., Ablin, A.R., D'Angio, G.J., Van Dongen-Melman, J., *et al.* (1999) Guidelines for assistance to terminally ill children with cancer: A report of the SIOP Working Committee on psychosocial issues in pediatric oncology. *Med. Pediatr. Oncol.* **32**, 44–48.

Meisel, A. (1991) Legal myths about terminating life support. *Arch. Intern. Med.* **151**, 1497–1501.

Morita, T., Tsunoda, J., Inoue, S., Chihara, S. (1999) Perceptions and decision-making on rehydration of terminally ill cancer patients and family members. *Am. J. Hosp. Palliat. Care* **16**, 509–516.

Morita, T., Tsunoda, J., Inoue, S., Chihara, S. (2000) Terminal sedation for existential distress. *Am. J. Hosp. Palliat. Care* **17**, 189–195.

Morita, T., Tsunoda, J., Inoue, S., Chihara, S. (2001) Effects of high dose opioids and sedatives on survival in terminally ill cancer patients. *J. Pain & Symptom Management* **21**, 282–289.

Mulhern, R.K., Lauer, M.E., Hoffmann, R.G. (1983) Death of a child at home or in the hospital: subsequent psychological adjustment of the family. *Pediatrics* **71**, 743–747.

Nelson, L.J., Rushton, C.H., Cranford, R.E., Nelson, R.M., Glover, J.J. (1995) Forgoing medically provided nutrition and hydration in pediatric patients. *J. Law Med. Ethics* **23**, 33–46.

Quill, T.E., Dresser, R., Brock, D.W. (1997) The rule of double effect – a critique of its role in end-of-life decision making. *N. Engl. J. Med.* **337**, 1768–1771.

Quill, T.E., Lo, B., Brock, D.W. (1997) Palliative options of last resort: a comparison of voluntary stopping eating and drinking, terminal sedation, physician-assisted suicide, and voluntary active euthanasia. *JAMA* **278**, 2099–2104.

Rousseau, P. (2001) Existential suffering and palliative sedation: a brief commentary with a proposal for clinical guidelines. *Am. J. Hosp. Palliat. Care* **18**, 151–153.

Rushton, C.H. (2001) Ethical decision making at the end of life. In Armstrong-Dailey, A., Zarbock, S. (Eds). *Hospice Care for Children* (2nd edn). Oxford: Oxford University Press, pp. 323–352.

Sirkiä, K., Saarinen, U.M., Ahlgren, B., Hovi, L. (1997) Terminal care of the child with cancer at home. *Acta Paediatr.* **86**, 1125–1130.

Spinetta, J.J. (1974) The dying child's awareness of death: a review. *Psychol. Bull.* **81**, 841–845.

Spinetta, J., Rigler, D., Karon, M. (1973) Anxiety in the dying child. *Pediatrics* **52**, 841–845.

Steif, B.L., Heiligenstein, E.L. (1989) Psychiatric symptoms of pediatric cancer pain. *J. Pain & Symptom Management* **4**, 191–196.

Stevens, M.M. (1998) Psychological adaptation of the dying child. In Doyle, D., Hanke, G.W.C., MacDonald, N. (Eds). *Oxford Textbook of Palliative Medicine* (2nd edn). New York: Oxford University Press, pp. 1057–1075.

Stevens, M.M., Dalla-Pozza, L., Cavalletto, B., Cooper, M.G., Kilham, H.A. (1994) Pain and symptom control in paediatric palliative care. *Cancer Surv.* **21**, 211–231.

Sullivan, M.D. (2001) Finding pain between minds and bodies. *Clin. J. Pain* **17**, 146–156.

Sullivan, R.J. Jr (1993) Accepting death without artificial nutrition or hydration. *J. Gen. Intern. Med.* **8**, 220–224.

Sulmasy, D.P., Pellegrino, E.D. (1999) The rule of double effect: clearing up the double talk. *Arch. Intern. Med.* **159**, 545–550.

Sulmasy, D.P., Ury, W.A., Ahronheim, J.C., Siegler, M., Kass, L., Lantos, J., *et al.* (2000) Responding to intractable terminal suffering [letter]. *Ann. Intern. Med.* **133**, 560–561.

Torelli, G.F., Campos, A.C., Meguid, M.M. (1999) Use of TPN in terminally ill cancer patients. *Nutrition* **15**, 665–667.

Weisdorf, S.A., Lysne, J., Wind, D., Haake, R.J., Sharp, H.L., Goldman, A., Schissel, K., *et al.* (1987) Positive effect of prophylactic total parenteral nutrition on long-term outcome of bone marrow transplantation. *Transplantation* **43**, 833–838.

Wesley, J.R. (1992) Efficacy and safety of total parental nutrition in pediatric patients. *Mayo Clin. Proc.* **67**, 672–675.

Wolfe, J. (2000) Suffering in children at the end of life: Recognizing an ethical duty to palliate. *J. Clin. Ethics* **11**, 157–163.

Wolfe, J., Klar, N., Grier, H.E., Duncan, J., Salem-Schatz, S., Emanuel, E.J., Weeks, J.C. (2000a) Understanding of prognosis among parents of children who died of cancer: impact on treatment goals and integration of palliative care. *JAMA* **284**, 2469–2475.

Wolfe, J., Grier, H.E., Klar, N., Levin, S.B., Ellenbogen, J.M., Salem-Schatz, S., Emanuel, E.J., Weeks, J.C. (2000b) Symptoms and suffering at the end of life in children with cancer. *N. Engl. J. Med.* **342**, 326–333.

Yanov, M.L. (2000) Responding to intractable terminal suffering [letter]. *Ann. Intern. Med.* **133**, 560.

PART TWO
PSYCHOSOCIAL ASPECTS

6

The Child's Subjective Experience of Cancer and the Relationship with Parents and Caregivers

DANIEL OPPENHEIM

Department of Paediatrics and Unit of Psycho-oncology, Institut Gustave Roussy, Villejuif, France

INTRODUCTION

The past few years have been marked by major improvements in the treatment of children with cancer. Nonetheless, it remains an overwhelming experience (Sanger, Copeland and Davidson 1991), which disturbs all their landmarks: the relation to their body, their family, the society they belong to, a sense of personal identity and of having a value. They are confronted with the question of death, and subsequently with the question of the meaning and the value of their life. They wonder: 'Why me? Why now? Who is responsible?', and cancer appears as a major ordeal. Treatment has two goals, curing children and helping them preserve their dynamics and faith in life.

We present how children experience being afflicted by and treated for a cancer, and what may remain of this experience. The situations are extremely diverse, as are the children, their families, their living conditions, the way they think and react, their illnesses, the countries they live in, the means paediatricians have at their disposal, etc. We intend to describe the major traits of this experience so that the children's words and behaviour can be easily understood, how they are accompanied throughout this difficult, painful journey and how we try to prevent and treat possible psychological and relational destabilisation.

Psychosocial Aspects of Pediatric Oncology. Edited by S. Kreitler and M. Weyl Ben Arush
© 2004 John Wiley & Sons Ltd: ISBN 0 471 49939 0

Caregivers take care of the children and their family (Grootenhuis *et al.* 1996), try to prevent and treat their disarray, and are attentive to the early signs of such confusion: difficulties in coping, anxiety (Last and Van Veldhuizen 1996), depression (Noll *et al.* 1999, Phipps and Srivastava 1997, Worchel *et al.* 1998), revolt, non-compliance (Kupst 1993, Spinetta *et al.* 2001), etc. However, they are also concerned for the future, and try to attenuate the risks of physical, cognitive, social and psychological sequels which may appear soon or long after the end of the treatment, at significant moments in their life: adolescence, undergraduate studies, entry into adulthood, becoming a parent, etc. Cancer is a long-lasting history, the effects of which may be positive or negative: this depends considerably on the way the child has lived through this intense experience.

THE CHILD, A MAJOR INTERLOCUTOR

Each child is unique. Children react according to their age, illness (disease site, constraints due to treatment, medical condition), their own and their family's lifestyle, way of thinking and behaving. Knowing these elements helps to foster relations of mutual confidence with the children and their parents, and may avoid pointless or dangerous conflicts.

As soon as children are able to speak, they can understand (Eiser and Havermans 1992) what they are going through: an illness, like those they know, but stronger, with longer and more unpleasant treatment. They accept its constraints more easily without becoming passive when they understand its characteristics, reasons and logic, when they continue to have confidence in their parents' ability to help and protect them and preserve the stability of the family, when the relation they have with the medical and nursing staff is good enough, which implies efficient treatment of pain.

The First Consultation

The first consultation closes the door on a period of anxiety and fear provoked by unnamed symptoms, to which it gives a cause ('a cancer') but not a reason ('why?'), opens the door to another period (the treatment is expected and feared), and introduces the child and his/her parents to the paediatric oncology setting. The paediatrician should therefore explain the diagnosis and treatment, but also its logic (Eden *et al.* 1994, Girgis and Sanson-Fisher 1995), maintaining a proper balance between stressing the risks involved and the need for good compliance, and expressing reasonable confidence in the outcome (not a promise nor a guarantee of success), or in the value of trying it. Grieving parents often ask: 'Was it worth it? Couldn't we have made better use of the time with our child, without all these sufferings?', and sometimes complain: 'The doctor was too optimistic, we feel as if we have been cheated'. Doctors should pay attention to the explanations given by the parents and by the child about the illness (Eiser, Havermans and Eiser 1995) and about the treatment. They may have their own theories that are conscious or not, private or shared by their family, their community, and that may be at variance with the medical theories and therefore likely to provoke conflicts. However, in all cases, these theories have a meaning and a value for them, and contribute to their sense of identity. The paediatrician as well as the social worker should know the social and practical living conditions of the family (distance from the ward, siblings and their age, income, social status, whom they can rely on, etc.): these elements can hinder the parents from supporting the child, and sometimes the cost and constraints of the treatment can provoke a relational or financial disaster for them, or the temptation to renounce treatment. The paediatrician should try to evaluate the quality of the relation between the child and the parents (if the child trusts them, and thus could trust the medical staff), and between the parents themselves.

The parents are shocked, unable to listen to the information, to understand its content. This information should therefore be reiterated later on, and not imparted just once. The parents and the child often understand these explanations via the screen of their fears, of their beliefs, of their knowledge, of the memories of other illnesses in the family history, and according to the place the child has in their lives. This explains the paradoxical questions or reactions they sometimes have (Koch *et al.* 1996). Their account (Mattingly 1984) of what has happened since the first symptoms provides precious information on their thoughts, their way of reacting, their relation with their community, with the caregivers and with the child, on their fears and expectations. They have to understand that cancer is not only an illness to be treated but an intense and complex period in their lives, which will last several months at least: therefore they must not try to be courageous little soldiers constantly and at all costs. They will share it with many people: medical and non-medical members of the staff, other parents and children, etc. They will have a special relation with the paediatrician who will keep track of the entire course of treatment, but also with many members of the team, who will liaise with their community caregivers.

The Course of Treatment

The course of treatment is a long journey, during which the parents and the child evolve. They discover the complex reality of what cancer means, its treatment, different from what they had imagined, and its consequences on their lives (school, friends, family and professional life), and also their unknown qualities and weaknesses. Their way of thinking about themselves, their plans and their past may evolve, old and unsolved questions may

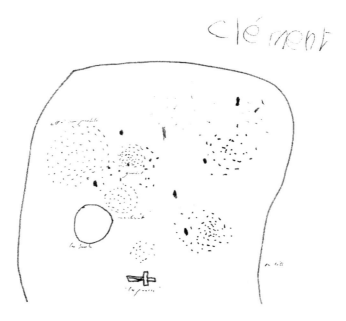

Figure 6.1 F., 7-year-old boy, treated for a brain tumour. He has illustrated the battle between good and evil elements in his brain

reappear, thrust into the present by the torturing question concerning the reasons for and the legitimacy of their choices: why are they living together?, why did they give birth to this child?, why have they educated him/her this or that way?, etc. This may explain moments of discouragement and revolt, which have their place during the course of treatment. The parents and the child should not be ashamed nor afraid of them, but should consider them as warning signs which offer them an opportunity to reflect upon themselves and upon coping with the treatment.

The parents and the children may be particularly disturbed when the treatment lasts longer than expected, or when it has to be changed, and the children try to perceive the meaning behind the change. High-dose chemotherapy and surgery are both feared and expected. These are powerful treatments, after which disappointment may ensue, because chemotherapy has to be pursued. The constraints generated by the treatment may affect family life: loss of a job, financial or marital difficulties, siblings' revolt. The children's drawings offer a precious insight into the evolution of their body image, their perception of the illness (Figure 6.1) and treatment (Figure 6.2), of themselves, of their relations with their parents and siblings, etc.

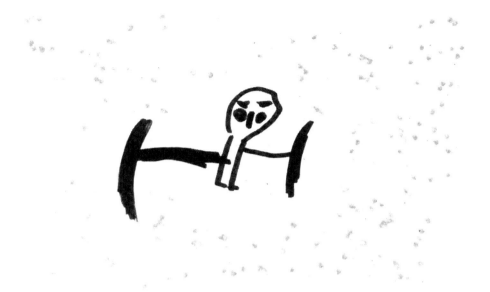

Figure 6.2 D., 7-year-old boy. He has drawn himself facing the ward and the treatment

The end of treatment is a very difficult moment that is awaited and feared. The child leaves the protected medical setting, but the exhausting fear of a relapse may hover. They have to return to 'normal life', explain to others what has happened, rekindle relations with friends and peers, and finally cope with physical or psychological sequels. Both the children and their parents wonder whether they are still the same, and how they have been transformed by the experience of illness (Figure 6.3). This last consultation, before follow-up, is an opportunity to receive an overall explanation of the treatment, to discuss exhaustively what has happened during that time. The satisfaction expressed by the paediatrician, the parents and the child may differ considerably, because their criteria, their aims in life, the personal cost they have accepted to pay for the treatment are different. This should be thoroughly discussed to avoid misunderstanding, mistrust, disappointment, anger, distress. The parents and the child may wonder whether the 'price' was not too high, when sequels appear intolerable. However, an automatic relation does not exist between the extent of such sequels and the feeling of distress (Figure 6.4): it depends on their values, their self-esteem, their plans, their social environment and their psychological traits. As during the first consultation, paediatricians should explain precisely the reasons for the choices they made, their point of view regarding the treatment and the child's situation; but they should be attentive to the parents' and the child's point of view.

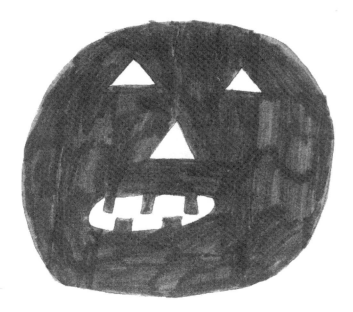

Figure 6.3 M., 10-year-old boy, treated for a brain tumour. In his drawing, his head is an empty Halloween pumpkin

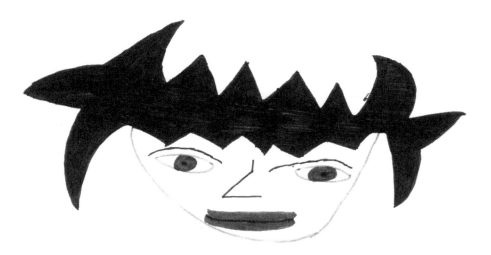

Figure 6.4 S., 12-year-old girl, treated for a brain tumour. She has portrayed the painful and burdensome sequels of her illness

The Period of Follow-up

The period of follow-up is a difficult one (Masera *et al.* 1996) of progressive rehabilitation (returning to school and to everyday life) (Larcombe and Charlton 1996), and assessment of the consequences of the treatment, for the child as well as for the parents (Kazak *et al.* 1998, Van Dongen Melman *et al.* 1995). They often fear the risk of relapse and do not know how to deal with it: should they strive to ignore it, or be attentive to the slightest signs? They may feel so different from who they were, so fragile, or invaded by a bitter feeling of injustice, which may develop into egotistical or even fraudulent behaviour: 'We have paid too much, we won't pay any longer, now it is the others' turn to pay'. They may feel ashamed of what happened, responsible for the cancer, as if they were not strong enough to cope with this ordeal (then compulsion to prove their courage and value may lead to risky behaviour), as if they will forever remain marked by a visible (when there are sequels) or invisible stain: some compare cancer to rape. They may also feel guilty about the difficulties their illness has caused their family (Barakat *et al.* 1997), and ashamed of these thoughts.

There may be negative psychological sequels (Gray *et al.* 1992): a loss of self-esteem (Figure 6.5), persistent anger against and mistrust of doctors and medicine or, on the contrary, excessive expectations, as if they could solve all the problems in their lives, and not only medical ones. They may feel fragile – their body (Pendley, Dahlquist and Dreyer 1997), themselves (Ropponen *et al.* 1992) – and thus stick to the safe nest of their family, sometimes with the complicity of their parents, or they may feel different from others, and trapped in loneliness. On the other hand, they may have discovered in themselves and in their parents or siblings unsuspected qualities, resources and strong ties, greater frankness, open-mindedness and attention to others, or new fields of interest (Greenberg and Meadows 1991), such as medicine or research. Paediatricians should then be attentive to the reasons for this vocation: it can express excessive identification with the caregivers, a criticism ('I will show you how you should treat children'), a determination to pay a debt, a temptation to remain where medical protection is present, an effort to at least discover what has happened. Some say: 'It was hard, I didn't choose it, but I do not regret it. It has given me strength, and new values'. The disturbing memory of what they have gone through may actively reappear, at significant moments: beginning or end of adolescence, undergraduate studies, parents' retirement or death, becoming parents, etc. Psychotherapeutic interviews may then be helpful.

A Relapse

A relapse is a difficult moment. The children may say: 'All those sufferings for nothing! I have been cheated', and be tempted to give up or to refuse treatment. They wonder whether they still have chances of being cured, although they may

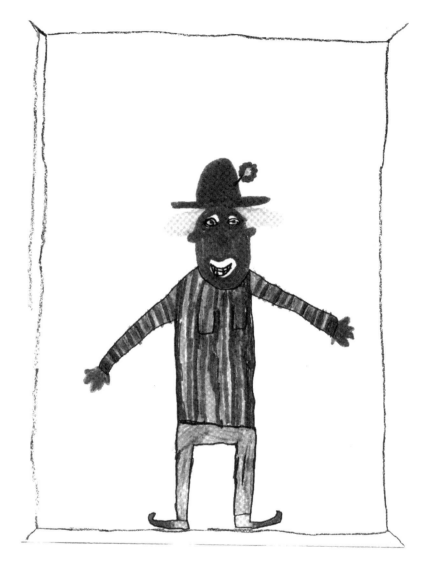

Figure 6.5 G., 8-year-old boy. In this drawing he is a clown, and he behaved accordingly

be smaller, or none whatsoever. All the worst memories of the first treatment reappear, and they must reappraise them in order to cope with the new one, and trust the paediatricians and their parents. The parents' reactions are diverse: they may seem totally surprised when relapse occurs because they had tried to ignore this risk, recognise an opportunity to fight anew, or take it as confirmation of the child's fatal fate of which they were certain right from the outset.

Terminal Illness

This difficult and important period (Masera *et al.* 1999, Whittam 1993) is still not always adequately managed (Wolfe *et al.* 2000). Staff need specific training (Papadatou 1997). The doctors do not have curative or palliative treatments to propose, the children cannot continue to do what they did before. Although nobody knows exactly when death will occur, death is inevitable even if the parents believe in a miracle (they are right when this belief alleviates their distress without separating them from reality). The children know, more or less, that they are going to die (Bluebond-Langner 1989), or that they are at a stage where death is highly probable (Figure 6.6), but they preserve a place for the belief that they may escape this outcome, or put this fact in a remote place in their mind. Clinical experience shows that they are not afraid of death, on certain conditions. When caregivers have been attentive to their physical needs (pain, discomfort, etc.) and to what they have said throughout the treatment, they do not fear loneliness. When they were able to rely sufficiently on their parents who did not change their behaviour and their relation with them considerably, when they remain the same for their parents, death will not mean oblivion: then, they are confident that they will preserve beautiful images of them, and not only the ones of the dreadful moments they sometimes went through. Sometimes parents say: 'My son/daughter has changed so much that we don't recognise him/her', and this terrible declaration means that they belong to separate worlds, that they practically have nothing left in common, even before death comes. When the parents say: 'All that done to reach this point . . . !' the children may fear that their parents are angry with them because of the sufferings they have caused, regret their treatment, and maybe their life. Thinking that one's life has been worthless is unbearable. When the parents say: 'If my son/daughter dies, we won't be able to live, life will be like hell', the child may feel guilty, and fear that his/her parents will die, and that nobody will be left to remember them and continue to love them; or that they will be replaced, not followed, by another child. When the parents criticise the caregivers excessively, the children may fear that these care providers will neglect them, or that their incompetence is responsible for their situation which could have been avoided. When the parents are attentive only to the physical manifestations of the disease and treatment, and not to the child's emotions, what he/she is expressing, when they are locked in despair, excessive anticipatory grief or intense depression, the child may feel dead already, and be afraid that death could be this dreadful loneliness. When the child is mute, the parents may perceive this silence as a reproach ('You are responsible for what is happening; I will die and you will go on living'), and this reactivates

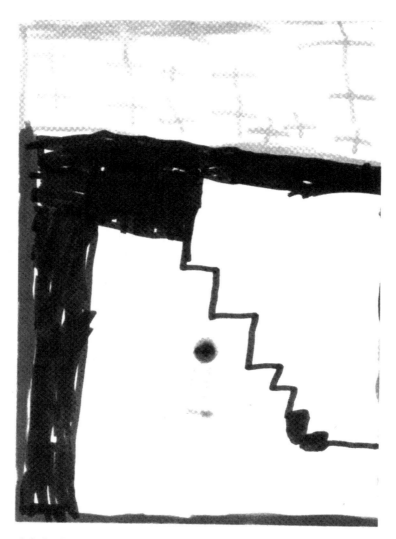

Figure 6.6 D., 7-year-old boy. He has drawn himself locked inside the ward and the treatment, with red crosses, signifying death, hovering above the building

their guilt and their feeling of powerlessness. However, they also fear the questions the children may ask: 'Am I really going to die?' So do the caregivers, and this explains why they partly avoid true dialogues with them. When the children ask this question, the parents can reply by the following question: 'Why are you asking this question?' and the child may then make them understand that it was because of excessive pain, or due to the death of another child, or because of provocation, or doubt, etc. Then, they may answer: 'The doctors said that the illness was too strong for their treatments. We believe them, but we nevertheless still have faith'. If the child wants to go on further: 'Will I die?', the parents may answer: 'We hope not. If that happens, it will cause us great sorrow, but life will go on. We will always think of you and of all the moments of happiness we have shared'.

During this period, the children try to strike a balance between their pains to keep in touch with others, and their need to go deeper into their shell; this should be distinguished from depression or anger, which can exist, of course. Caregivers should therefore be trained to recognise and understand the child's and the parents' thoughts, emotions and fears, and their own. They may thus be able to help parents maintain their relations with the child and their parental role until the last moment, even when he/she is unconscious: they can try to understand the meaning of the slightest movement or attitude of his/her body and face. This implies treating pain and delirium, and explaining it to parents, and to siblings. They should also be helped to maintain their parental role towards the siblings, to be attentive to their distress, their emotions such as anger against doctors, jealousy towards the sick child, guilt about being the one who will live, fear of the future (do they run the same risk, what will the family become, what will be their place in it, etc.?). When the siblings hear: 'It is always the best one who dies', they feel worthless, think that success is dangerous, and wonder: 'Maybe my parents would have preferred that I die?' The siblings' distress can be expressed in paradoxical ways: they may refuse to be present beside their brother or sister (they should not be falsely accused of egoism – they feel helpless), or, on the contrary, remain at his/her bedside, as if they do not trust their parents' ability to take care of the dying child, or in order to sacrifice themselves, etc. They may try to be as perfect as an angel, to compete with him/her, or on the contrary play the role of the black sheep, by behaving badly at home or in school, or by naughty remarks. Parents should not say: 'You are an egotistical monster', but rather, 'We know you are a good girl/boy, you love him/her, you are suffering so much, but you could and should behave differently. We love you just as much'. This may avoid sometimes long-lasting sequels, such as depression, even suicide, a lack of self-esteem, persistent guilt, with negative effects on their academic achievements and their emotional, family and social life: 'If parents suffer so much when a child is severely ill, I will never have children', or 'I cannot succeed because I will be accused of taking advantage of his/her death, because he/she cannot be outdistanced, because success leads to death, etc.'.

Parents are often locked in the present, unable to think of the future or remember the past (before this phase, before the illness). Some feel incapable of being alone beside the child, while others practically forbid the caregivers to come and take care of him/her, as if they were saying: 'The child is ours, we know better than you what is good for him/her; you have done enough harm'.

Some overtly express their emotion, while others hide and control it: their distress may be deeper. Caregivers can assist the child and the family by helping them to remain as close and as mutually understanding as possible, to preserve their ties – not only those related to the present, but also to the past they have shared, and to their future – by helping the child to express his/her feelings, demands, doubts, and by helping the family to understand his/her slightest signs of expression.

Grieving

Everywhere, the death of a child is one of the most terrible experiences for a parent (Davies *et al.* 1998). Initially, they are in a state of shock, 'emptied' (Martinson, Davies and McClowry 1991), they cannot believe the child's death and act as if he/she was not dead. They are afraid of the risk of forgetting, are persecuted by insistent, terrifying images of his/her last moments, disturbing 'flashbacks' which come at any moment, and therefore are tempted to expunge their memory. They remember that they were torn between the dual temptation of endless treatments (to defer the moment of his/her death as much as possible, and of their unimaginable distress) and of euthanasia (to put a stop to the child's sufferings as well as their own distress), they do not know which would have been the best 'choice', and feel guilty about these thoughts. They are tempted to both get rid of all the child's belongings and to transform his/her room into a museum full of untouchable things. Mothers may say they will never have children again, because the risk of experiencing such agonies again is unthinkable and, at the same time, they express their yearning for a pregnancy to fill the intolerable void in themselves, to replace the lost child immediately. They feel they have lost their reasons for living, their identity, reduced to that of 'parents of a child who was treated for cancer and who is dead', their youth, their value, their beauty, their sexual desire. The relations in the couple become difficult, but this ordeal may strengthen it, and they often are incapable of noticing the siblings' grief (Pollack 1985) (Figure 6.7) – changes in schooling, in mood or behaviour, such as solitude, violence or excessive gentleness – or of helping them. They fear all anniversary dates (dates of birth, illness, death, etc.), all the family gatherings, because they reactivate the obviousness of the child's absence. They continue to search for the cause of his/her death, for a culprit: doctors, themselves and all the wrong choices they have made, the paucity of medical means, of research, etc. They feel different from all others whose children are alive, who are incapable of understanding what they feel.

Some elements may serve to assuage the intensity and the excessive duration of grief. With adequate, true information imparted by a referee paediatrician (a responsible interlocutor, whom they know well) throughout treatment, the parents may be able to strike a balance between excessive fears and blind optimism. Then death will not be a total surprise. They may acknowledge that

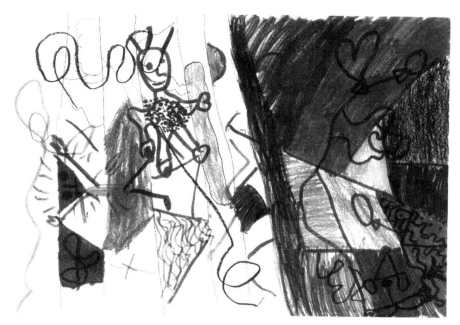

Figure 6.7 A., 6-year-old girl. Her sister died two and a half years earlier, and she is still grieving. She has drawn her room, which is in a mess, like her mind and the deceased sibling is present

they have not been cheated, that they have done all they could do, that nobody is responsible for the child's death, neither the caregivers nor themselves. The caregivers and the psychotherapist will have helped them to understand the child's statements and behaviour, particularly during the last days of life, so that they are not overburdened by the guilt of having misunderstood or ignored the child's demands, fears, joys, messages of anger and/or love, but know that the true relation between them existed until the last moment. They will be more able to cope with the child's death if they have sufficiently overcome former griefs (their own parents, a sibling, a grandparent, a dear friend, etc.) before it happens: the psychotherapist should be attentive to this point from the outset.

The process of grief (Freud 1957) is a normal, unavoidable process, which may last several months or years, during which the parents gain a wider and deeper consciousness of the place the child had in their life, of the meaning and value of their own life, regain a different memory of and attachment to the child, with less sufferings and less enslavement to him/her, but without forgetting, become open again to new attachments and new goals. They regain their faith in themselves, in others, in the price and value of living without guilt, the sad feeling of betraying the dead child. They may say that they found enrichment in such a painfully paid experience, and that they are more open to others.

THE CHILDREN'S MAJOR LANDMARKS

The children's major landmarks (their body, their place in their family and in society, a sense of identity and of having a value, the meaning and value of their life) are more or less disturbed during the experience of cancer.

The Body

The children wonder whether they can still rely on it; whether the various impairments (hair loss, fatigue, pain, modifications, etc.) will remain or cease; whether they are still the same, still beautiful, still recognise themselves, whether their friends, their parents still recognise them, and what image they have of them now. The disorders in their unconscious body image may be perceived in their drawings, in excessive fears (of vein punctures, of nursing, of clinical examinations, of surgery). Psychotherapy and relaxation may be helpful. The body is a key to their identity: 'Who am I now?' Gym, sports activities, camps, may help the children maintain confidence in their body and in themselves.

The Family

The children are attentive to the style of education adopted by the family, its cultural, ideological or religious habits and beliefs, to the diverse internal (between parents and children, parents and grandparents, in the couple, between the siblings) and external relations (friends, colleagues, neighbours), to accounts of its history. All these elements are affected and disturbed by the experience of cancer, and are the basis for many questions: the search for a cause and a culprit – parents wonder whether they are responsible, because they were too young, or too old, or were experiencing a crisis, have educated the child too severely, or on the contrary because they made the wrong choices in their life, etc. The experience of cancer may exacerbate past or present family conflicts (between parents and grandparents, between the father's and the mother's side, etc.), or it may lead to a truce and solutions, and greater solidarity. These elements may sometimes explain paradoxical reactions or behaviour such as non-compliance or excessive pessimism on the part of the parents or the child. Helping them to cope with dysfunction, unsolved conflicts and questions, and with cancer are all necessary, and should be undertaken together.

Siblings

Siblings suffer a lot (Cohen *et al.* 1994, Zeltzer *et al.* 1996), feel neglected, or guilt about the child's illness (because of jealousy, because they were the parents' favourite, etc.). They may become excessively obedient, sacrifice their school interests, their activities with their friends, their success: the sick child could be jealous, or sad about the difference between them, or may be suffering from a feeling of injustice. On the contrary, they may exacerbate their jealousy and play the 'role' of the black sheep in the family: irrespective of what they do, the sick child will always be the good one, simply because he/she is severely sick. These attitudes may remain intact for many years, even when they become adults, and even more so if the child dies (Davies 1991).

The Parents

The parents should be helped to maintain their social relations, their professional activities, their parental role, which is not always easy. If not, the child may feel guilty about their financial difficulties, their bitter loneliness, that their siblings have been neglected, even if they claim the constant presence of their parents, and disturbed when the usual rules of education are abandoned ('He/she is suffering too much, may die, we will not add educational constraints'), when their humanistic or religious beliefs ('We were good and honest people, have faith, and our child can die!') are also abandoned, when they say they regret his/her birth ('All that to reach this point!'). The children may think that they had been cheated by the educational constraints they have accepted – who could they trust now? – or that their case is inevitably desperate if their parents give up all rules and demands. When the parents are locked in an unfinished process of grieving for their own parents, or a childish relationship with them that prevents them from imagining their death, then they will not be able to face the idea of their child's possible death. Helping them to overcome this former grief and to cope with the child's cancer and his/her possible death goes hand in hand.

The Place in Society

Cancer, because of its appalling image and of the constraints imposed by treatment drives the children and their families into isolation. They must be helped to preserve their place in society: learning is a right and a duty, at school or at home, and it helps to continue to associate with one's peers; maintaining links with friends is easier if they know how to discuss their illness, their treatment, their future, if they find alternative activities with equivalent demands on them (a chess competition instead of a basketball competition) when they are unable to pursue their hobbies. They pay special attention to the way people look at them, and dislike pity, voyeurism, false sympathy, useless emotion, avoidance, but they need to be helped to conquer their anger, sadness, scorn for such attitudes, and to develop a tolerant and nevertheless lucid opinion of others.

The Quest for a Cause and a Meaning

The children wonder whether it is not a punishment (but for whose fault? – theirs?, their parents'?), the effect of jealousy, of a spell, etc. They may share their parents' or the community's psychosomatic and etiological theories, or develop their private ones. This effort to find a meaning to their illness, to give a meaning to their life, to stress their cultural identity, is extremely valuable. These theories should not be mocked, nor approved as scientifically sound, but should open the way for fruitful dialogues accompanying their efforts to muster enough regard for their family history, their own history, their place in their parents' desire, their reflections on life and death: the time the illness lasts can also be a rich period of maturation. Such dialogues avoid the risk of passivity or loss of self-esteem ('There is nothing to understand, doctors are the only ones who know, trying to understand is useless etc.'), and the risk of non-compliance when the gap between the family's theories and the medical ones is too large ('I do not accept their theories and their practical consequences. The doctors are asking me to choose between my parents' theories and theirs. How can I betray my parents?'). Some 'psychosomatic theories' ('If you love and support him/her enough, if you have enough faith and desire, he/she will be cured') may pointlessly make the parents or the child feel guilty if the treatment turns out to be unsuccessful ('We did not love or support him/her enough'). Even when the parents strongly believe in their theories, they may accept and feel a sense of relief that a judge releases them temporarily from their parental responsibility of accepting an aspect of the treatment. Rivalry should not exist between caregivers and parents: sometimes the parents behave as if the child is theirs and that only they know what is good for him/her. On the contrary, they should be collaborators and the children should not be torn between the two groups. Therefore, when points of view are drastically different, caregivers should accept certain compromises with the parents in the interest of the child, provided they do not seriously compromise his/her chances of being cured. These situations raise complex and difficult clinical, psychological, ethical and legal problems that each member of staff should be trained to discuss.

What is Death for a Child?

Death is a complex reality, not just a word or a biological reality. Children differentiate dying and being dead. They may fear dying because of the risk of physical pain, of loneliness, etc. They have already seen how death has occurred in the ward, or in their family, and how their own pain and physical sufferings were treated.

Death is the unknown. To humanise and tame this terrifying unknown, they wonder what the dead become after death. The question of memories and traces of them takes precedence over the question of the body: will they be forgotten, or replaced by a brand new child? What images of themselves and what moments will remain (their beauty and qualities or the last horrible moments, the joys they have given to their parents and shared with them, or the constraints and sufferings caused by their illness, etc.). They wonder what their loved ones will become? Will they go on living, or will they be blocked in endless grief (they may feel guilty about that), will they also die (then, who will remember them: death may appear as a terrifying black and void hole)? They may have heard their parents say: 'If he/she dies, we will never have any more children, it's so hard'; or 'we will not be able to live: he/she is our entire life'. They also try to tame this unknown with fantasies: images of death (skeletons, monsters, witches, etc.), stories of the living-dead, legends that reassure that death is not 'for real', that one can return from the dead, have several lives, like in electronic games, etc. They feel more secure when they can express these thoughts to their parents, and know that these thoughts belong to our common cultural background.

Death is also linked to several specific and disturbing experiences that the children may go through during treatment, or may have undergone during their early development, and which may be perceived as partial experiences of death. This is the loss of temporal landmarks (death is eternity where they are excluded from the time that is shared by everyone) that is not rare in BMT units: the children no longer know when the treatment started nor when it will end, every moment, every day is similar to the other ('We live minute by minute'), time is passing in the absence of progress, devoid of any rhythm. Their past is out of reach or forbidden because a comparison with the present is so painful, and the future is unimaginable. The loss of bodily landmarks (when you are dead you become a skeleton and dust) is caused by intense pain, excessive fatigue, mucositis, diarrhoea, surgery, or corticoids, etc. The children may lose the feeling that their body is protecting them from the outside, that it is a unit and not a patchwork, that they reside in their body which belongs to them. These body transformations, the dramatic changes in their psychological traits may lead to the loss of their identity. They no longer recognise themselves, nor do they know who they are now. Death is nowhere, is the hereafter. The risks of losing their family (when their parents have resigned themselves to a dismal outcome, locked in excessive anticipatory grief, or have shifted all their hopes onto their siblings) and their place in society (when the links with school and friends have vanished) are thus highly distressing. Death is extreme loneliness: the children may feel this loneliness when the parents are physically absent, because of intense phobia, because they cannot stand looking at them, or are present but psychically and emotionally absent because of severe depression. They also feel profoundly incapable of thinking (when you are dead, you do not think; death is unimaginable, unthinkable). This occurs when they are too tired, too depressed, or too frightened to think and fancy, because the slightest thought will lead to the idea of their death, or because they have been told tactlessly that they will surely die: there is no longer room for hope and for imagining another outcome.

If the children are helped to overcome this dreadful situation, they continue to have faith in themselves and in their value, in their parents and caregivers, and they know that their life has been worth living, that their parents do not regret their birth, that they will not be left alone facing death, nor be forgotten if death does eventually and unfortunately occur. If these experiences are brief or are treated adequately, the children are less terrified by the idea of their own possible death.

When children or adolescents talk about death, they are not always depressed, nor sure that they will die: they need to tame the images and the thoughts of their possible death through dialogue. Terrifying fantasies are preferable to being unable to think and to imagine death.

A Sense of Personal Identity

The experience of severe illness forces the children and the parents to think about themselves, about the meaning of their lives, their values and objectives in life. All these aspects help to preserve or otherwise to dissolve the children's sense of identity, of having a value, their faith in the medical outcome but also in their place in a loving family and a humane society.

SOME SPECIFIC SITUATIONS

Babies

The parents of babies are often young and lack experience. Cancer may exacerbate their fear of taking care of the child, undermine their confidence in their capabilities and legitimacy as parents. In such cases, nurses can offer them advice and support, without judging their abilities, by simply explaining that if the children do not accept the food they are giving, this does not mean that they are angry with them nor that they do not love them any more. If they give them a poor welcome this usually signifies that he/she has missed them. Such advice may obviate conflicts in the couple, between the parents and the grandparents, or between the parents and the child, which could lead to neglect or ill-treatment. But babies have a tremendous capacity for adaptation and their development is stimulated by confronting them with other children and many attentive adults. Preserving the child's usual environment (babies keep their cuddly toys, a handkerchief with the mother's odour when they are in the ward, the nurses talk to them about their parents), and the way they usually take care of them, which is difficult, are helpful and will allow them to maintain confidence in themselves and in the staff.

Adolescents

Adolescence is a long and difficult journey, and even more so when confronted with cancer (Allen, Newman and Souhami 1997, Whyte and Smith 1997). Adolescents have to accomplish a double task: surmounting cancer, and living through adolescence. They have to become acquainted with a body that is changing because of puberty and because of cancer and its treatments (Pendley, Dahlquist and Dreyer 1997): they may consider it as dirty, repellent, hostile, incomprehensible, foreign, the cause of pain or shame. Preserving the ties with their peers helps them to maintain confidence in their value and beauty, provides support for their efforts to achieve their autonomy and avoids regression to a childish relationship with their parents. Usually, their revolt, a symbolic struggle between life and death, is a means of 'discovering' that their parents are mortal and not almighty gods, just like they are. When confronted with cancer, adolescents and their parents may consider that death is for real, and may choose to avoid this fake battle even though it is vital for successfully coping with adolescence. This revolt may shift towards the caregivers, and be expressed as non-compliance with or opposition to the treatment. Caregivers should try to separate what applies to the parents, to themselves, and what expresses a real or imaginary difficulty in bearing the treatment, in believing in its success, in considering it worth the sufferings they are experiencing. Alopecia, emaciation, and passivity may hinder the quest for their sexual identity, especially if there are more women than men in the staff. The proposal of sperm or ovary conservation may plunge them prematurely into questions about adult sexuality and parenthood. Adolescents often prefer to express their questions and their fears with their behaviour rather than with words and caregivers should be trained to understand this trait.

Social and Cultural Specificity

Paediatric cancers are not related to social, environmental or cultural specificity. The intensity of the situations and the rigorous constraints of the protocols mask cultural and social differences. However, they may partly explain certain uncommon or paradoxical forms of behaviour of the parents or of the children, and especially non-compliance because they do not understand or do not have confidence in the treatment, because its cost and constraints could be disastrous to the financial status or the equilibrium of the family, because they feel they are not respected in their specific beliefs concerning illness. Some children behave as if they have to choose between the caregivers' culture, language, way of thinking – and thus have the best chances of being cured – and those of their parents, in order not to betray them. Caregivers should therefore try to know, understand and respect, the cultural characteristics of the families, inasmuch as there is no contradiction between these features and the treatment. However, this cultural specificity may be associated with social difficulties that should not be smothered.

High-dose Chemotherapy and BMT or SCT

These are intense and distressing remedies (Andrykowsky 1994) that the parents fear because of their constraints and high risks and anticipate (Dermatis and Lesko 1990, Kodish *et al*. 1991) because they are efficient treatments, and sometimes the sole remaining treatment available – the last chance, so to speak. Because of the duration and of the isolation involved, the parents as well as the children may lose their temporal and social landmarks. Having photographs of their family and home, writing a diary, filling in a calendar, having regular activities (playing, learning, drawing, listening to the news, etc.) are helpful ways of coping with this situation. Parents often shun discussions because they are afraid of thinking, because all their thoughts will be frightening, and might cause their fragile equilibrium to collapse. Many parents want to forget everything as soon as they are outside the high-dose chemotherapy unit, as if it had never happened. Some adolescents say they want to sleep all the time (time goes by faster) or to 'shoot up' analgesics (but add that coming back to reality is dreadful). It is difficult, but useful, to carefully help the parents and the children (drawings are more readily accepted) to express their emotions, fear, anger, disarray, hope, etc. and their physical sensations. In this manner, they will not be passive, and later on this period will not be perceived as a distressing and disturbing black hole in their memory and in their life. Helping them to talk about the past (before entering the BMT unit, before the illness) and about the future (what they intend to do afterwards, what are the children's plans in the short and long term) is useful. Parents may be excessively present and stimulating, or inadequate when they feel impotent and useless, find the child's sufferings and reproaches unbearable and are obsessed by his/her possible death. Understanding the child's behaviour and reactions sufficiently helps them to preserve their parental role, towards him/her as well as towards the siblings, thus avoiding guilt and excessive jealousy. Leaving the unit is dramatically awaited and feared: 'Outside is remote from medical protection and fraught with microbes and danger' there is nothing to and they need to be reassured the something can be done in the case of a relapse or failure. This fear may last a long time (Sormanti, Dungan and Rieker 1994). Parents may shift from being excessively obedient and confident to showing outright mistrust, and the staff must be aware of their extreme sensibilities, and be attentive to the risk of conflicts, sometimes due to misinterpreted words or attitudes, or fear of mistakes the caregivers might make.

Pain

The younger the children, the more likely their pain may be overlooked. These last ten years, the evaluation (Poulain, Pichard and Gauvain 1994) and treatment of pain have improved considerably. Several scales are used daily: the NFCS (facial expressions) up to 18 months, the Amiel Tison score up to 3 years old, the Objective Pain Scale from 2 months until adolescence, the CHEOP scale up to 6 years, the DEGR scale from 2 years of age. Between 4 and 6 years old, a Visual Analogue Scale (VAS) is associated with a facial expression scale. After the age of 6, the VAS and vocabulary scales are validated. If pain is suspected, the currently well-codified clinical examination must reveal what type of pain. There are four major types of level II analgesics. From the age of one month, the child may receive practically all of the opioids (WHO level III) administered to adults. Controlled analgesia is useful, with the help of the nurse or the parents before 6 years of age and administered by the children themselves thereafter. Thus, the early and excessive use of steroids, notorious for their adverse effects, has diminished. Loco-regional and complementary methods (Wood, Vieyra and Poulain 2000) are useful, especially when the parents can employ them and thus regain contact with the child's body and confidence in themselves.

If pain is insufficiently recognised and treated, the children may lose confidence in the staff, like their parents, and may sometimes lose confidence in their parents. This may lead to non-compliance with or opposition to treatment, or a long-lasting distressful memory of the treatment. Pain gives rise to some common symptoms with depression (tears, fatigue, a feeling of helplessness, psychomotor atonia, etc.) but may also contribute to its onset. Adolescents have a complex and ambivalent attitude towards major analgesics. Some say they accept a certain amount of pain, because they want to remain totally lucid, while other adolescents use these drugs to place a distance between them and the difficult reality they are living.

Surgery

Surgery is expected (the image of removing the disease seems magical, and explains some of the difficulties in accepting subsequent chemotherapy) and feared: anaesthesia, pain, scars, imaginary or realistic sequels, intrusion in the body, fantasy of a gaping body. Caregivers should discuss these fears, explain why surgery is planned and the operative procedure, its place in the course of the treatment, evaluate the sequels in light of the child's activities and plans, but they must also try to understand what is unconsciously behind these fears. Excessive fears may be caused by a weak body image, by a reasonable or unconscious fear of his/her parents, sometimes by a persistently painful memory of past operations. Relaxation and psychotherapeutic interviews may be helpful.

Brain Tumours

The children may experience these lesions more intensely than tumours at other sites, because the brain is more difficult to imagine than the other organs, as it is associated with the activity of thinking, and producing some of the most disturbing symptoms such as motor, sensorial or cognitive impairments, or headache, vomiting which may for several weeks be explained by psychological reasons that can cause the parents to feel guilty, and lose confidence in the psychologist's expertise. Both the children and parents know about the risk of cognitive sequels and express anxiety about this outcome. The children may experience fear of losing all their qualities (becoming incapable of doing the physical or intellectual activities they used to do, when their younger siblings are now doing better than them), and their identity (they no longer recognise themselves, and wonder whether this state will be lifelong) (Figure 6.8). Early neurosurgery is a bleak introduction to the treatment, especially when a coma, akinetic muteness or motor impairment ensue. However, on the contrary, it may magically suppress the first painful symptoms for a while. Unfortunately, how the children and the parents experience this important period is still rather obscure.

More precise information is known about sequels, which are mostly cognitive (Ris and Noll 1994, Mulhern *et al.* 1998), and neuropsychological evaluation is part of the clinical picture (Kieffer-Renaux *et al.* 2000). It assesses overall (IQ, verbal, performance) or specific cognitive impairment (oral and written language, motor skills, alertness and attention, praxis and gnosis, memory, treatment of information, logical reasoning, behaviour and mood, visual–spatial abilities). It takes into account the child's medical and personal history, socio-cultural environment, the child's personality and family dynamics. This evaluation is confronted with the child's, the parents', the paediatricians', the teachers' and the psychologist's points of view. This evaluation offers the children and their parents precious explanations for the reasons for academic and behavioural difficulties: all of this is not entirely their fault, they are not lazy, nor silly and can be helped through adapted rehabilitation. It helps the teachers to have a better appraisal of the children (neither neglect nor pity, neither extreme tolerance nor anger), to adapt their teaching methods, and to define the best choices for their academic studies. Thus the children may regain confidence in themselves, their parents have a

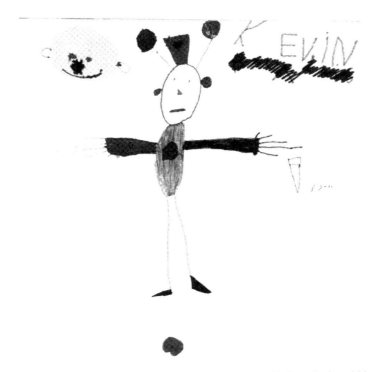

Figure 6.8 K., 8-year-old boy, treated for a brain tumour. He has depicted himself with asymmetric arms, a wedge entering his head, a black hole in his chest, his heart lying on the floor

better appraisal of their abilities, find it easier to accept the reality of cognitive impairment and are less divided between the temptation to keep them in 'normal schools' for as long as possible until a major failure and transferring them to a specific school for mentally retarded children. The children can then adapt themselves better to their impairments, overcome the impression of a split in their life, re-acquire a sense of personal identity and of having a value, their place in the family, in school, in society.

THE CAREGIVING TEAM

The caregiving team must be competent. If not, when the children and their parents get angry with the caregivers, they will not be able to distinguish between real and imaginary reasons and the caregivers will not be able to overcome their distress or guilt at not having cured the children. The care-providers should be aware of the major orientations in the ward: the position adopted by the staff regarding euthanasia and endless treatments, the type of patients treated there, the balance between routine practice and research, between caregivers and other professionals (teachers, clowns, etc.). This nurtures solidarity between them and the feeling of belonging to the same group. Regular meetings are useful to discuss the most difficult and disturbing situations that the staff have experienced from a medical point of view but also the emotional, relational and ethical aspects. This helps prevent burn-out (Grootenhuis *et al.* 1996, Spinetta *et al.* 2000). The presence of parents and siblings should be facilitated together with support to ease social, financial and lodging difficulties when necessary. Caregivers should regularly explain what they are doing and the ward's major orientation so that the parents can fully assume their role and help forge a therapeutic alliance between the children, the staff and themselves. (Masera *et al.* 1998).

The children should be helped to remain children, or adolescents in order to be able to cope with the illness and the treatment. This means dialogues and true information, which is not excessive, brutal or unilateral. They need to keep on learning – in order not to lose their place in society, their confidence in their intelligence, their hope of academic and social success, their faith in their future – playing, creating, fancying, meeting together, continuing to have confidence in their beauty and in their body. Therefore teachers, teachers of art (Sourkes 1991), clowns (Oppenheim, Simonds and Hartmann 1997), a place where they can play, relax, etc. are necessary.

The psychotherapist members of staff strive (Oppenheim and Hartmann 2000) to develop prevention and early treatment of psychological difficulties before the most insignificant signs become evident symptoms, to acquire a more profound and broader experience, and to transmit it to the staff. They should be familiar to the children and the parents who will henceforth rarely say: 'We don't need psychological help, we are not crazy!'

For their own sake and that of the children, caregivers should remain reasonably proud of their work and of belonging to a proud, competent team. If not, they will be more fragile when criticism comes from colleagues or when they are the target of pertinent or unjust remarks of the parents', or as a result of the children's sufferings and sometimes their death. Risks of doubt, discouragement, guilt, conflicts and burn-out are permanently present (Grootenhuis *et al.* 1996). The children and the parents may need to revolt against them (a form of resistance to illness) because they are ambivalent (they trust and fear them: 'They have the life and the death of our child in their hands'), they want to assert their liberty, check the caregivers' solidity and confidence in themselves and in the staff. Caregivers should therefore be trained and helped by the psycho-oncologist, during clinical discussions and specific training, such as Balint groups, to understand these behaviours and their various causes (conscious and unconscious, based on reality and/or fantasy) and meanings, and to manage these situations. This avoids pointless conflicts and fatigue for everybody.

CONCLUSION

Being afflicted by and treated for a cancer is a most intense, dangerous and overwhelming experience, where medical, psychological, social and cultural elements coexist. It is the cause of sufferings and disarray, but also an edifying experience, where the children and the parents may discover the strength and richness of their relationship, their unexpected qualities, new interests and plans, may solve old problems, and gain a more open and confident view on others. Caregivers share the responsibility for whether this experience leaves long-lasting distress or not, even when physical or cognitive sequels occur.

ACKNOWLEDGEMENT

Thanks to Lorna Saint Ange for her help with the translation.

REFERENCES

Allen, R., Newman, S.P., Souhami, R.L. (1997) Anxiety and depression in adolescent cancer: findings in patients and parents at the time of diagnosis. *Eur. J. Cancer* **33**, 1250–1255.

Andrykowsky, M.A. (1994) Psychosocial factors in bone marrow transplantation: a review and recommendation for research. *BMT* **13**, 357–375.

Barakat, L.P., Kazak, A.E., Meadows, A.T., *et al.* (1997) Families surviving childhood cancer: a comparison of post traumatic stress symptoms with families of healthy children. *J. Pediatr. Psychol.* **22**, 843–859.

Bluebond-Langner, M. (1989) Worlds of dying children and their well siblings. *Death Studies* **13**, 1–16.

Cohen, D.S., Friedrich, W.N., Jaworski, T.M., *et al.* (1994) Pediatric cancer: predicting sibling adjustment. *J. Clinic Psychol.* **50**, 303–319.

Davies, B. (1991) Long-term outcome of adolescent sibling bereavement. *J. Adolesc. Research* **6**, 83–96.

Davies, B., Deveau, E., deVeber, B., *et al.* (1998) Experiences of mothers in five countries whose child died of cancer. *Cancer Nurs.* **21**, 301–311.

Dermatis, H., Lesko, L.M. (1990) Psychological distress in parents consenting to child's bone marrow transplantation. *Bone Marrow Transplant* **6**, 411–417.

Eden, O.B., Black, I., Mackinlay, G.A., Emery, A.E. (1994) Communication with parents of children with cancer. *Palliat. Med.* **8**, 105–114.

Eiser, C. (1996) Comprehensive care of the child with cancer: obstacles to the provision of psychosocial support in paediatric oncology: a comment. *Psychol. Health Med.* **1**, 145–147.

Eiser, C., Havermans, T. (1992) Children's understanding of cancer. *Psycho-Oncology* **1**, 169–181.

Eiser, C., Havermans, T., Eiser, J.R. (1995) Parent's attribution about childhood cancer: implications for relationships with medical staff. *Child Care Health Development* **21**, 31–42.

Elliott, R., Fischer, C.T., Rennie, D.L. (1999) Evolving guidelines for publication of qualitative research studies in psychology and related fields. *Br. J. Clin. Psychol.* **38**, 215–229.

Freud, S. (1957) Mourning and melancholia. In Freud, S., *The Complete Works*, std. edn, Vol. 14, Strachey, J. (Ed.). London: Hogarth Press & Institute of Psycho-Analysis, pp. 243–258.

Girgis, A., Sanson-Fisher, R.W. (1995) Breaking bad news: consensus guidelines for medical practitioners. *J. Clin. Oncol.* **9**, 2449–2456.

Gray, R.E., Doan, B.D., Shermer, P., *et al.* (1992) Psychologic adaptation of survivors of childhood cancer. *Cancer* **70**, 2713–2721.

Greenberg, H.S., Meadows, A.T. (1991) Psychosocial impact of cancer survival on school age children and their parents. *J. Psychosocial Oncol.* **9**, 43–56.

Grill, J., Kieffer Renaux, V., Bulteau, C., *et al.* (1999) Long-term intellectual outcome in children with posterior fossa tumors according to radiation doses and volumes. *Int. J. Radiation Oncol. Biol. Phys.*, **45**, 137–145.

Grootenhuis, M.A., Last, B.F. (1997) Adjustment and coping by parents of children with cancer: a review of the literature. *Support Care Cancer* **5**, 466–484.

Grootenhuis, M.A., Van der Wel, M., De Graaf Nijkerk, J., Last, B.F. (1996) Exploration of a self protective strategy in pediatric oncology staff. *Med. Ped. Oncol.* **27**, 40–47.

Houtzager, B.A., Grootenhuis, M.A., Last, B.F. (1999) Adjustment of siblings to childhood cancer: a literature review. *Support Care Cancer* **7**, 302–320.

Kameny, R.R., Bearison, D.J. (1999) Illness narratives: discursive constructions of self in pediatric oncology. *J. Pediatr. Nurs.* **14**, 73–79.

Kazak, A.E., Stuber, M.L., Barakat, L.P., *et al.* (1998) Predicting posttraumatic stress symptoms in mothers and fathers of survivors of childhood cancer. *J. Am. Acad. Child Adolesc. Psychiatry* **37**, 823–831.

Kieffer-Renaux, V., Bulteau, C., Grill, J., Kalifa, C., Viguier, D., Jambaque, I. (2000) Patterns of neuropsychological deficits in children with medulloblastoma according to craniospatial irradiation doses. *Dev. Med. Child Neurol.* **42**, 741–745.

Koch, U., Haerter, M., Jakob, U., Siegrist, B. (1996) Parental reactions to cancer in their children. In Baider, L., Cooper, C.L. (Eds), *Cancer and the Family*, Chichester, John Wiley, pp. 149–170.

Kodish, E., Lantos, J., Stocking, C., *et al.* (1991) Bone marrow transplantation for sickle cell disease – a study of parents' decisions. *N. Engl. J. Med.* **325**, 1349–1353.

Kupst, M.J. (1993) Family coping. Supportive and obstructive factors. *Cancer* **71**(10 Suppl.), 3337–3341.

Larcombe, I., Charlton, A. (1996) Children's return to school after treatment for cancer: study days for teachers. *J. Cancer Educ.* **11**, 102–105.

Last, B.F., Van Veldhuizen, A.M. (1996) Information about diagnosis and prognosis related to anxiety and depression in children with cancer aged 8–16 years. *Eur. J. Cancer* **32A**, 290–294.

Manne, S.L., Lesanics, D., Meyers, P., *et al.* (1995) Predictors of depressive symptomatology among parents of newly diagnosed children with cancer. *J. Pediatr. Psychol.* **20**, 491–510.

Martinson, I.M., Davies, B., McClowry, S. (1991) Parental depression following the death of a child. *Death Studies* **15**, 259–267.

Masera, G., Chesler, M., Jankovic, M., *et al.* (1996) SIOP Working Committee on Psychosocial Issues in Pediatric Oncology: guidelines for care of long-term survivors. *Med. Pediatr. Oncol.* **27**, 1–2.

Masera, G., Spinetta, J.J., Jankovic, M., *et al.* (1998) Guidelines for a therapeutic alliance between families and staff: a report of the SIOP Working Committee on Psychosocial Issues in Pediatric Oncology. *Med. Pediatr. Oncol.* **30**, 183–186.

Masera, G., Spinetta, J.J., Jankovic, M., *et al.* (1999) Guidelines for assistance to terminally ill children with cancer: a report of the SIOP Working Committee on Psychosocial Issues in Pediatric Oncology. *Med. Pediatr. Oncol.* **32**, 44–48.

Mattingly, C. (1994) The concept of therapeutic 'emplotment' *Soc. Sci. Med.* **38**, 811–822.

Mulhern, R.K., Kepner, J.L., Thomas, P.R., Armstrong, F.D., Friedman, H.S., Kun, L.E. (1998) Neuropsychologic functioning of survivors of childhood medulloblastoma randomized to receive conventional or reduced-dose craniospinal irradiation: a Pediatric Oncology Group study *J. Clin. Oncol.* **16**, 1723–1728.

Noll, R.B., Kulkarni, R. (1989) Cognitive and motor development of infants coping with cancer: longitudinal observations. *Infant Mental Health J.* **10**, 252–262.

Noll, R.B., Garstein, M.A., Vanatta, K., *et al.* (1999) Social, emotional and behavioral functioning of children with cancer. *Pediatrics* **103**, 71–78.

Oppenheim, D. (1999) *Ne jette pas mes dessins à la poubelle. Dialogues avec Daniel, traité pour cancer, entre sa 6ème et sa 9ème année.* Paris, Seuil, 223 pages.

Oppenheim, D., Hartmann, O. (2000) Psychotherapeutic practice in paediatric oncology: four examples. *Br. J. Cancer* **82**, 251–254.

Oppenheim, D., Simonds, C., Hartmann, O. (1997) Clowning on children's wards. *Lancet* **350**, 1838–1840.

Papadatou, D. (1997) Training health professionals in caring for dying children and grieving families. *Death Study* **271**, 575–600.

Pendley, J.S., Dahlquist, L.M., Dreyer, Z.A. (1997) Body image and psychosocial adjustment in adolescent cancer survivors. *J. Pediatr. Psychol.* **22**, 29–43.

Phipps, S., Srivastava, D.K. (1997) Repressive adaptation in children with cancer. *Health Psychol.* **16**, 521–528.

Pollack, G.H. (1985) Childhood siblings loss: A family tragedy. *Psychiatr. Ann.* **16**, 309–314.

Poulain, P., Pichard Léandri, E., Gauvain Piquard, A. (1994) Assessment and treatment of pain in children. *Eur. J. Palliat. Care* **1**(1), 31–35.

Ris, M.D., Noll, R.B. (1994) Long-term neurobehavioral outcome in pediatric brain-tumor patients: review and methodological critique *J. Clin. Exp. Neuropsychol.* **16**, 21–42.

Ropponen, P., Siimes, M.A., Rautonen, J., Aalberg, V. (1992) Psychosocial problems in male childhood malignancy survivors. *Acta Psychiatr. Scand.* **85**, 143–146.

Sanger, M.S., Copeland, D.R., Davidson, E.R. (1991) Psychosocial adjustment among pediatric cancer patients: a multidimensional assessment. *J. Pediatr. Psychol.* **16**, 463–474.

Sawyer, S.M., Bowes, G. (1999) Adolescence on the health agenda. *Lancet* **354**(Suppl. II), 31–34.

Sormanti, M., Dungan, S., Rieker, P.P. (1994) Pediatric bone marrow transplantation: psychosocial issues for parents after a child's hospitalization. *J. Psychosoc. Oncol.* **12**, 23–42.

Sourkes, B.M. (1991) Truth to life: art therapy with pediatric oncology patients and their siblings. *J. Psychosoc. Oncol.* **9**, 81–96.

Spiegel, L. (1998) Pediatric psychopharmacology. In Holland, J.C. *Psycho-oncology*, New York: Oxford University Press, pp. 954–961.

Spinetta, J.J., Jankovic, M., Eden, T., *et al.* (1999) Guidelines for assistance to siblings of children with cancer: report of the SIOP Working Committee on Psychosocial Issues in Pediatric Oncology. *Med. Pediatr. Oncol.* **33**, 395–398.

Spinetta, J.J., Jankovic, M., Ben Arush, M.W., *et al.* (2000) Guidelines for the recognition, prevention and remediation of burnout in health care professionals participating in the care of children with cancer: report of the SIOP working committee on psychosocial issues in pediatric oncology. *Med. Pediatr. Oncol.* **35**, 122–125.

Spinetta, J.J., Masera, G., Eden, T., *et al.* (2002) Refusal, non-compliance, and abandonment of treatment in children and adolescents with cancer: prevention and resolution. *Med. Ped. Oncol.* **38**, 114–117.

Stommel, M., Given, C.W., Given, B.A. (1993) The cost of cancer home care to families. *Cancer* **71**, 1867–1874.

Van Dongen Melman, J.E., Pruyn, J.F., De Groot, A., *et al.* (1995) Late psychosocial consequences for parents of children who survives cancer. *J. Pediatr. Psychol.* **20**, 567–586.

Whittam, E.H. (1993) Terminal care of the dying child. Psychosocial implications of care. *Cancer* **71**(Suppl.), 3450–3462.

Whyte, F., Smith, L. (1997) A literature review of adolescence and cancer. *Eur. J. Cancer Care* **6**, 137–146.

Wolfe, J., Grier, H.G., Klar, N., *et al.* (2000) Symptoms and suffering at the end of life in children with cancer. *N. Engl. J. Med.* **342**, 326–333.

Wood, C., Vieyra, M., Poulain, P. (2000) Non-pharmacological methods for the treatment of pain in children. In Simpson, K.H., Budd, K. (Eds). *Cancer Pain Management. A comprehensive approach*. Oxford University Press, pp. 74–83.

Worchel, F.F., Nolan, B.F., Willson, V.L., *et al.* (1998) Assessment of depression in children with cancer. *J. Pediatr. Psychol.* **13**, 101–112.

Zeltzer, L.K., Dolgin, M.J., Sahler, O.J.Z., *et al.* (1996) Siblings adaptation to childhood cancer collaborative study: health outcomes of siblings of children with cancer. *Med. and Ped. Oncol.* **27**, 98–107.

7

Quality of Life in Children with Cancer: Definition, Assessment and Results

SHULAMITH KREITLER

*Psychooncology Unit, Tel-Aviv Medical Center, Israel
and Department of Psychology, Tel Aviv University*

MICHAL M. KREITLER

Psychooncology Unit, Tel-Aviv Medical Center, Israel

In the closing pages of their basic text on pediatric psychooncology Bearison and Mulhern (1994, pp. 220–221) deplore the absence of valid quality of life (QOL) measures for children with cancer and urge their development. At the time this state of affairs contrasted blatantly with the prominence of interest in QOL of adult patients. Furthermore, despite a recommendation by the National Cancer Institute to include quality-of-life assessment as part of clinical trials in general (Nayfield *et al.* 1992), such assessments have not become an integral part of clinical trials in children. Out of published reports of 70 Phase III clinical trials from the Pediatric Oncology Group and Children's Cancer Group only 3% included QOL data (Bradlyn, Harris and Spieth 1995). Yet, in recent years there has been increased interest in this domain, with several research centers focusing on the development of assessment instruments and reporting data on the level of the children's QOL.

Psychosocial Aspects of Pediatric Oncology. Edited by S. Kreitler and M. Weyl Ben Arush
© 2004 John Wiley & Sons Ltd: ISBN 0 471 49939 0

DEFINITION OF QOL

Definition of QOL

QOL is defined as the individuals' perception of their functioning and wellbeing in different domains of life (Fayers and Machin 2000) or more specifically, the individuals' evaluation of their position in life, in the context of the culture and value systems in which they live, and in relation to their goals, expectations, standards and concerns (WHOQOL Group 1995). These definitions emphasize the individuals' overall evaluations of their satisfaction or happiness in major domains of life. Historically these evaluations were known as 'life satisfaction' or 'subjective wellbeing', and are now referred to as 'global QOL' or 'overall QOL'. They refer to all domains that make up one's QOL or contribute to it rather than only health.

Related Constructs

QOL as defined above has to be distinguished from other related constructs. Major among these are the following:

(a) Health status and perceived health status (or health perceptions): Health status is the person's relative status of health or illness, considering the presence of biological or physiological dysfunction, symptoms and functional impairment. Most definitions of health status refer to physical function, sensation, self-care and dexterity, cognition, pain and discomfort, and psychological wellbeing. The Health Utilities Index Mark 2 (HUI2) and the Health Utilities Index Mark 3 (HUI3) are common tools for assessing health status in pediatric oncology (Feeny et al. 1992, 1995). The Lansky play performance scale (Lansky et al. 1987) is a health status measure in children with cancer which closely parallels the standard health status Karnovsky scale used with adult cancer patients.

    Perceived health status is the individual's subjective ratings of his or her health status. Though the two may coincide, they are not necessarily identical (Wilson and Cleary 1995). Symptoms and health perceptions are often included in HRQL.

(b) Health-related quality of life (HRQL): It refers to the individual's satisfaction or happiness with domains of life insofar as they are affected by one's health (e.g., disease and its treatments). Most conceptualizations of HRQL refer to the effects of disease in general (generic HRQL) or a particular disease or treatment (condition-specific HRQL) on physical, social, emotional and cognitive functioning (Ware 1995). The four listed domains are the basic ones defined by the European Organization for the Research and Treatment of Cancer (EORTC) (Sprangers et al. 1993).

(c) Mood: Emotional responses, usually negative ones, mainly depression, anxiety or anger that are often reported as part of QOL or the related constructs. The rationale is that emotions of this kind may result from or affect functional performance, health status and HRQL (Wilson and Cleary 1995).

(d) Symptoms: Patients' reports of physical symptoms in general or those that are of particular interest in view of their disease or treatments they get, such as fatigue or nausea in cancer.

(e) Disease severity: Scales of disease severity reflect the overall degree of severity of the patient's disease, which may be based on any or all of the following: objective symptoms, physicians' ratings and also on patients' reports.

(f) Functional status: Refers to the individual's ability to perform regular activities required to meet basic needs, fulfill one's roles and maintain wellbeing (Leidy 1994; Wilson and Cleary 1995). It may include both functional capacity (based on actual assessment of capacity or on others' ratings) as well as functional performance (based on self-reports), which may or may not overlap.

In some cases the boundaries between the constructs are difficult to draw and get blurred for theoretical or methodological reasons, such as between health status and HRQL or disease severity and functional status.

Major Characteristics of QOL

The standard approaches to QOL highlight the following characteristics of QOL (Niv and Kreitler 2001):

(a) QOL is a *subjective* construct, reflecting the individual's view of his or her wellbeing and functioning;

(b) QOL is a *phenomenological* construct, providing a surface image of the situation, without explaining how or why it arose;

(c) QOL is an *experiential or evaluative* construct, which presents judgments without any attempt to relate them to objectively verifiable facts;

(d) QOL is a *dynamic* construct, expected to be sensitive to significant changes in the individual's state;

(e) QOL is a *multidimensional* construct, based not merely on a single global measure but on evaluations in specific domains that have been identified as major constituents of QOL;

(f) QOL is a *quantifiable* construct, which may be assessed so that it provides scores comparable across different individuals or across different states or time points in the same individual.

The characterization of QOL would not be complete without specifying the negative features. Accordingly, QOL is not identical with (a) quantity of life (i.e., duration of life, survival), (b) health status, (c) functional status, and (d) disease severity.

ASSESSING QOL: GENERAL ISSUES

Goals

A major consideration in assessing QOL is the purpose. The basic question is 'why do we need to assess the QOL of pediatric oncology patients?' One often-mentioned answer is that this would enable us to identify the needs of the large numbers of survivors of pediatric cancer who may be impaired due to the highly toxic treatments they have undergone (Feeny et al. 1999). To this we may add that it is important to learn through QOL assessments also about the needs of children while they are undergoing the difficult oncological treatments. Hence, QOL assessments would enable us to address, anticipate and possibly remediate the difficulties of the disease and its treatments (Monaco 1999).

Another important goal would be to complement the information we usually get about the effects of treatments. While most of this information reflects medically objective facts relevant for the cure, QOL focuses attention on additional effects that may reflect the costs of the cure in terms of impairments and suffering. Accordingly, QOL assessments provide a broader basis for evaluating treatments and for comparing them. Sometimes integrating the medical and QOL information sources enables evaluating the net effect of a treatment, which may be lower than the initially assumed one. Further, QOL information may help researchers set new goals for developing treatments which would reduce impairment of QOL without compromising clinical efficacy. In this context it is of interest to note that radiation to the brain was administered as a regular prophylaxis therapy to patients with acute lymphoblastic leukemia but when QOL assessments identified serious sequelae of this therapy (Green, Zevon and Hall 1991, Mostow et al. 1991), radiation-sparing was developed as well as chemotherapy substituting for radiotherapy whenever possible (Feeny et al. 1999).

Again, in cases of doubt about whether to apply a given treatment, QOL information may help physicians and parents reach a decision, balancing probable cure effects against likely damage to QOL. When there is no possibility of choosing among treatments, information about the likely QOL effects of the particular treatment may help in planning adequate interventions for moderating these likely effects or even preparing the children in advance with prophylactic measures (Lauria et al. 1996).

An important argument for assessing QOL has been put forward by Guyatt (1999) who considers the assessment as an anchor for examining psychosocial and demographic correlates of good and poor QOL. Information about the correlates could help both in identifying beforehand children at risk for low-level QOL and in better planning of interventions for improving QOL.

It is customary to view QOL assessments as contributing also to screening, describing the beneficial effects of treatments, assisting in the management of individual patients, and contributing to decisions about clinical policy and resource allocation (Osoba 1995, Parsons and Brown 1998).

Finally, QOL assessments communicate to the child an important message – that regardless of how difficult the treatment that has to be applied is, the medical staff does not lose sight of the basic fact that the patient is first and foremost a human being.

Difficulties in Assessing QOL in Children; or QOL by Whom – Children or Parents?

One major problem investigators have confronted is the assumed limited ability of children to report about their QOL. The severity of this problem increases the younger the child is, especially when the child is less than 5 years old. But even for children above 5 years there is evidence for a tendency to avoid reliance on children as the source of information. One often-mentioned argument is that children are limited or unable to understand, value and identify factors that 'contribute or detract from HRQL' (Mulhern *et al.* 1989) or point out major functional domains for children (e.g., school, social relations) (Watson *et al.* 1999). Further, even if one accepts the claim of someone like Eiser (1996) that only the children themselves can provide a 'real' measure of their HRQL, it is doubtful whether they are a reliable source of information (Watson *et al.* 1999). Several investigators openly state that parents of children are a better source of information about the children's HRQL, both from the point of view of reliability (presumably because they are adults) and from the point of view of validity because parents 'are usually the most knowledgeable about the child's behavior across time and situations' (Watson *et al.* 1999) and are 'believed to be very familiar with their child's life' (Goodwin, Boggs and Graham-Pole 1994). In order to further bolster the status of adults as the source of information about the child's QOL Watson *et al.* (1999) claim that it is no use bothering with the child's views since anyway 'it is almost always the parents' view of their child's symptoms and behavior which is crucial in determining what is done about any health problem' at least up to the child's early adolescence. Further, it has always been the doctors who in the course of regular history-taking and monitoring of clinical progress have asked patients, or in the case of children, their parents, about how they feel on a number of health-related dimensions (Watson *et al.* 1999). The implied conclusion is that there is no special reason to change this age-honored procedure.

Because of the importance of the issue we will bring further examples of arguments along these lines. For one, children may be too ill to respond (Levi and Drotar 1999). Or, the child develops and his or her ability to respond to

QOL questionnaires changes continuously, which may necessitate flexibility in the approach to assessment and presumably impair psychometric standards (Kamphuis 1987). Again, assessing the child's views alongside those of the parents or healthcare providers may reveal discrepancies which are difficult to resolve (Mulhern *et al.* 1989). Finally, understanding the child's experience of the disease and the treatment can best be done by qualitative means which do not provide psychometrically acceptable results and may at best be viewed as 'curiosity-based research' (Guyatt 1999).

Another area of concern is determining the reference point for evaluating the QOL of the child: other children with a similar illness receiving a similar treatment, children who have completed treatment or children who have never experienced either the disease or the treatment (Mulhern *et al.* 1989).

One result of this distrust of children's reports is that in pediatric oncology assessments of HRQL have inadvertently slipped over from the subjective to the objective view, referring more to facts. This has rendered the situation even more difficult and resulted in justifying the use of proxy sources of information. Replacing the subjective by the objective was bolstered by the argument that some problems are better observable by others than by the patient, for example, vomiting as against nausea. This may or may not be true, but vomiting and nausea are not identical. And the discrepancy between the subjective and objective grows when we deal with emotional and behavioral problems (Eiser and Jenney 1996).

When the patients are adolescents, it is impossible to justify bypassing their views. The usual practice is not to rely on the patients' reports but to use parallel forms – one for the parents and one for the adolescents, 'to allow them to report their own views alongside parental ratings', whereby it is implicitly clear that the parental one is the real and crucial report, the so-called 'gold standard' of QOL. This practice is further supported by the argument that multiple sources of information are necessary and advisable.

We have dwelt on this issue of assessing the children's QOL by proxy reports because of its importance and its implications for the whole field. It is evident that many of the arguments against questioning children do not hold water. Most of them apply equally to assessing QOL with adult patients, such as the need to rely on multiple sources of information, being too sick to respond, the difficulty in choosing adequate control groups, or subjectivity in responses. None of these arguments has deterred assessing QOL in adults.

No doubt parents are an available and cooperating source of information. But are they a source that could replace the source provided by the children themselves? The evidence shows that this is not so. For example, on the subscales of the Behavioral, Affective and Somatic Experiences Scale the correlations between the responses of the children (less than 6 to above 12 years of age) and the parents were significant but low ($r = 0.29$ to 0.57) and actually not very different than those between the responses of the parents and the nurse ($r = 0.19$ to 0.62) (Phipps *et al.* 1999).

On 10 of the 11 subscales of the Child Health Questionnaire the correlations between the responses of adolescents in treatment (10–18 years old) and their parents were significant but in the low to medium range except in regard to the Role/Social–Physical and Self-Esteem, in which the adolescents reported significantly higher scores than their parents. Hence, the parents reported a stronger impact of the illness on the adolescents' physical functioning, social and school activities and self-esteem than the adolescents themselves did. The relations between the adolescents' and parents' reports were lower for the group in treatment. The investigators conclude that the parents' reports cannot be assumed to reflect accurately the adolescents' views in all domains, including some key areas (Sawyer *et al.* 1999). Also, in another study with the Children Health Questionnaire, greater discrepancies between the reports of parents and children were found in the cancer group (mean age 13.2, $SD = 2.6$ years) than in the healthy children's group (Levi and Drotar 1999). The sick children reported significantly less bodily pain/distress, better general health perceptions, fewer limitations in performing activities requiring a lot or some energy, walking or climbing stairs, fewer limitations in the kind of school activities they could complete and the amount of time spent on that due to physical health (see also Canning, Canning and Boyce 1992). Similarly, on the PCQL-32 (Vance *et al.* 2001), children 6–12 years old reported higher scores on three scales (physical, psychological, disease-related) and lower on social functioning than their parents. The reports of children and parents were mostly not correlated.

In a study with children 6 to 16 years old, Challinor *et al.* (1999) found on the Behavioral Assessment System for Children questionnaires, that the scores of parents and children on the scale of somatization were not related at all, while the scores on the scales of anxiety and depression were correlated but those of parents were higher than those of children. Notably, also in another study the scores of parents and children for depression on the Child Behavior Checklist were not correlated and the parents reported higher levels of depression for the children than the children themselves (Worchel *et al.* 1988). A similar pattern emerged in a study with children in the age range of 8 to 18 years on the Child Heath Questionnaire: on 50% of the items there were significant differences in the responses of the parents and the children, with the parents reporting typically higher levels of distress and restrictions for the children than the children themselves (Levi and Drotar 1999). Similar findings were reported for a sample of children aged 5–12 undergoing bone marrow transplantation: the scores of parents on QOL and mental health were lower than of the children (Parsons *et al.* 1999).

In a systematic review of the literature, Eiser and Morse (2001) examined the interrelations between parent and child reports of HRQL in the case of chronically sick children on the basis of 14 studies using 10 separate measures of HRQL. In regard to domains of HRQL they found a tendency for somewhat greater agreement in regard to observable behaviors, such as physical functioning, and lower for less observable ones, such as emotions and social functioning. They also found that parents tended to report lower levels of functioning, more distress and in general a greater impact of the illness on the child's performance than the children did.

Another study of relevance for the present context found serious discrepancies between the importance assigned by pediatricians and sick children even to physical symptoms. For example, the pediatricians overestimated the importance of diarrhea and underestimated the importance of 'worries about future health problems' (Loonen, Derkx and Griffith, 2002). The conclusion is that even the views of experts in a disease and in treating children cannot replace the views of the children themselves.

In sum, though there is some relation between the reports of parents and children on the children's QOL, the discrepancies are too large to justify substituting parents' reports for children's reports. Discrepancies are to be expected also in view of the fact that the reports of parents and children are based partly on different kinds of data (observations and communication versus subjective personal experience, respectively) (Zeltzer *et al.* 1991). The discrepancies tend to be particularly large in regard to content domains that are of greatest interest to the clinician and not accessible through direct observation (viz. emotional and social functioning) and in regard to the groups of children that are of greatest interest in this context (viz. sick children versus healthy children, and children in treatment versus children off treatment). Typically parents tend to report higher levels of distress and impairment than the children. This gap may be due, on the one hand, to the anxiety and stress of the parents evoked by the children's disease, and, on the other hand, to the tendencies of children to cope by minimizing their reported distress and also to protect their parents. Explanations of this kind do not, however, change the basic fact that to assess QOL of children in the original and basic sense of the term one has to deal with the children themselves.

In this context there arise problems that need to be confronted. For example, the issues and the questions need to be formulated in a manner that is understandable and meaningful to the children but also meaningful to the medical staff; special procedures for ensuring reliability need to be undertaken; and time needs to be invested in administering the questionnaires to the children.

Major Decisions or Choices

In constructing or selecting an assessment tool of QOL it is necessary to make some decisions. The first and foremost one concerns the source of the information: Who will answer the questions about the child's QOL? The major options are the child, one or both parents, or a member of the medical staff (e.g., the physician, a nurse). This issue has been discussed in the previous section in regard to using parents' reports instead of the children's. The conclusion was that parents' reports cannot replace children's reports and, if they are collected at all, then they are to be considered as a separate source of data in its own right. The same applies in regard to other sources of information, such a siblings, members of the medical staff, teachers, or friends.

A related question has to do with the assessment tool that will be selected even when the source of information is the patient: Will it be a tool designed for adults or for children. There are evident disadvantages to administering to children, or even adolescents, tools designed for adults, because they are likely to be inappropriate in regard to format, style, and contents (e.g., items referring to fertility, sexuality, marital relations). Yet, it seems that this was done in some studies, e.g., Bradlyn *et al.* (1993) used the Quality of Well-Being Scale completed by parents in regard to their sample of children 4–18 years old; Zebrack and Chesler (2001) used the Quality of Life – Cancer Survivors scale for adults in their sample of 16–29-year-olds.

An important choice of a different order concerns the manner of getting the desired information. There are several options. One is a questionnaire that may be administered to the child by an adult or that the child answers by himself or herself. Another option is an interview, which may be conducted according to predetermined guidelines or may follow the material the children produce spontaneously in response to a general question about things that matter to them (Clay 1999). Other options, more limited in their range of application, are requesting the children (or other informants) to keep a diary, or behavioral observations of the children according to some time-sampling procedure.

A third choice concerns the form of the questions, in the case where the questionnaire option is selected. The usual options are ratings, category ratings (e.g., Likert-type scale with descriptive headings for each category), rating scale with faces expressing degree of acceptance or satisfaction, 'eggs scale' which is a rating scale with different quantities of 'eggs' representing degrees of acceptance (see Appendix), linear visual analog scale, feeling thermometer, or open-ended questions. A related choice concerns the form of response required from the child. The child may express his or her preferences or responses verbally, graphically, by pointing, by tapping, by drawings, by coloring the appropriate category, by sorting cards representing the choices, and so on.

Another important choice concerns the range of applicability of the assessment tool. The basic choice in this respect refers to whether the tool is specific or general (generic). If it is specific it is a tool designed, for example, for a specific disease or class of diseases, for children who got a specific treatment, for children who have survived a particular disease, for children with a particular impairment, for a particular age group, and so on. If it is a generic tool its range of applicability is not restricted by any defining criteria or other specifications. The main advantage of a specific tool resides in the targeted information that it provides but which restricts the range of possible comparisons, whereas the main advantage of the general tool is that it is not restricted in its applicability and allows comparisons of groups of a great variety. The advantages of both approaches are combined in the modular approach, advocated by the European Organization for Research and Treatment of Cancer (EORTC), which is based on using a generic core measure of HRQL and supplemental modules designed for discrete subgroups (Sprangers *et al.* 1993).

A further choice related to the generality issue concerns the basic contents structure of the tool. Each question may be phrased in general referring directly to the domain of interest (e.g., level of anxiety) or may refer to the impact of health (i.e., the disease, treatment) on the domain of interest (e.g., how did the disease or the treatment one got affect one's level of anxiety). The former type of question is characteristic for global QOL, whereas the latter type of question is characteristic for health-related QOL.

Another aspect of generality refers more closely to the type of evaluations requested of the participants: the evaluations may be only specific (e.g., referring to depression, food, sleep) or may refer also to the totality of one's QOL. Historically, QOL was assessed by means of global evaluations, which were replaced by specific evaluations. Aggregating the scores of the specific evaluations yields a total score for QOL. This, however, does not obviate the need or possibility of including also a global question about QOL. Hence, the choice is in fact between basing the global QOL on aggregate scores, on global evaluations or on both.

A further major decision concerns the domains (also called scales, subscales, factors or dimensions) which are to be included in the QOL assessment tool. The nature or contents of the domains and the manner in which they have been derived and defined are major features differentiating among the assessment tools (see Major Assessment Tools of Pediatric QOL). Options for the derivation of the domains include interviewing children, doctors, nurses, parents, or teachers; checking developmental criteria and functions; or preparing downgraded versions of accepted adult questionnaires (e.g., Quality of Well-Being Scale, see Bradlyn *et al.* 1993).

The format of the scores on the QOL tool is related to the issue of global evaluation as against aggregate score for QOL as well as to the representation of the domains in the questionnaire. Scores can be given per item, per groups of items (viz. domains or scales) and for the sum of all items, as well as for a combination of these options.

MAJOR ASSESSMENT TOOLS OF PEDIATRIC QOL

In recent years several assessment tools of pediatric QOL have been developed. We will present briefly several of the better known. All tools fulfill the basic psychometric standards concerning reliability and validity. The first four tools (nos. 1–4) are parental proxy measures, the next five (nos. 5–9) are designed to be completed by both parents and children, and the last three (nos. 10–12) are designed only for children.

(1) *The Miami Pediatric Quality of Life Questionnaire* (MPQOLQ) (Armstrong *et al.* 1999). It was developed specifically for assessing HRQL of pediatric oncology patients. It was constructed on the basis of extensive in-depth interviews with 30 families whose children represented three age groups (preschool, school age, adolescents) and both minimal and severe treatment regimens. Consideration was given both to objective indices of function and psychological adjustment as well as to their subjective importance. The published parent form of the MPQOLQ includes 56 items to which the parents respond twice, first on a five-point Likert scale comparing one's child with other same-aged healthy children (1 = much less than other children the same age, 5 = much more than other children the same age), and then on a 5-point Likert scale rating the importance of the item (1 = not at all important, 5 = extremely important), used to assign weights to the objective scale responses, ranging from 0.8 to 1.2, respectively. Three principal factors with unique loadings were identified by factor analysis: social competence (10 items; e.g., attends school, enjoys activities with same-aged peers), emotional stability (12 items; e.g., cries, has emotional highs and lows); and self-competence (18 items; e.g., motivated to achieve in life, acts independently). It provides three scores for each of the three subscales and a total QOL Index based on all items. The MPQOLQ has good reliability and discriminant validity in regard to diagnostic groups and treatments.

(2) *The Pediatric Oncology Quality of Life Scale* (POQOLS) (Bijttebier *et al.* 2002, Goodwin, Boggs and Graham-Pole 1994): This is a QOL instrument designed to be completed only by the parent and is specific only for children. It is adapted to children of a wide range of age (from preschool to adolescence). It has 21 items, based on written suggestions by parents and physicians. On the basis of factor analysis, three subscales were defined: physical restrictions (nine items, e.g., 'My child has been physically able to perform as usual'); emotional distress (seven items, e.g., 'My child has anger outbursts'); discomfort from medical treatment (five items, e.g., 'My child has complained of pain from medical procedures'). The responses are provided on Likert-type scales with seven options, ranging from 'never' to 'very often'. The POQOLS provides four scores: one for each of the three scales and an overall summated score of QOL. It is not related to age or gender and hence has a broad range of applicability

without the need for specific forms for different age groups. It has high internal consistency (despite having three scales) and inter-rater reliability. In addition, the scores of the POQOLS demonstrated good concurrent and discriminant validity as assessed by relations with measures, such as The Child Behavior Checklist (Achenbach and Edelbrock 1983) and The Play Performance Scale for Children (Lansky *et al.* 1987). The correspondence to child report is good for physical restrictions but not for emotional distress or discomfort due to medical treatment (Boggs and Durning 1998).

(3) *Watson et al.'s measure of HRQL* (Watson *et al.* 1999). It was constructed following the recommendations of the EORTC Quality of Life Study Group. The first to be developed was the form for parents. The preliminary form includes 66 items in the following scales: functional status (six items, e.g., feeding, dressing, mobility, social roles, playing), global health (two items), physical symptoms (26 items, e.g., fatigue, nausea, pain), emotional status (12 items, e.g., tense, irritable, worried), social functioning (four items, e.g., ability to make friends), cognitive functioning (five items, e.g., maintain attention to tasks), behavioral problems (12 items, e.g., enuresis, sleep disorder), school/educational problems (one item). The time period of the questionnaire is one week prior to assessment. Each item has four Likert-type response options. The measure provides scores for each scale and a global QOL score. It can be applied in regard to children from 2 to 19 years of age. Preliminary data showed satisfactory reliability and validity.

(4) *Play Performance Scale for Children* (PPSC) (Mulhern *et al.* 1990). A parental rating scale of child play behavior used as a measure of the children's QOL. The ratings of parents and doctors were correlated significantly for children who were hospitalized, children who received therapy as outpatients, and those who had completed treatment. The parental ratings were highly correlated with ratings on visual analog scales of QOL, mood, physical comfort and the Vinland Adaptive Behavior Scales.

(5) *Pediatric Quality of Life Inventory (PedsQL^{TM} 4.0) Generic Core Scales and The PedsQL^{TM} Condition-Specific Modules* (Varni *et al.* 2002, Varni, Seid and Rode, 1999). These scales were developed over several years in an iterative process on the bases of former versions (Varni *et al.* 1998a, 1998b). The reliability (internal consistency, test–retest), validity (discriminative, construct) and sensitivity are high. Following the EORTC approach, the assessment model includes generic core scales and modules for specific symptoms or diagnostic groups.

(a) *The PedsQL 4.0 Generic Core Scales*: ThePedsQL includes parallel child (for ages 5–7, 8–12, 13–18 years) and parent forms (in regard to children aged 2–4, 5–7, 8–12, 13–18 years). The PedsQL comprises 23 items in four scales: physical functioning (eight items), emotional functioning (five items), social functioning (five items), and school functioning (five items; in the parent form for 2–4 there are only three items in this scale). The following is an example of an item in the social functioning scale from the children 8–12 form: 'In the past one month, how much of a problem has this been for you . . . : How I get along with others (problems with . . .). It is hard to keep up when I play with other kids'. The items are essentially identical and comparable. The Standard Version asks how much of a problem each item has been in the last month, the Acute Version – in the past 7 days. A five-point Likert response scale is used in the child self-reports from age 8 to 18 and in all parent reports (ranging from $0 =$ never a problem, to $4 =$ almost always a problem). For the young child (ages 5–7 years) the Likert scale has been shrunk to three degrees ($0 =$ not at all a problem, $2 =$ sometimes a problem, $4 = $ a lot of a problem, with each category anchored to a happy to sad face). The items are reverse scored, summed, divided by the number of answered items and transformed linearly to a 0–100 scale ($0 = 100$, $1 = 75$, $2 = 50$, $3 = 25$, $4 = 0$). The higher scores reflect higher levels of HRQOL. There are five scores: one for each of the four scales and a Total score. In some cases two component summary scores are computed: the Physical Health Summary Score (based on eight items; identical to the score of Physical Functioning scale) and Psychosocial Health Summary Score (based on the mean of the 15 items of the three remaining scales of emotional, social and school functioning).

(b) *The PedsQL^{TM} Condition-Specific Modules*: Two of the modules are of relevance in the present context. In both the format (structure of parallel forms for child and parent and for the different age groups), instructions, Likert-type response scales and scoring method are identical to those of the PedsQL 4.0 Generic Core Scales.

One is the *PedsQL Multidimensional Fatigue Scale*. It includes a total of 18 items in three subscales: general fatigue, sleep/rest fatigue, and cognitive fatigue, with six items in each. It provides four scores, one of each subscale and a Total fatigue score based on all three subscales.

The other scale is *The PedsQL 3.0 Cancer Module*. It includes a total of 27 items in eight scales: pain and hurt (two items), nausea (five items), procedural anxiety (three items), treatment anxiety (three items), worry (three items), cognitive problems (five items), perceived physical appearance (three items), and communication (three items). It provides nine scores, one for each of the subscales and a Total score based on all subscales.

(6) *Child Health Questionnaire* (CHQ) (Landgraf, Abetz and Ware 1996). It is a multidimensional profile of HRQL, emphasizing physical and psychosocial functioning and wellbeing, which was developed specifically for children and adolescents, and hence it assesses several concepts not included in assessment tools of QOL in adults: the child's self-esteem and behavior as well as the effect

the child's HRQL has on the parents and the family. The original form included 98 items (CHQ-PF98), the shorter commonly used form includes 50 (CHQ-PF50) (also CHQ-PF28, and CHQ-10 are currently available). In the form for parents there are currently 14 scales (number of items per scale 1–6): physical functioning, role/social–physical, general health perceptions, bodily pain, parental time impact, parental emotional impact, role/social–emotional, role/social–behavioral, self-esteem, mental health, general behavior (i.e., aggressive, immature), family activities, family cohesion, change in health over last year. In the form for children there are 10 scales: physical functioning, bodily pain, limitations in schoolwork and activities with friends due to physical health, general health perceptions, change in health, limitations in schoolwork and activities with friends due to emotional/ behavioral difficulties, mental health, general behavior, and self-esteem. The responses are given in terms of Likert scales and the scores are summed across the scales. Raw scores are converted to a 0–100 scale with higher scores denoting better functioning and wellbeing. Internal consistency, reliability and validity are satisfactory. There are validated translations into other languages, including Spanish, Dutch, German and French. The CHQ has been tested successfully also outside the US in the UK, Canada and Germany (Landgraf *et al.* 1998).

(7) *The Behavioral, Affective and Somatic Experiences Scale* (BASES) (Phipps *et al.* 1994, 1999, 2002). It was developed specifically for assessing acute and short-term outcomes in patients undergoing bone marrow transplantation and may be appropriate for patients undergoing very intense chemotherapy. It was designed to be sensitive to acute changes in HRQL and is adapted for repeated-measures designs. It consists of five subscales, labeled: Somatic Distress (i.e., disease state and physical symptoms), Mood Disturbance (i.e., psychological functioning), Compliance, Quality of Interactions (i.e., social functioning), and Activity (i.e., functional status). Examples for Somatic Distress items include nausea, appetite loss, fatigue/malaise; examples for Mood Disturbance include sad/subdued, fearful/anxious, angry/irritable. Four of the subscales (all except Compliance) correspond to commonly accepted 'core' domains of HRQL.

The BASES includes separate versions for the nurse, parent, and the patient. In the nurse's and parent's versions there are 38 items (11, 8, 14, 4, and 1 in the five subscales, respectively). The two versions are almost identical except for the rewording of a few technical terms in the parent's version (e.g., mouth sores for mucositis). All items are weighed equally. A five-point Likert scale is used for all items but the description of the five anchor points differs by scale. The nurse or parent are requested to rate the child's behavior in the last shift or day, respectively. The child's version includes only 14 items (with 3, 3, 4, 2, and 2 items in the five scales, respectively). It is appropriate for children from the age of 5 onward, though some may need the items read to them or other assistance. The BASES yields five scores, one for each scale. In some cases scores for separate items are also considered separately. The scale scores of the three versions of the BASES have shown good reliability, both in terms of internal consistency and inter-rater and cross-informant consistency, good discriminatory validity and good sensitivity to changes in the course of hospitalization for bone marrow transplantation.

(8) *Child Health Rating Inventory (CHRI) and the Disease Impairment Inventories – Bone Marrow Transplant* (DSII-BMT) (Parsons *et al.* 1999). These two inventories conform to the EORTC approach. The CHRI is a generic tool, with 20 items, supplemented by the DSII-BMT which is a disease-specific module, with 10 items. Each of the 30 items starts with the stem 'How much has not feeling well gotten in the way . . . ' followed by a description of some function. Response options are presented pictorially using a five-point Likert scale, and the child is instructed to select the 'kid most like you'. The items of the CHRI were combined conceptually and empirically into seven dimensions (two to seven items per dimension): physical function, role function, mental health, overall quality of life, social/personal resources, cognitive function, and energy. The CHRI yields seven scores, one per each dimension. The items of the DSII-BMT were combined into four dimensions: problems, body image, worry/distress, and self-esteem/isolation. The scores represent each of the dimensions as well as the sum of all four dimensions, converted into a homogeneous scale 0–100. There are two further forms of the questionnaire – for parents and for physicians, designed to parallel closely the item content of the child's questionnaire. The form for parents includes a section on their rating of the child's health status and another section on the parent's own health and functioning. Similarly, the physicians' form requests rating the child in each of the functional domains. All disease-specific items had the additional response option of 'check here if this hasn't happened to you'.

(9) *The Behavioral Assessment System for Children* (BASC) (Reynolds and Kamphaus 1992). This is a five-component questionnaire designed to assess the emotional and behavioral status of children aged 4 to 18 years. There are separate forms to be completed by teachers, parents and the children/adolescents themselves. The teacher and parent forms include three age levels: 4–5, 6–11, and 12–18 years. The form for children/adolescents includes one for the age group 6–11, and another for the age group 12–18. The items refer to observations of positive or negative behaviors that are rated by teachers and parents, and to positive or negative feelings and self-perceptions that are rated by the children/adolescents. Higher scores indicate pathology, except on the adaptation scale where lower scores indicate pathology. Three of the five subscales are considered as particularly relevant for children with cancer or other chronic diseases and indicative of their HRQOL: somatization, anxiety and depression. There exists a large body of normative data about the scores of healthy children on the BASC. Reliability and validity are very good.

(10) *The Minneapolis-Manchester Quality of Life* (MMQL) *Instrument* (Bhatia *et al.* 2002). The MMQL is a patient self-report instrument designed to assess HRQL of survivors of childhood cancer. It is being developed for three age groups: youth (8–12 years), adolescents (13–20) and young adults (21–45). The published form is designed for adolescents. The first is interview-based, the last two are self-administered. It includes seven scales: physical functioning (functional status in the activities of daily life); psychological functioning (emotional functioning including stress and worry); social functioning (interpersonal relationships); cognitive functioning (sequelae of disease and treatment); body image (self-perception of one's body and serves as indicator of self-esteem); outlook on life (satisfaction with current and future life situations); and intimate relations (interpersonal relations with focus on intimacy). All items were scored using the Likert method of summated ratings, with four- or five-point response scales. The MMQL has good reliability (internal consistency, Cronbach's $\alpha = 0.78$, test–retest stability over at least 2 weeks ranged from 0.60 to 0.90, $p < 0.05$, for the different scores) and good validity, both discriminative validity (it discriminated between patients currently in therapy, those who have completed therapy and healthy) and construct validity (as manifested in its significant correlations with the CHQ scales).

(11) *Discrepancy Quality of Life* (Disquol) (Eiser *et al.* 1999, Vance *et al.* 2001). This is a generic computer-administered measure of HRQL suitable for children 6–12 years old. It is a child-centered measure in its theoretical background and methodology. The adopted theoretical model is based on Calman's (1984) approach that HRQL should measure the potential for growth by assessing the difference between the individual's goals and actual experience at a given point in time. The items are presented in a social context in view of the assumption that children 6–12 years old are sensitive to social restrictions and how they are perceived by other children (Eder, 1990). There are 12 items referring to situations that occur commonly for sick children. Each item is presented by means of a picture and a brief verbal description of the target child. For example, 'X [the actual names used are gender-specific] finds it hard to go to sleep at night. Then he feels tired in school the next day', 'Here is a picture of Y having a good time at the swimming pool'. The other items refer to the tendency to feel aches and pain, becoming sick more often than one's friends, on the playground getting tired sooner than others, not being able to eat at a birthday party like the others for fear of feeling ill, succeeding at school, feeling fit and healthy for sports and games, dealing with parental restrictions, not being asked out to play and difficulty in making friends with other kids. The picture on the screen is shown together with a visual analog scale anchored first on 'not like me' (rated 0) to 'exactly like me' (rated 100), and then, when administered again, on 'don't want to be like that' (rated 0) to 'really want to be like that' (rated 100). To each item the child is requested to

give two answers, first in terms of resemblance at present, and then in terms of desire or wish for resemblance to the target child. The response is given by clicking with the mouse on the right point on the scale. By summing the child's ratings across items, the scale yields three scores (all in the range of 0–100): actual self, ideal self, and the discrepancy representing the actual minus ideal self scores. The higher the discrepancy score, the higher HRQL. The reliability is medium (0.50–0.55). The validity is good as manifested in correlations between the three scores and scores on the PCQL-32, especially for the discrepancy score and social functioning.

(12) *The Children's Quality of Life measure* (CQL) (Kreitler and Kreitler, 2003a) (see Appendix). This is a generic tool developed for children in general, both healthy and not healthy, based on the following assumptions. First, a measure for children should be addressed to children in contents, form and format, as closely as possible. Secondly, a measure of QOL should address the construct of QOL in contents, form and format, as closely as possible. Thus, in regard to the first assumption, concerning contents, the only criterion for selecting items was the views of the children, the meanings they assigned to quality of life, rather than the views of parents, educators, or experts on development and on health. An effort was made to select for the CQL items that refer to themes of interest and importance to children, as determined on the basis of extensive interviews with children from the ages of 3 to 18. Further, the different versions of the questionnaire were presented to children of the relevant age groups for evaluation and discussion, in single sessions and in groups. Concerning form, the response alternatives are quantifiable but present only three options, which is what the children chose as most appropriate and easiest to handle. Further, the response alternatives are presented in three convergent forms: in graphic illustrative form (the degrees or extent are exemplified by a different number of heaped up 'eggs'), by brief verbal descriptions, and by location from left to right. The verbal descriptions accompanying the items may differ across items because the clarity and appropriateness of the response alternatives as judged by the children played a more important role than homogeneity of format. The children can respond to the items by pointing at the preferred option, crossing it out, underlining it, encircling it, or by coloring it, whichever they prefer and decide on the spot. No homogeneity of response formats is required from the child. Concerning format, the items are precise, specific, concrete and easily understandable.

In regard to the second assumption, concerning contents, an effort was made to include only items that refer directly to subjective or experiential features, with a minimum of evaluation. The respondent is led to focus mainly on phenomenologically presented aspects, without dealing with judgments of causes and consequences. Therefore, the CQL does not include items that require the respondent to judge the extent to which his/her activity or state have been affected by his/her state of health or medical treatments. To our mind, judgments of this kind, which constitute the basis for HRQL measures, reflect one's *evaluation* of the impact of health, but cannot replace objective measures of the impact of health or subjective measures of QOL. Concerning form and format, the CQL items are highly specific and concrete. Thus, they refer to friends, having a special friend and to feeling lonely rather than to one's social state; or again, they refer to feeling successful rather than being a good student. Further, the CQL includes domains of QOL that are not included in any of the standard measures, for example, interest in what goes on around oneself, nutrition, accommodation, and being able to do things for one's siblings.

The present version of the CQL is the result of an iterative process over the last 8 years. It has been administered to samples of over 4000 healthy children in the various age levels from 3 to 18, and to childen with various diseases, mainly oncological samples, children with asthma, diabetes, or various neurological disorders. Up to now versions in three languages have been prepared and tested (Hebrew, Arabic, English). The Russian version is in the process of testing. The CQL may be administered in individual sessions or in groups of any size. Children of any age that require help may have the questions read to them. The standard version does not refer to any specific time period. Temporal or other specifications can be added, according to the interests of the investigator or practitioner, for example, 'please respond according to your state now, today, at present/in the last week/in the last month/in the course of the treatments/since you have become sick' etc. The CQL may be administered repeatedly, as needed.

Two parallel forms of questionnaires are of special interest in the present context. They consists of two proxy versions of the CQL in which another person, who may have some contact or relation with the child (e.g., parent, sibling, physician, nurse, friend), responds to each of the items (a) about the child and (b) as he/she thinks the child himself/herself would supposedly respond or would have supposedly responded in given circumstances. These two proxy versions differ. The first involves changing the items of the CQL so that they refer to the child (e.g., 'The child (name may be specified) is worried about his/her health', 'The child is satisfied with the food that he/she usually eats'). In the second proxy version the items remain unchanged and the proxy respondent completes them as if he/she were the child. Notably, in most studies of HRQL in children, the two proxy versions are not held apart, e.g., sometimes the second version is used but the first is assumed.

It may be of interest to note that the CQL resembles in the content of some of its items the Adult Quality of Life (AQL) (Kreitler and Kreitler 2003b) and hence may be compared with it in some respects.

The present standard version of the CQL has 55 items, each with three response alternatives, scored 1 to 3, where 3 represents the better score from the

Table 7.1 Summary of items and scales of the CQL

Item or Scale	Description
Q1	Health worries
Q2	Feeling healthy
Q3	Having pain
Q4	Extent of pain
Q5	School attendance
Q6	Fulfilling duties at school
Q7	Attending classes at school
Q8	Activity during recess at school
Q9	Activity in the schoolyard
Q10	Playing outdoors
Q11	Playing at home
Q12	Mobility
Q13	Fulfilling duties at home
Q14	Doing things for one's parents
Q15	Doing things for one's siblings
Q16	Stressing out because of not doing everything required
Q17	Doing things one is not good at
Q18	Doing things one really likes doing
Q19	Existence of something that bothers the child
Q20	Talking about his/her problems with his/her family
Q21	Financial situation from the child's point of view
Q22	Accommodation
Q23	Nutrition
Q24	Having friends
Q25	Having one special friend
Q26	Having fun with friends or family
Q27	Ability to keep busy, not to be bored
Q28	Interest in what is going on around him/her
Q29	Liking the way one looks
Q30	Taking care of the way one looks
Q31	Ability to solve problems
Q32	Feeling successful
Q33	Feeling of being in control
Q34	Managing by oneself
Q35	Ability to concentrate
Q36	Memory
Q37	Ability to think and understand
Q38	Nervousness
Q39	Being oriented
Q40	Sadness
Q41	Loneliness
Q42	Sleep difficulties
Q43	Tiredness, fatigue
Q44	Guilt
Q45	Anger
Q46	Fear

(continued)

Table 7.1 *(continued)*

Item or Scale	Description
Q47	Confusion
Q48	Feeling safe
Q49	Jealousy
Q50	Worthlessness
Q51	Feeling miserable
Q52	Hopefulness
Q53	Happiness and enjoyment
Q54	Motivation
Q55	Having something to live for
Q56	Life satisfaction
Family functioning scale	Items Q13, Q14, Q15, Q26
School functioning scale	Items Q5, Q6, Q7, Q8, Q9
Negative feelings scale	Items Q16, Q17, Q38, Q39, Q40, Q41, Q44, Q45, Q46, Q47, Q49, Q50, Q51
Positive feelings scale	Items Q26, Q48, Q53, Q56
Confusion scale	Items Q39, Q47
Cognitive functioning scale	Items Q28, Q35, Q36, Q37
Health worries scale	Items Q1, Q2
Pain scale	Items Q3, Q4
Friends scale	Items Q24, Q25, Q26
Body image scale	Items Q29, Q30
Mastery and independence scale	Items Q27, Q31, Q33, Q34
Play scale	Items Q10, Q11
Stress scale	Items Q16, Q17, Q19
Basic needs scale	Items Q12, Q21, Q22, Q23, Q42, Q48
Motivation scale	Items Q52, Q54, Q55

Note. This table represents the 56 items and 15 scales of the CQL questionnaire that was used in the studies reported in chapter 7. In the scales some items are included in more than one scale (Q17, Q26, Q39, Q47, Q48), some are not included in any scale (Q18, Q20, Q32, Q43). This version of the CQL includes one item – no. 8 – that was inserted specifically on the request of the children with cancer. It is not included in the standard version of the CQL which is presented in the Appendix. Therefore, from Q9 onward there is a 1-step discrepancy between the description of the items in the table and the standard version of the CHQ in the Appendix. For the additional item see end of Appendix. The preliminary version of the Children's Quality of Life (CQL-0) questionnaire included only 49 items (missing items: Q8, Q16, Q17, Q18, Q19, Q32, Q49).

point of view of QOL. The items are grouped into 15 scales. The scales represent grouping by contents that has been fully confirmed by factor analyses of data in various age levels (the scales are presented and defined in Table 7.1). There are three kinds of scores: (a) scores for each item separately (range 1–3), which may be important for detecting particular problems, e.g., in sleep; (b) scores for each of the 14 scales; and (c) an overall global score based on summing the responses to all items. In rough terms, scores 56–93 represent low level of QOL, 94–131 a medium level, and 132–168 a high level. Table 7.2 presents basic descriptive and reliability information about the CQL and the scales in the pediatric oncology sample used for the study reported in this chapter.

Table 7.2 The means, SDs and reliabilities of the scales of the CQL

Scale	No. of items	Mean of scale[a]	SD of scale[a]	Item mean[b]	Item SD[b]	Cronbach's alpha
Family	4	9.953	1.833	2.488	0.093	0.692
School	5	13.161	2.129	2.632	0.042	0.759
Negative feelings	13	32.478	4.098	2.498	0.243	0.826
Positive feelings	4	11.016	1.368	2.754	0.049	0.691
Confusion	2	5.113	0.949	2.557	0.036	0.646
Cognitive functioning	4	10.757	1.332	2.689	0.063	0.538
Health worries	2	4.694	0.981	2.347	0.504	0.450
Pain	2	4.832	1.037	2.416	0.061	0.714
Friends	3	7.798	2.530	2.599	0.315	0.303
Body image	2	5.417	0.811	2.709	0.069	0.392
Mastery and inde-pendence	4	9.698	1.455	2.424	0.102	0.552
Play	2	4.674	1.086	2.337	0.030	0.384
Stress	3	6.787	1.441	2.262	0.109	0.546
Basic needs	6	16.199	1.565	2.700	0.101	0.452
Motivation	3	8.457	0.827	2.819	0.125	0.462
Total QOL	56	142.559	12.828	2.546	0.229	0.881

[a]Represents the mean and SD across participants but not items.
[b]Represents the mean and SD across participants and items.

REPRESENTATIVE FINDINGS ON THE QOL OF CHILDREN WITH CANCER

This section is devoted to reviewing major findings concerning the QOL of children with cancer, focusing on the periods of diagnosis, active treatment and follow-up, but excluding studies of pediatric cancer survivors as well as children undergoing bone marrow transplantation which are dealt with in other chapters in the book (Chapters 11, 10). Since we are dealing with a newly developing field, it is not surprising that in many cases findings about the QOL of the children constitute part of the development of the assessment tool.

Using the *MPQOLQ*, Armstrong *et al.* (1999) found that children with brain tumors scored lower than those with leukemias/lymphomas on the Total Index, social competence and self-competence (though not on emotional stability). There were no significant differences between leukemia/lymphomas and solid tumors. Children who had received whole-brain radiation (mostly those diagnosed with ALL or high-grade brain tumors) scored significantly lower on the Total Index, social competence and self-competence than those who did not (but there was no difference on emotional stability). Physician's global ratings of HRQL were not related to any of the four scores of QOL.

Analyzing the data on the *POQOLS* (Bijttebier *et al.* 2001) showed high intercorrelations among all three scale scores (physical restrictions, emotional distress and discomfort from medical treatment). This indicates that at least in this oncology sample QOL is a general global characteristic. The scores do not differ for the different ages (2.8 to 19.7) and the genders. Comparing children out of treatment with those on intensive treatment showed that the latter had lower scores on the scales physical restrictions and discomfort from medical treatment, but did not have more emotional distress. Comparing only patients of leukemia and lymphoma differing in treatment status (off-treatment, on maintenance treatment and on intensive treatment) showed that those in intensive treatment scored higher on physical restrictions, but not higher on emotional distress, or on discomfort from medical treatment, and did not have an overall worse QOL. Comparing children with different diagnoses showed that those with leukemia or lymphoma had less emotional discomfort, less discomfort from treatment and overall better QOL than those with solid tumors (brain, solid, neuroblastoma). Time since diagnosis was correlated with physical restrictions, so that the longer the time, the fewer physical restrictions the child was reported to have.

On Watson's *et al.*'s (1999) *HRQL* (parental form), comparing the reports on children with a variety of cancer diagnoses on- and off-treatment showed that in the course of treatment the children had more physical symptoms, but had *higher* scores on emotional status (suggested explanation: this is due to a decline of the distress they have had earlier during diagnosis), and *better* cognitive functioning (suggested explanation: 'settling down to things' and persisting are perhaps easier for the children because they are busy with physical effects of treatment). However, there were no differences on functional status, global health, social functioning, behavioral problems and global QOL.

Quite a different assessment tool, based on observing the children's play activities (*PPSC*; Mulhern *et al.* 1990), showed that the ratings of the children's QOL were most influenced by the child's physical symptoms. There were significant differences between inpatients and outpatients, but not between outpatients receiving therapy and those patients who had completed therapy.

The *PedsQL 4.0 Generic Core Scales* were administered to a pediatric oncology sample that included 339 patients of both genders (mean age 8.72 years, range 2–18) with ALL, brain tumors, Hodgkin and non-Hodgkin lymphomas, Wilms' tumor and other cancers, with no co-morbidity, newly diagnosed and with recurrent disease, on- and off-treatment, with short or long remissions. Their scores on the Acute Version were compared with those of 157 healthy children (age range 2–18), and on the Standard Version with the scores of 730 healthy children (Varni *et al.* 2002). In general, the oncology sample as a group had lower scores on all four scale scores of physical, social, emotional and school functioning as well as on the total score. However, there were many exceptions to this general description.

In the Generic scales, child report, Acute Version, the oncology sample did not get lower scores than the healthy sample on the total score in the case of children older than 12 off-treatment, on the scale of physical health in the case of children younger or older than 12 off-treatment, on the scale of emotional functioning in the case of children older than 12 off-treatment, on the scale of social functioning in the case of children older than 12 off-treatment, and on the scale of school functioning in the case of children younger or older than 12 off-treatment. Further, in the case of children younger than 12 there were no differences between the groups on-treatment and off-treatment on either of the scores, in contrast to the case of children older than 12 where there were significant differences between the on- and off-treatment groups on the total score and on the scores of the scales of physical and emotional functioning.

Examining the findings on the Generic scales, parent report, Acute Version shows that in the case of children younger or older than 12, the on- and off-treatment groups scored in all cases less than the healthy controls. However, the on- and off-treatment groups did not always differ from each other; for example, they did not differ significantly in the scores of the scales of psychosocial health, social functioning and school functioning.

On the condition-specific module of *Multidimensional Fatigue* (child-report version) the findings are also not homogeneous. Thus, on the total score, the sick children on-treatment as well as the younger than 12 off-treatment (but not the older ones) scored lower than the healthy controls; on the scales of general fatigue and sleep/rest fatigue, the children on-treatment scored lower than those off-treatment older than 12 and also lower than the healthy controls; on the scale of cognitive fatigue only the children on-treatment scored lower than the healthy controls but not those off-treatment, regardless of whether they are older or younger than 12.

The results on the parent-report version of the *Multidimensional Fatigue Scale* show that on the total score and on all scales all children with cancer, regardless of age and of treatment status, scored less than the healthy controls. However, only on two of the scales (i.e., general fatigue and sleep/rest fatigue) the on-treatment children scored less than the off-treatment children, regardless of age. On total fatigue and cognitive fatigue, for example, there were no differences between the on- and off-treatment children younger than 12.

On the other condition-specific *Cancer Module*, the child form, there were no significant differences between children on- and off-treatment on five of the eight scales, regardless of age; on the scales of worry, nausea and treatment anxiety, the on-treatment children scored lower than the off-treatment ones but only in the case of children older than 12.

On the parental form of the *Cancer Module*, the on-treatment children scored lower than the off-treatment ones on five scales (pain, nausea, procedural anxiety, treatment anxiety and worry), but not always in regard to both age groups (in the case of pain, only older children; in the case of nausea, procedural anxiety and worry, both age groups; in the case of treatment anxiety, only the younger children).

Some studies report results with pediatric oncology samples using The Pediatric Quality of Life Inventory (a previous version of the generic PedsQL scale). Thus, in one study 28 children with brain tumors were compared with 28 children with other types of cancer, matched in demographic and medical characteristics (Stephenson 2003). The group with brain tumors reported lower overall HRQOL as well as lower HRQOL in the domains of physical functioning, psychological functioning and social functioning. Another study (Varni, Seid and Rode 1999) compared 125 on-treatment pediatric patients with 156 patients off-treatment (all diagnostic groups, age range 8–18 years) and found that they differed significantly only on the scale of physical functioning, but not on psychological and social functioning.

On the *PCQL-32* children 6–12 years old (8.92 mean), diagnosed with ALL in different stages of disease and treatment, had the highest scores in social functioning (mean = 0.89), followed in a descending order by psychological functioning (mean = 0.76), overall QOL (mean = 0.70), cognitive functioning (mean = 0.63), physical functioning (mean = 0.60), and disease and treatment problems (mean = 0.58). Parents rated the children lower than they themselves did (Vance *et al.* 2001).

On the *CHQ* (Sawyer *et al.* 1999) parents' reports showed that adolescents (mean age 13.6, SD = 2.2 years) with cancer were rated significantly lower than healthy controls on seven of the 12 scales: physical functioning, role/social–physical, general health perceptions, family activities, role/social–emotional/ behavioral, parental impact – emotional, and self-esteem. There were no significant differences on pain, parental impact – time, mental health, behavior and family cohesion. Within the cancer group, the lowest scores were on the scales that rated the emotional impact that the adolescent's illness had on parents (the extent to which they were worried and concerned) and on the parents' perceptions of their adolescents' general health. These findings seem to tell us more about the parents than about the adolescents. On the bases of their own reports, adolescents with cancer scored significantly higher than healthy controls, on the scales of mental health and role/social behavioral and lower on the scales self-esteem and general health perceptions. The latter scale yielded the lowest scores they reported.

Further, the self-report form showed that adolescents in active treatment had significantly lower scores than the adolescents off-treatment only on two scales: physical functioning and general health perceptions. However, the parent-report ratings indicated that adolescents in active treatment scored significantly lower than those off-treatment on seven of the 12 scales: physical functioning, role/social–physical, bodily pain, family activities, role/social– emotional, parental impact – time, and parental impact – emotional.

The adolescents' self-reports yielded significant correlations between time since cancer diagnosis and the scales physical functioning, role/social–physical and general health perceptions. The parents' reports showed significant correlations between time since diagnosis and seven scales: physical functioning, role/social–physical, bodily pain, family activities, role/social–emotional/behavioral, parental impact – time, parental impact – emotional. These findings suggest that parents assign a greater impact to the disease and the treatments than the adolescents tend to.

Comparisons of CHQ (self-report form) scores of sick and healthy adolescents were carried out also in the framework of another study (Bhatia *et al.* 2002). The sample included 268 adolescents with cancer (median age 16.4, range 13–20.9) of both genders, diagnosed with a variety of cancer diagnoses (45.15% leukemia, 22.01% lymphomas), partly on- and partly off-therapy for 1 year. The investigators reported that the CHQ discriminated successfully between the cancer patients on- and off-therapy on the scales of global health, physical functioning, bodily pain, self-esteem, general health perceptions, and family activities.

The *BASC* (Reynolds and Kamphaus, 1992) was administered to children (about 9 years old, range 6–14), mostly with ALL, who had not undergone cranial irradiation, and were partly on- and partly off-treatment (Challinor *et al.* 1999). Parents (mostly mothers) reported for the children higher depression levels than the teachers and the children themselves. Again, the teachers and the parents reported for the children higher somatization levels than the children themselves. In regard to anxiety, the parents reported for the children higher levels than the teachers and the children. The reports of the parents and the children correlated moderately and significantly in regard to anxiety and depression but not in regard to somatization. All three scales correlated significantly and positively in each respondent group (i.e., children, parents, and teachers).

In all three subscales the scores were on the whole within the normal range. Yet, on the basis of the scores, a certain percentage of the children could be identified as 'at risk': in regard to somatization 30.8–46.5%, in regard to anxiety 11.6–32.3%, in regard to depression 11.6–20.9%. In each case the highest numbers were those based on the parents' reports. There was agreement among the three types of respondents about who was 'at risk' in regard to anxiety and depression but not in regard to somatization. Gender, treatment status, and cranial irradiation had no influence on who was identified as 'at risk'. This was true also of age, except in regard to anxiety: more adolescents than children were rated by their parents in the 'at risk' range.

The *MMQL Instrument* (Bhatia *et al.* 2002) was administered to 268 adolescents with cancer (median age 16.4, range 13–20.9) of both genders, diagnosed with a variety of cancer diagnoses (45.15% leukemia, 22.01% lymphomas), partly on- and partly off-therapy for 1 year. The control participants were 129 healthy adolescents with similar demographic characteristics. The comparisons showed that the cancer patients as a group had significantly lower scores on 4 of the 8 scales: physical functioning, cognitive functioning, psychological functioning, and social functioning. There were no significant differences between the sick and healthy adolescents on the scales of body image, outlook on life, and intimate relations, as well as on the overall global score. Notably, patients on-therapy differed from those off-therapy in their lower scores on physical functioning, psychological functioning, and outlook on life and *higher* scores on social functioning (probably because of the social support they were getting in the course of therapy). It is of special interest to note that healthy adolescents and cancer patients off-treatment did not differ significantly in half of the scales (psychological functioning, body image, outlook on life and intimate relations) as well as on the global score of QOL.

The *Disquol* (Eiser *et al.* 1999) was administered to children (age range 6–12), diagnosed with ALL, in different stages of disease and treatment (Vance *et al.* 2001). The results showed that older children had higher scores on actual self and smaller discrepancy scores, namely, lower HRQL. In general, the children's discrepancy scores were lower when the parents were depressed.

Findings with a new pilot version of a QOL measure developed for pediatric oncology (*PEDQOL*) ($\alpha > 0.60$) were reported for 49 children off-treatment in the age range of 8 to 18 years (51% had leukemia or lymphoma and 49% solid tumors) (Calaminus *et al.* 2000). The authors reported that there was a greater impairment of QOL in the leukemia/lymphoma patients than in those with solid tumors. The affected QOL domains included autonomy, emotional functioning, cognition and familial interactions. Those with solid tumors had less impairment, which was evident particularly in physical functioning and body image.

Findings with the CQL[1]

The CQL (preliminary version with 49 items) was administered first to a small sample of children with cancer ($n = 35$) and matched healthy children ($n = 40$) in order to test the applicability and sensitivity of this tool in the context of pediatric oncology. The oncology sample included children in the age range of 9 to 14 with a variety of diagnoses, in different disease stages, with longer or shorter disease duration, some in treatment (hospitalized or as outpatients) and some off-treatment. Administering the questionnaire showed that it was easy for the children to complete and that it seemed relevant and even interesting to them. We will mention some of the findings that were of particular importance in demonstrating sensitivity of the CQL in relevant respects about which we could set up hypotheses.[2] Comparing sick and healthy children showed that the sick children had significantly lower scores on the scales of school functioning

---

[1] The studies involving the CQL were carried out together with Professor Myriam Ben Arush.
[2] The items of the CQL mentioned in the text or the tables as Q1 etc. are described in Table 7.1.

(especially Q5, Q7, and Q8), play (especially Q10), mastery and independence (especially Q34), cognitive functioning (especially Q31), basic needs (especially Q12), positive feelings (especially Q53, Q56), and negative feelings (especially Q46, Q51). Lower scores denote lower QOL in all cases, including negative feelings. These findings support the hypothesis that the effect of disease on the children is negative and pervasive. Another meaningful comparison in the present context focuses on children in treatment and off-treatment. Despite the small number of cases, the results showed that children in treatment had lower scores in the scales of friends, cognitive functioning, negative feelings and basic needs. Of particular interest is the finding that in regard to the children in treatment, the inpatients differed from the outpatients in their higher scores on the scale of basic needs (especially Q42, and Q48). In an interview after the study the inpatients explained that during the treatment they felt more secure in the hospital where they could be sure that a doctor or nurse would be always available to offer professional help in any eventuality. Or, in the words of one child: 'At home if something happens and I feel sick, my parents don't know what to do and start arguing about whether to bring me to the hospital'.

These preliminary findings were sufficiently encouraging to enable us to proceed with the main part of the project. We will report major findings obtained with the CQL in a sample of 217 children with cancer. The children were of both genders (108 boys, 109 girls), ranged in age from 6 to 18 (M = 14.93, SD = 3.75), were mostly born in Israel (76%) and included children of the major pediatric oncological diagnoses (see Table 7.5), in the major disease stages (13.85%, 41.45%, 27.15%, and 17.55% in stages 1 to 4, respectively), partly on-treatment (35.81%) and partly off-treatment (64.19%). An overall view of the scale means (Table 7.2) shows that from the point of view of QOL the five highest relative scores are in the domains of motivation (M = 2.819) and positive feelings (M = 2.754) followed by body image (M = 2.709), basic needs (M = 2.700) and cognitive functioning (M = 2.689). In contrast, the five lowest relative scores of QOL are in the domains of mastery and independence (M = 2.424), pain (M = 2.416), health worries (M = 2.347), play (M = 2.337), and stress (M = 2.262). The latter are the QOL domains hit the hardest in children with cancer.

In order to learn more about the grouping of the domains of QOL in children with cancer, a factor analysis of the scale scores was performed (Table 7.3). It shows that the scales form three factors. The first and major one is defined by high saturations on the scales of negative feelings, confusion and stress and may be labeled Emotional Distress. The second factor is defined by high saturations on the scales of positive feelings, body image, basic needs and motivation for living, and may be labeled Coping with the Disease. The third factor is defined by high saturations on the scales of pain, school and family and may be labeled Themes of Concern or Worry. Since the three factors accounted only for 51.27% of the variance, it is of interest to examine which of

Table 7.3 Results of factor analysis on the scales of the CQL

Scales of CQL	Factor I	Factor II	Factor III	**Communalities**
Family functioning			0.563	**0.459**
School functioning			0.612	**0.434**
Negative feelings	0.890			**0.865**
Positive feelings		0.665		**0.639**
Confusion	0.803			**0.660**
Cognitive functioning				**0.409**
Health worries				**0.539**
Pain			0.623	**0.436**
Friends				**0.228**
Body image		0.647		**0.447**
Mastery and independence				**0.431**
Play				**0.404**
Stress	0.756			**0.642**
Basic needs		0.508		**0.540**
Motivation		0.630		**0.558**
Eigenvalue	3.010	2.359	2.321	
Per cent of explained variance	20.071	15.725	15.473	
Suggested title of factor	**Emotional distress**	**Coping with the disease**	**Themes of concern or worry**	

Note. The factor analysis was done by the varimax method with Kaiser normalization. The numbers in the factor columns are factor loadings. Only loadings > 0.500 are presented.

the scales contribute most to the pool of variance not accounted for (namely, have communalities < 0.50). These are the scales of friends, play, cognitive functioning, body image, mastery, school, family and even pain, which may be assumed to reflect tendencies shaped primarily by determinants beyond the disease, such as the child's personality and environment.

In order to find out about the structure of the whole field of QOL in a pediatric oncology sample, a factor analysis (with varimax rotation) of the items of the CQL was carried out. It yielded 18 factors (with eigenvalues ranging from 4.80 to 1.33, and per cent of variance ranging from 8.58 to 2.37) accounting for 65.26% of the variance. The factors from 1 to 18 represented the following sequence of domains: 1. Negative feelings, 2. School functioning, 3. Pain, 4. Motivation for living and coping, 5. Fulfilling duties at home, 6. Positive feelings, 7. Mastery and control, 8. Life at home (accommodation, playing, discussing problems), 9. Cognitive functioning (solving problems, being oriented), 10. Health and despair (health worries, feeling of health and low hopefulness), 11. Jealousy in regard to health, 12. Food and eating, 13. Cognitive functioning (memory and thinking), 14. Having close friends, 15. Spending money on taking care of one's appearance, 16. Doing things that one likes, 17. Being bothered and worried about something, and 18. Having friends for keeping busy and active. Although the listed series of 18 factors may not have sufficient stability and reliability, it serves to illustrate an important feature of the structure of QOL in the pediatric oncology sample. The field of QOL seems to consist of a pattern of specific factors, each of which is clearly focused on a definite theme and accounts for a small amount of variance.

Three sets of comparisons of CQL items and scale scores were performed. *The first set of comparisons referred to demographic variables.* Comparisons in terms of age yielded significant results for 20 items (Q2, Q3, Q11, Q19, Q20, Q22, Q25, Q26, Q29, Q32, Q35, Q38, Q40–Q43, Q47, Q51, Q53, Q56), and 7 scales (school, negative feelings, positive feelings, health, body image, play, stress) as well as for the total QOL score. In all cases except one (Q25) the QOL of children younger than 15 was better than that of children older than 15. Comparisons in terms of gender, yielded significant results for 12 items (Q7, Q8, Q10, Q12, Q22, Q25, Q32, Q40, Q41, Q43, Q46, Q50) and one scale (negative feelings) as well as for the total QOL score. In all except two cases (Q12, Q25) boys had higher QOL scores than girls. Comparisons in terms of country of birth yielded significant results for eight items (Q4, Q16, Q17, Q31, Q38, Q39, Q48, Q50) and three scales (negative feelings, mastery and independence and stress). In all except one case (Q4), children born in Israel had higher QOL scores than children born in other countries who immigrated to Israel. In sum, the results indicate first, that the CQL questionnaire is sensitive to demographic characteristics, and second, that in the case of children with cancer QOL is higher for younger than for older children, for boys than for girls, and for Israeli-born children than for children who have immigrated to Israel.

The second set of comparisons referred to treatment variables (Table 7.4). The results yield specific information about the extent and nature of the effects of treatments on QOL variables. The comparisons in terms of current status (i.e., remission versus on-treatment) yielded significant differences in regard to 18 items, seven scales and the total score of QOL. The results show, as expected, that the scores of the children in remission reflect higher QOL than the scores of the children on-treatment in all except two cases: the motivation scale, probably because they do not have to deal any more with the difficult side-effects of the treatments, and communication within the family (Q20), probably because there is less need for the support of the family and greater need for maintaining broader social ties.

Other comparisons were made in terms of specific current treatments, chemotherapy versus other treatments, and the estimate of chemotherapy load (heavy, medium or light). As expected, the comparisons in terms of the chemotherapy load showed that in the majority of cases (13 of 15 items with significant results and in the overall QOL), the lowest QOL characterized the group getting 'heavy' chemotherapy. There are three notable exceptions: in the scales of pain, body image and motivation the children with the lightest load

Table 7.4 Significant results of comparisons of CQL variables – items and scale scores – in groups defined by treatment characteristics

QOL variables	Treatment variables	Means	SDs	t or F values	Significant differences between means
Current treatment					
Q1	Radiation	2.00	2.00	2.410*	
	Chemotherapy	1.69	1.69		
	Endocrinal	1.67	1.67		
	Pills	2.50	2.50		
	Tamoxifen	2.50	2.50		
	No treatment	2.06	2.06		
Q3	Radiation	3.00	0.00	5.500***	Tam < endo,
	Chemotherapy	2.14	0.64		chemo, none,
	Endocrinal	2.00	1.00		rad, pills
	Pills	3.00	0.00		
	Tamoxifen	1.00	0.00		
	No treatment	2.43	0.54		
Q4	Radiation	2.67	0.58	7.983***	
	Chemotherapy	2.06	0.72		
	Endocrinal	2.50	0.71		
	Pills	3.00	0.12		
	Tamoxifen	1.00	0.00		
	No treatment	2.59	0.52		
Q5	Radiation	3.00	0.00	24.615***	Chemo < none,
	Chemotherapy	1.83	0.79		rad, tam
	Endocrinal	2.33	0.58		
	Pills	2.50	0.71		
	Tamoxifen	3.00	0.00		
	No treatment	2.86	0.38		
Q6	Radiation	2.67	0.58	6.240***	
	Chemotherapy	2.30	0.84		
	Endocrinal	2.33	1.15		
	Pills	2.50	0.71		
	Tamoxifen	3.00	0.00		
	No treatment	2.90	0.48		
Q7	Radiation	3.00	0.00	6.223***	
	Chemotherapy	2.17	0.83		
	Endocrinal	2.33	0.58		
	Pills	2.00	1.41		
	Tamoxifen	3.00	0.00		
	No treatment	2.79	0.54		

(continued)

Table 7.4 *(continued)*

QOL variables	Treatment variables	Means	SDs	t or F values	Significant differences between means
Q8	Radiation	2.67	0.58	2.490*	
	Chemotherapy	1.96	0.60		
	Endocrinal	2.00	0.00		
	Pills	2.50	0.71		
	Tamoxifen	1.50	0.71		
	No treatment	2.39	0.72		
Q9	Radiation	3.00	0.00	3.387**	
	Chemotherapy	2.30	0.82		
	Endocrinal	3.00	0.00		
	Pills	3.00	0.00		
	Tamoxifen	3.00	0.00		
	No treatment	2.82	0.00		
Q12	Radiation	3.00	0.00	7.617***	Tam < chemo,
	Chemotherapy	2.53	0.56		endo, none,
	Endocrinal	2.67	0.58		rad, pills
	Pills	3.00	0.00		
	Tamoxifen	1.50	0.71		
	No treatment	2.85	0.38		
Q13	Radiation	2.67	0.58	2.749*	
	Chemotherapy	2.11	0.78		
	Endocrinal	2.33	0.58		
	Pills	2.50	0.71		
	Tamoxifen	3.00	0.00		
	No treatment	2.55	0.66		
Q14	Radiation	2.33	0.58	5.280***	
	Chemotherapy	2.00	0.68		
	Endocrinal	3.00	0.00		
	Pills	2.00	1.41		
	Tamoxifen	3.00	0.00		
	No treatment	2.53	0.61		
Q15	Radiation	2.33	0.58	2.405*	
	Chemotherapy	2.09	0.69		
	Endocrinal	3.00	0.00		
	Pills	2.00	1.41		
	Tamoxifen	3.00	0.00		
	No treatment	2.41	0.63		

(continued)

Table 7.4 *(continued)*

QOL variables	Treatment variables	Means	SDs	t or F values	Significant differences between means
Q16	Radiation	3.00	0.00	1.100	Endo < rad
	Chemotherapy	2.17	0.83		
	Endocrinal	1.67	1.15		
	Pills	2.00	0.00		
	Tamoxifen	2.50	0.71		
	No treatment	2.24	0.64		
Q17	Radiation	2.50	0.71	1.633	Pills < tam
	Chemotherapy	2.30	0.70		
	Endocrinal	2.00	1.00		
	Pills	1.50	0.71		
	Tamoxifen	3.00	0.00		
	No treatment	2.41	0.59		
Q20	Radiation	2.67	0.58	2.977*	Tam < none,
	Chemotherapy	2.31	0.62		chemo, pills,
	Endocrinal	2.67	0.58		rad, endo
	Pills	2.50	0.71		
	Tamoxifen	1.00	0.00		
	No treatment	2.02	0.71		
Q25	Radiation	1.67	1.15	1.888	Tam < endo
	Chemotherapy	2.17	0.77		
	Endocrinal	3.00	0.00		
	Pills	2.00	1.41		
	Tamoxifen	1.00	0.00		
	No treatment	2.27	0.77		
Q26	Radiation	3.00	0.00	1.083	Tam < rad, pills
	Chemotherapy	2.69	0.52		
	Endocrinal	2.50	0.71		
	Pills	3.00	0.00		
	Tamoxifen	2.00	0.00		
	No treatment	2.70	0.53		
Q28	Radiation	3.00	0.00	0.849	Pills < rad
	Chemotherapy	2.67	0.48		
	Endocrinal	2.50	0.71		
	Pills	2.00	1.41		
	Tamoxifen	2.50	0.71		
	No treatment	2.67	0.57		

(continued)

Table 7.4 *(continued)*

QOL variables	Treatment variables	Means	SDs	*t* or F values	Significant differences between means
Q31	Radiation	2.67	0.58	1.617	Pills < none, chemo, endo, rad
	Chemotherapy	2.47	0.51		
	Endocrinal	2.50	0.71		
	Pills	1.50	0.71		
	Tamoxifen	2.00	0.00		
	No treatment	2.46	0.55		
Q34	Radiation	3.00	0.00	3.561**	Pills, chemo < rad
	Chemotherapy	2.03	0.56		
	Endocrinal	2.50	0.71		
	Pills	2.00	0.00		
	Tamoxifen	2.50	0.71		
	No treatment	2.35	0.51		
Q35	Radiation	2.67	0.58	0.758	Endo < tam
	Chemotherapy	2.67	0.53		
	Endocrinal	2.00	0.00		
	Pills	2.50	0.71		
	Tamoxifen	3.00	0.00		
	No treatment	2.64	0.55		
Q36	Radiation	3.00	0.00	1.145	Pills < rad, tam
	Chemotherapy	2.72	0.51		
	Endocrinal	2.50	0.71		
	Pills	2.00	1.41		
	Tamoxifen	3.00	0.00		
	No treatment	2.74	0.52		
Q37	Radiation	3.00	0.00	5.057***	Endo, pills < none, rad, tam
	Chemotherapy	2.61	0.49		
	Endocrinal	2.00	0.00		
	Pills	2.00	0.00		
	Tamoxifen	3.00	0.00		
	No treatment	2.83	0.38		
Q38	Radiation	2.33	0.58	1.327	Pills < tam
	Chemotherapy	2.08	0.69		
	Endocrinal	2.50	0.71		
	Pills	1.50	0.71		
	Tamoxifen	3.00	0.00		
	No treatment	2.08	0.65		

(continued)

Table 7.4 *(continued)*

QOL variables	Treatment variables	Means	SDs	t or F values	Significant differences between means
Q42	Radiation	3.00	0.00	4.309***	Tam < chemo,
	Chemotherapy	2.47	0.61		none, rad, endo,
	Endocrinal	3.00	0.00		pills
	Pills	3.00	0.00		
	Tamoxifen	1.00	0.00		
	No treatment	2.57	0.54		
Q44	Radiation	3.00	0.00	1.606	Endo < rad,
	Chemotherapy	2.54	0.56		pills, tam
	Endocrinal	2.00	0.00		
	Pills	3.00	0.00		
	Tamoxifen	3.00	0.00		
	No treatment	2.66	0.51		
Q45	Radiation	2.67	0.58	1.749	Pills < rad, tam
	Chemotherapy	2.06	0.71		
	Endocrinal	2.00	0.00		
	Pills	1.50	0.71		
	Tamoxifen	3.00	0.00		
	No treatment	2.22	0.65		
Q53	Radiation	3.00	0.00	1.868	Tam < chemo,
	Chemotherapy	2.73	0.57		none, rad, endo,
	Endocrinal	3.00	0.00		pills
	Pills	3.00	0.00		
	Tamoxifen	2.00	0.00		
	No treatment	2.83	0.42		
School scale	Radiation	14.25	0.44	11.642***	
	Chemotherapy	11.13	2.55		
	Endocrinal	12.00	2.00		
	Pills	12.50	2.12		
	Tamoxifen	13.50	0.71		
	No treatment	13.69	1.69		
Negative feelings scale	Radiation	36.74	2.40	2.175*	Endo, chemo,
	Chemotherapy	31.41	4.66		pills < tam
	Endocrinal	30.95	1.77		
	Pills	31.50	0.71		
	Tamoxifen	38.50	0.71		
	No treatment	32.63	4.00		

(continued)

Table 7.4 *(continued)*

QOL variables	Treatment variables	Means	SDs	t or F values	Significant differences between means
Positive feelings scale	Radiation	11.67	0.58	1.171	Tam < pills
	Chemotherapy	10.77	1.36		
	Endocrinal	11.09	1.01		
	Pills	12.00	0.00		
	Tamoxifen	9.50	0.71		
	No treatment	11.10	1.39		
Cognition scale	Radiation	11.67	0.58	2.337*	Pills < chemo, none, tam, rad
	Chemotherapy	10.67	1.39		
	Endocrinal	9.59	1.42		
	Pills	8.50	2.12		
	Tamoxifen	11.50	0.71		
	No treatment	10.87	1.28		
Health scale	Radiation	5.00	0.00	2.949*	
	Chemotherapy	4.19	0.98		
	Endocrinal	4.33	1.15		
	Pills	5.50	0.71		
	Tamoxifen	5.00	1.41		
	No treatment	4.82	0.95		
Pain scale	Radiation	5.67	0.58	8.651***	Tam < chemo, endo, none, rad, pills
	Chemotherapy	4.21	1.25		
	Endocrinal	4.49	1.31		
	Pills	5.73	0.38		
	Tamoxifen	2.00	0.00		
	No treatment	5.01	0.88		
Mastery scale	Radiation	10.67	1.53	1.635	Pills < tam, rad
	Chemotherapy	9.35	1.35		
	Endocrinal	9.90	0.17		
	Pills	8.00	1.41		
	Tamoxifen	10.50	0.71		
	No treatment	9.83	1.45		
Play scale	Radiation	4.67	0.58	1.178	Tam < endo, pills
	Chemotherapy	4.57	1.02		
	Endocrinal	5.33	0.58		
	Pills	5.50	0.71		
	Tamoxifen	3.34	1.89		
	No treatment	4.72	1.10		

(continued)

Table 7.4 *(continued)*

QOL variables	Treatment variables	Means	SDs	t or F values	Significant differences between means
Basic needs scale	Radiation	17.00	1.00	2.786*	Tam < none, endo, rad, pills
	Chemotherapy	15.73	1.40		
	Endocrinal	16.44	1.26		
	Pills	17.50	0.71		
	Tamoxifen	13.79	0.29		
	No treatment	16.40	1.50		
QOL	Radiation	146.67	14.57	5.892***	Endo < rad
	Chemotherapy	125.39	15.95		
	Endocrinal	113.00	46.94		
	Pills	140.50	0.71		
	Tamoxifen	137.00	1.41		
	No treatment	139.97	16.37		

Chemotherapy vs. other treatments

Q9	Chemotherapy	2.36	0.81	− 2.727**	
	Other treatments	2.87	0.35		
Q31	Chemotherapy	2.49	0.51	2.544*	
	Other treatments	2.07	0.59		
Q35	Chemotherapy	2.67	0.53	2.574*	
	Other treatments	2.27	0.46		
Q37	Chemotherapy	2.64	0.49	2.082*	
	Other treatments	2.33	0.49		
Cognitive scale	Chemotherapy	8.05	1.15	2.859**	
	Other treatments	7.07	1.10		

Chemotherapy estimation[a]

Q5	Light	2.81	0.40	3.268*	Heavy < light
	Medium	2.76	0.56		
	Heavy	2.46	0.82		
Q8	Light	2.42	0.99	2.804*	Heavy < medium
	Medium	2.48	0.59		
	Heavy	2.08	0.75		
Q9	Light	2.79	0.93	3.397*	Heavy < medium
	Medium	2.91	0.36		
	Heavy	2.53	0.71		

(continued)

Table 7.4 *(continued)*

QOL variables	Treatment variables	Means	SDs	t or F values	Significant differences between means
Q12	Light	2.89	0.31	3.465*	Heavy < light
	Medium	2.78	0.54		
	Heavy	2.60	0.50		
Q13	Light	2.79	0.50	5.646**	Heavy < light
	Medium	2.48	0.67		
	Heavy	2.21	0.84		
Q15	Light	2.21	0.69	2.971*	
	Medium	2.52	0.64		
	Heavy	2.25	0.59		
Q17	Light	2.63	0.49	2.268*	Heavy < light
	Medium	2.43	0.64		
	Heavy	2.30	0.56		
Q28	Light	2.64	0.62	3.704*	Heavy < medium
	Medium	2.87	0.34		
	Heavy	2.61	0.59		
Q29	Light	2.96	0.19	3.106*	Heavy < light
	Medium	2.77	0.47		
	Heavy	2.72	0.45		
Q30	Light	2.54	0.69	4.571*	Heavy < medium
	Medium	2.75	0.48		
	Heavy	2.37	0.70		
Q34	Light	2.50	0.58	3.034*	Heavy < light
	Medium	2.42	0.56		
	Heavy	2.20	0.51		
Q35	Light	2.46	0.64	5.584**	Light < medium
	Medium	2.83	0.38		
	Heavy	2.66	0.48		
Q40	Light	2.54	0.64	3.274*	Heavy < light
	Medium	2.39	0.56		
	Heavy	2.29	0.68		
Q48	Light	2.82	0.48	2.819*	Heavy < medium
	Medium	2.88	0.33		
	Heavy	2.66	0.53		

(continued)

Table 7.4 *(continued)*

QOL variables	Treatment variables	Means	SDs	t or F values	Significant differences between means
Q50	Light	2.96	0.19	6.005**	Heavy < light, medium
	Medium	2.98	0.14		
	Heavy	2.79	0.41		
Pain scale	Light	3.00	0.12	34.964***	
	Medium	5.65	0.41		
	Heavy	5.27	1.07		
Body image scale	Light	2.00	0.12	10.500*	
	Medium	5.50	0.84		
	Heavy	5.00	1.53		
Motivation scale	Light	5.00	0.12	75.571***	
	Medium	8.83	0.41		
	Heavy	8.29	1.50		
QOL	Light	142.54	14.99	4.822**	Heavy < light, medium
	Medium	140.14	16.19		
	Heavy	137.68	18.45		
Current status					
Q1	Remission	2.06	0.68	8.001**	
	Treatment	1.76	0.60		
Q2	Remission	2.76	0.49	8.371**	
	Treatment	2.51	0.65		
Q3	Remission	2.43	0.55	8.338**	
	Treatment	2.16	0.66		
Q4	Remission	2.59	0.52	31.346***	
	Treatment	2.04	0.73		
Q5	Remission	2.86	0.38	91.867***	
	Treatment	2.00	0.84		
Q6	Remission	2.89	0.49	32.584***	
	Treatment	2.33	0.81		
Q7	Remission	2.78	0.54	28.292***	
	Treatment	2.21	0.83		
Q8	Remission	2.40	0.71	9.842**	
	Treatment	2.00	0.58		
Q9	Remission	2.83	0.53	13.543***	
	Treatment	2.42	0.75		
Q10	Remission	2.41	0.74	10.250**	
	Treatment	1.98	0.83		
Q12	Remission	2.84	0.39	23.779***	
	Treatment	2.48	0.62		

(continued)

Table 7.4 *(continued)*

QOL variables	Treatment variables	Means	SDs	t or F values	Significant differences between means
Q13	Remission	2.54	0.66	9.729**	
	Treatment	2.19	0.76		
Q14	Remission	2.53	0.62	16.811***	
	Treatment	2.10	0.71		
Q18	Remission	2.71	0.47	4.126*	
	Treatment	2.52	0.67		
Q19	Remission	2.24	0.76	5.415*	
	Treatment	1.93	0.79		
Q20	Remission	2.04	0.70	4.243*	
	Treatment	2.27	0.64		
Q37	Remission	2.80	0.40	7.424**	
	Treatment	2.61	0.49		
Q56	Remission	2.78	0.47	7.475**	
	Treatment	2.56	0.59		
Family scale	Remission	10.17	1.79	3.238***	
	Treatment	9.22	1.82		
School scale	Remission	13.69	1.69	6.297***	
	Treatment	11.33	2.46		
Health scale	Remission	4.82	0.94	3.574***	
	Treatment	4.26	0.99		
Pain scale	Remission	5.01	0.89	4.011***	
	Treatment	4.23	1.26		
Mastery scale	Remission	9.81	1.45	2.092*	
	Treatment	9.32	1.40		
Basic needs scale	Remission	16.34	1.53	2.478*	
	Treatment	15.72	1.61		
Motivation scale	Remission	8.39	0.89	-3.263**	
	Treatment	8.70	0.48		
QOL	Remission	138.94	18.07	15.797***	
	Treatment	127.51	16.40		

Note. The fifth column reports t values (based on t-tests) or F values (based on analyses of variance) in line with the performed comparison. The last column reports differences between pairs of means, according to the Duncan test. Because of the importance of comparing different kinds of treatments, significant pair comparisons are reported for the 'Current treatment' variable even in cases when the overall F-value was not significant. For the description of the items (Q1 to Q56) and the scales see Table 7.1.
[a]Based on the consensual independent evaluations by 3 pediatric oncologists.
*$p<0.05$, **$p<0.01$, ***$p<0.001$.

had the lowest scores. Interviewing the children showed that being prepared for 'light' treatment they did not expect pain, changes in appearance or need for special motivation.

Except for the comparison of chemotherapy vs. other treatments, each of the other comparisons yielded significant results in an appreciable number of items (range 15 to 18) and scales (range 3 to 7). This in itself indicates how pervasive are the effects of oncological treatments on the children's QOL. QOL variables that yielded significant results in at least three of the comparisons are limited to items concerning school (Q5, Q8, Q9), mobility (Q12), fulfilling duties at home (Q13), ability to think and understand (Q37), the pain scale and the overall QOL. However, QOL variables that yielded significant results in two of the comparisons cover a much broader range, spanning health concerns (Q1, Q3, Q4, health scale), school (Q6, Q7, school scale), functioning at home (Q14, Q15, Q20), cognition (Q28, Q31, Q37, cognitive functioning scale), mastery (Q34, mastery scale), basic needs scale, motivation scale, and specific emotions (viz. life satisfaction and anger).

It is also of interest to note that specific aspects of QOL are affected significantly only in particular contexts. Thus, the motivation scale had significant effects in the comparisons based on chemotherapy estimate, when it plays a larger role in the moderate and heavy treatment loads than the light one, or in the remission vs. on-treatment comparison, when it plays a lesser role in the off-treatment group. Again, the body image scale yielded significant results specifically in the context of comparisons based on chemotherapy estimate because different loads of chemotherapy may affect differently one's external appearance. Finally, it is of special interest that, only in the context of remission vs. treatment, a significant effect was noted for the theme of being bothered by something (Q19). It seems to be the task of the caregivers to find out what this thing is.

Further, comparisons of particular treatments (see 'current treatment') reveal two notable trends: one concerns tamoxifen, the other concerns pills. Tamoxifen affects QOL aspects more adversely than other treatments in regard to pain (Q3 and pain scale), mobility, discussing problems with one's family, sleep, enjoyment, having fun with family and friends, play, one's special friend, and ability to concentrate. Also pills affect adversely QOL but in other domains: interest in what is going on, cognition (ability to solve problems, memory, and ability to think and understand), doing things one is not good at, and negative emotions (especially, anger and nervousness). Findings of this kind may serve as guidelines for psychological interventions designed to help the child cope.

Finally, the results concerning emotional effects are instructive. The effect on negative emotions is evident in the comparisons of different kinds of treatments (negative feelings scale, and nervousness, stressfulness, and doing things one is not good at) and in the chemotherapy estimate (sadness, worthlessness). The effects on positive emotions refer to reductions in life satisfaction, feeling safe, enjoyment, and having fun with family and friends. The results are interesting both in what they include (i.e., reductions in positive feelings and not only increases in the negative ones) and in what they do not include (e.g., anger, sadness, guilt, fear).

The third set of comparisons referred to disease-related variables (Table 7.5). Examining the effects of different diagnoses (see comparisons of 'Diagnosis') reveals that the kind of disease the child has is of prime importance in regard to his or her QOL. There were significant effects in regard to 33 items (out of 56) and 8 out of 15 scales as well as the total score of QOL. More specifically, there is clear evidence that children with leukemia had the lowest levels of QOL in many domains (18 items and 8 scales). Furthermore, comparing leukemia with lymphoma shows clearly that in all 19 scores with significant results (11 items, 8 scales), leukemia patients scored lower on QOL than lymphoma patients. Further, concerning the diagnosis of lymphoma, there were significant differences only in three scores. Comparing lymphoma with sarcoma, which is another frequent diagnosis, shows that sarcoma patients scored significantly lower than lymphoma patients on 13 of the 15 variables that yielded significant results, including the scales of school, pain and play. Comparing the diagnoses of head and brain tumors showed differences in seven QOL variables, in five of which children with head tumors scored lower than those with brain tumors (e.g., having fun with friends and family, taking care of one's appearance). Comparing each of these diagnoses – head and brain tumors – with the diagnosis of solid tumors in the body show unclear results: children with head tumors scored lower than children with solid tumors in the body in four QOL variables (basic needs scale, and home life), but higher in three variables (memory, ability to think and anger). Comparing brain tumors with solid tumors in the body yielded differences only in four QOL variables but three of them indicate that the solid tumors children had lower QOL scores in regard to food, appearance and feeling miserable. Surprising findings were obtained by comparing children with malignant and non-malignant diseases: in five variables the scores for malignancy were higher, in three they were lower. It is likely that the decline in QOL of the children with non-malignant diseases is due to the lower levels of support they often get.

Stage of disease is another aspect of diagnosis which plays an important role in regard to QOL. It yielded significant results in 23 out of 56 items, and in 7 out of 15 scales. Some of the more notable findings are that children with a stage IV disease had the lowest QOL only in some of the variables and these are highly meaningful ones: existence of something that bothers the child, external appearance, managing alone, sadness, loneliness, guilt, confusion, fear and misery (Q19, Q29, Q34, Q40, Q41, Q46, Q47, Q51, scales of health, negative feelings, stress and confusion). The list of domains in which children with stage I disease scored lowest on QOL is different: health worries (Q1, health scale),

Table 7.5 Significant results of comparisons of CQL variables – items and scale scores – in groups defined by disease characteristics

QOL variables	Disease variables	Means	SDs	t or F values	Significant differences between means
Diagnosis					
Q1	Lymphoma	1.95	0.69	2.315*	Leuk <lymph,
	Sarcoma	2.10	0.62		solid, sarc, head
	Brain tumors	1.83	0.58		Brain <head
	Solid tumors in the body	2.00	0.64		
	Head (not brain) tumors	2.40	0.70		
	Non-malignant tumors	1.91	0.83		
	Leukemia	1.45	0.52		
Q2	Lymphoma	2.81	0.39	1.816	Brain <lymph
	Sarcoma	2.63	0.61		
	Brain tumors	2.33	0.78		
	Solid tumors in the body	2.73	0.52		
	Head (not brain) tumors	2.60	0.70		
	Non-malignant tumors	2.64	0.67		
	Leukemia	2.73	0.47		
Q4	Lymphoma	2.63	0.54	1.927	Leuk <lymph
	Sarcoma	2.39	0.68		
	Brain tumors	2.36	0.50		
	Solid tumors in the body	2.42	0.50		
	Head (not brain) tumors	2.50	0.71		
	Non-malignant tumors	2.27	0.79		
	Leukemia	2.10	0.57		
Q5	Lymphoma	2.78	0.50	2.674*	Leuk <nm,
	Sarcoma	2.63	0.69		brain, head,
	Brain tumors	2.58	0.51		sarc, lymph,
	Solid tumors in the body	2.85	0.36		solid
	Head (not brain) tumors	2.60	0.70		
	Non-malignant tumors	2.56	0.13		
	Leukemia	2.09	1.04		
Q7	Lymphoma	2.69	0.55	2.004	Leuk <solid
	Sarcoma	2.60	0.67		
	Brain tumors	2.50	0.67		
	Solid tumors in the body	2.96	0.69		
	Head (not brain) tumors	2.60	0.70		
	Non-malignant tumors	2.56	0.73		
	Leukemia	2.27	0.79		

(continued)

Table 7.5 *(continued)*

QOL variables	Disease variables	Means	SDs	t or F values	Significant differences between means
Q8	Lymphoma	2.40	0.63	1.916	Head < nm,
	Sarcoma	2.13	0.63		solid
	Brain tumors	2.20	0.79		
	Solid tumors in the body	2.56	0.92		
	Head (not brain) tumors	1.90	0.88		
	Non-malignant tumors	2.50	0.53		
	Leukemia	2.30	0.48		
Q9	Lymphoma	2.86	0.46	2.202*	
	Sarcoma	2.52	0.67		
	Brain tumors	2.75	0.45		
	Solid tumors in the body	2.96	0.71		
	Head (not brain) tumors	2.75	0.71		
	Non-malignant tumors	2.67	0.71		
	Leukemia	2.76	0.53		
Q12	Lymphoma	2.93	0.31	8.404***	Sarc < head,
	Sarcoma	2.43	0.56		nm, solid,
	Brain tumors	2.92	0.29		brain, lymph
	Solid tumors in the body	2.87	0.35		
	Head (not brain) tumors	2.80	0.63		
	Non-malignant tumors	2.82	0.40		
	Leukemia	2.70	0.48		
Q14	Lymphoma	2.43	0.63	1.709	Nm < sarc,
	Sarcoma	2.38	0.61		lymph, leuk,
	Brain tumors	2.67	0.78		solid, head,
	Solid tumors in the body	2.57	0.73		brain
	Head (not brain) tumors	2.60	0.70		
	Non-malignant tumors	1.90	0.74		
	Leukemia	2.45	0.69		
Q16	Lymphoma	2.16	0.71	2.173*	Brain,
	Sarcoma	2.44	0.57		leuk < sarc
	Brain tumors	1.83	0.58		
	Solid tumors in the body	2.23	0.73		
	Head (not brain) tumors	2.33	0.87		
	Non-malignant tumors	2.18	0.60		
	Leukemia	1.90	0.57		

(continued)

Table 7.5 *(continued)*

QOL variables	Disease variables	Means	SDs	t or F values	Significant differences between means
Q17	Lymphoma	2.42	0.60	2.299*	Brain < nm.
	Sarcoma	2.46	0.53		solid, lymph,
	Brain tumors	1.83	0.58		sarc, head
	Solid tumors in the body	2.37	0.67		
	Head (not brain) tumors	2.67	0.50		
	Non-malignant tumors	2.36	0.81		
	Leukemia	2.22	0.67		
Q18	Lymphoma	2.64	0.51	2.001	Leuk < solid,
	Sarcoma	2.59	0.63		brain
	Brain tumors	2.92	0.29		
	Solid tumors in the body	2.87	0.35		
	Head (not brain) tumors	2.56	0.53		
	Non-malignant tumors	2.73	0.47		
	Leukemia	2.40	0.52		
Q20	Lymphoma	1.99	0.68	1.938	Head, lymph,
	Sarcoma	2.08	0.78		nm < brain
	Brain tumors	2.58	0.51		
	Solid tumors in the body	2.23	0.57		
	Head (not brain) tumors	1.80	0.79		
	Non-malignant tumors	2.00	0.63		
	Leukemia	2.18	0.40		
Q22	Lymphoma	2.78	0.48	7.384***	Head <
	Sarcoma	2.77	0.46		leuk < nm, sarc,
	Brain tumors	3.00	0.00		lymph, solid,
	Solid tumors in the body	2.93	0.25		brain
	Head (not brain) tumors	1.90	0.88		
	Non-malignant tumors	2.73	0.65		
	Leukemia	2.36	0.81		
Q23	Lymphoma	2.81	0.42	1.045	Nm < brain
	Sarcoma	2.75	0.50		
	Brain tumors	3.00	0.00		
	Solid tumors in the body	2.73	0.45		
	Head (not brain) tumors	2.70	0.67		
	Non-malignant tumors	2.55	0.69		
	Leukemia	2.73	0.65		

(continued)

Table 7.5 *(continued)*

QOL variables	Disease variables	Means	SDs	t or F values	Significant differences between means
Q26	Lymphoma	2.73	0.50	2.805*	Head < lymph,
	Sarcoma	2.75	0.43		sarc, solid,
	Brain tumors	2.82	0.40		brain
	Solid tumors in the body	2.80	0.41		
	Head (not brain) tumors	2.20	0.79		
	Non-malignant tumors	2.45	0.82		
	Leukemia	2.45	0.69		
Q27	Lymphoma	2.63	0.51	2.027	Leuk < brain,
	Sarcoma	2.57	0.65		solid, sarc,
	Brain tumors	2.45	0.52		head, lymph
	Solid tumors in the body	2.53	0.63		
	Head (not brain) tumors	2.60	0.70		
	Non-malignant tumors	2.36	0.67		
	Leukemia	2.00	0.63		
Q29	Lymphoma	2.87	0.33	2.567*	Leuk < solid,
	Sarcoma	2.68	0.50		nm, head,
	Brain tumors	2.82	0.60		brain, lymph
	Solid tumors in the body	2.72	0.45		
	Head (not brain) tumors	2.80	0.63		
	Non-malignant tumors	2.73	0.47		
	Leukemia	2.36	0.67		
Q30	Lymphoma	2.65	0.60	2.093*	Head < sarc,
	Sarcoma	2.63	0.55		leuk, lymph,
	Brain tumors	3.00	0.00		solid, nm, brain
	Solid tumors in the body	2.73	0.45		
	Head (not brain) tumors	2.20	0.92		
	Non-malignant tumors	2.82	0.40		
	Leukemia	2.64	0.50		
Q33	Lymphoma	2.44	0.52	1.102	Head < solid
	Sarcoma	2.43	0.59		
	Brain tumors	2.36	0.67		
	Solid tumors in the body	2.59	0.57		
	Head (not brain) tumors	2.10	0.57		
	Non-malignant tumors	2.27	0.47		
	Leukemia	2.40	0.70		

(continued)

Table 7.5 *(continued)*

QOL variables	Disease variables	Means	SDs	t or F values	Significant differences between means
Q34	Lymphoma	2.43	0.57	2.578*	Leuk < lymph
	Sarcoma	2.30	0.46		
	Brain tumors	2.09	0.30		
	Solid tumors in the body	2.10	0.48		
	Head (not brain) tumors	2.20	0.79		
	Non-malignant tumors	2.36	0.50		
	Leukemia	2.00	0.45		
Q35	Lymphoma	2.71	0.51	2.389*	Head < solid,
	Sarcoma	2.65	0.51		sarc, lymph
	Brain tumors	2.45	0.52		Leuk < lymph
	Solid tumors in the body	2.63	0.61		
	Head (not brain) tumors	2.20	0.79		
	Non-malignant tumors	2.55	0.52		
	Leukemia	2.27	0.47		
Q36	Lymphoma	2.73	0.50	3.128**	Nm < lymph,
	Sarcoma	2.77	0.53		brain, sarc,
	Brain tumors	2.73	0.65		solid, head
	Solid tumors in the body	2.83	0.38		Leuk < sarc,
	Head (not brain) tumors	3.00	0.00		solid, head
	Non-malignant tumors	2.27	0.79		
	Leukemia	2.36	0.50		
Q37	Lymphoma	2.83	0.38	2.697*	Leuk < sarc,
	Sarcoma	2.72	0.45		nm, solid,
	Brain tumors	2.82	0.40		brain, lymph,
	Solid tumors in the body	2.73	0.45		head
	Head (not brain) tumors	3.00	0.00		
	Non-malignant tumors	2.73	0.47		
	Leukemia	2.36	0.50		
Q41	Lymphoma	2.66	0.55	1.447	Head < lymph
	Sarcoma	2.63	0.55		
	Brain tumors	2.64	0.50		
	Solid tumors in the body	2.63	0.49		
	Head (not brain) tumors	2.20	0.92		
	Non-malignant tumors	2.36	0.81		
	Leukemia	2.45	0.52		

(continued)

Table 7.5 *(continued)*

QOL variables	Disease variables	Means	SDs	*t* or F values	Significant differences between means
Q44	Lymphoma	2.66	0.53	1.329	Nm,
	Sarcoma	2.73	0.45		leuk < head
	Brain tumors	2.64	0.50		
	Solid tumors in the body	2.57	0.57		
	Head (not brain) tumors	2.90	0.32		
	Non-malignant tumors	2.45	0.52		
	Leukemia	2.45	0.69		
Q45	Lymphoma	2.24	0.68	1.520	Nm < sarc
	Sarcoma	2.30	0.67		
	Brain tumors	2.00	0.00		
	Solid tumors in the body	2.13	0.57		
	Head (not brain) tumors	2.20	0.79		
	Non-malignant tumors	1.73	0.79		
	Leukemia	2.09	0.54		
Q48	Lymphoma	2.80	0.43	1.920	Leuk < brain,
	Sarcoma	2.81	0.39		head, lymph,
	Brain tumors	2.73	0.65		sarc, solid
	Solid tumors in the body	2.87	0.35		
	Head (not brain) tumors	2.80	0.63		
	Non-malignant tumors	2.55	0.52		
	Leukemia	2.38	0.52		
Q50	Lymphoma	2.91	0.29	1.693	Leuk < nm,
	Sarcoma	2.91	0.28		solid, head,
	Brain tumors	2.91	0.30		lymph, brain,
	Solid tumors in the body	2.87	0.35		sarc
	Head (not brain) tumors	2.90	0.32		
	Non-malignant tumors	2.82	0.60		
	Leukemia	2.56	0.53		
Q51	Lymphoma	2.94	0.25	2.574*	Leuk < head,
	Sarcoma	2.83	0.38		sarc, solid,
	Brain tumors	3.00	0.00		lymph, brain,
	Solid tumors in the body	2.87	0.35		nm
	Head (not brain) tumors	2.80	0.63		
	Non-malignant tumors	3.00	0.00		
	Leukemia	2.56	0.53		

(continued)

Table 7.5 *(continued)*

QOL variables	Disease variables	Means	SDs	*t* or F values	Significant differences between means
Q53	Lymphoma	2.81	0.40	1.957	Head < solid,
	Sarcoma	2.84	0.41		brain
	Brain tumors	2.91	0.30		
	Solid tumors in the body	2.90	0.30		
	Head (not brain) tumors	2.50	0.85		
	Non-malignant tumors	2.64	0.68		
	Leukemia	2.56	0.53		
Q54	Lymphoma	2.92	0.27	1.824	Leuk < brain,
	Sarcoma	2.93	0.31		lymph, sarc, nm
	Brain tumors	2.92	0.29		Head < nm
	Solid tumors in the body	2.83	0.38		
	Head (not brain) tumors	2.70	0.67		
	Non-malignant tumors	3.00	0.00		
	Leukemia	2.63	0.74		
Q56	Lymphoma	2.77	0.45	2.245*	Leuk < sarc,
	Sarcoma	2.76	0.43		lymph, brain,
	Brain tumors	2.83	0.58		solid
	Solid tumors in the body	2.83	0.38		Head < brain,
	Head (not brain) tumors	2.40	0.97		solid
	Non-malignant tumors	2.59	0.58		
	Leukemia	2.33	0.71		
School scale	Lymphoma	13.53	1.69	3.377**	Leuk < lymph,
	Sarcoma	12.68	2.12		solid
	Brain tumors	12.64	1.94		Head, brain,
	Solid tumors in the body	14.22	2.54		sarc < solid
	Head (not brain) tumors	12.45	2.26		
	Non-malignant tumors	12.97	2.56		
	Leukemia	11.89	2.13		
Positive feelings scale	Lymphoma	11.11	1.27	3.726**	Head, leuk <
	Sarcoma	11.16	1.16		lymph, sarc,
	Brain tumors	11.27	1.05		brain, solid
	Solid tumors in the body	11.40	0.90		Nm < brain,
	Head (not brain) tumors	9.90	2.88		solid
	Non-malignant tumors	12.23	1.63		
	Leukemia	9.95	1.33		

(continued)

Table 7.5 *(continued)*

QOL variables	Disease variables	Means	SDs	*t* or F values	Significant differences between means
Cognition scale	Lymphoma	10.99	1.17	2.952**	Leuk < brain, sarc, head, solid, lymph
	Sarcoma	10.77	1.45		
	Brain tumors	10.65	1.15		
	Solid tumors in the body	10.90	1.27		
	Head (not brain) tumors	10.80	1.55		
	Non-malignant tumors	10.00	1.48		
	Leukemia	9.45	1.13		
Health scale	Lymphoma	4.76	0.91	1.397	Brain, leuk < head
	Sarcoma	4.73	1.05		
	Brain tumors	4.17	0.94		
	Solid tumors in the body	4.73	0.94		
	Head (not brain) tumors	5.00	1.05		
	Non-malignant tumors	4.55	1.21		
	Leukemia	4.18	0.75		
Body image scale	Lymphoma	5.52	0.69	1.831	Head, leuk < brain
	Sarcoma	5.30	0.92		
	Brain tumors	5.78	0.59		
	Solid tumors in the body	5.46	0.77		
	Head (not brain) tumors	5.00	1.15		
	Non-malignant tumors	5.55	0.52		
	Leukemia	5.00	1.00		
Mastery scale	Lymphoma	9.97	1.37	1.848	Leuk < lymph
	Sarcoma	9.75	1.37		
	Brain tumors	9.39	1.23		
	Solid tumors in the body	9.61	1.52		
	Head (not brain) tumors	9.40	2.01		
	Non-malignant tumors	9.18	1.54		
	Leukemia	8.67	1.62		
Stress scale	Lymphoma	6.84	1.41	1.855	Brain < sarc, head
	Sarcoma	7.02	1.25		
	Brain tumors	5.75	1.42		
	Solid tumors in the body	6.77	1.59		
	Head (not brain) tumors	7.08	1.79		
	Non-malignant tumors	6.64	1.50		
	Leukemia	6.11	1.52		

(continued)

Table 7.5 *(continued)*

QOL variables	Disease variables	Means	SDs	t or F values	Significant differences between means
Basic needs scale	Lymphoma	16.52	1.34	4.280***	Head,
	Sarcoma	15.90	1.62		leuk < lymph,
	Brain tumors	16.69	0.90		brain, solid
	Solid tumors in the body	16.73	1.44		Nm < brain,
	Head (not brain) tumors	15.00	2.11		solid
	Non-malignant tumors	15.55	1.81		
	Leukemia	15.10	1.58		
QOL	Lymphoma	138.86	17.75	1.822	Leuk < lymph,
	Sarcoma	133.67	20.23		solid
	Brain tumors	135.08	25.60		
	Solid tumors in the body	141.27	9.98		
	Head (not brain) tumors	135.90	22.58		
	Non-malignant tumors	133.41	14.25		
	Leukemia	123.55	14.98		
Stage of disease					
Q1	I	1.81	0.60	4.075**	I, IV < II
	II	2.17	0.65		
	III	2.02	0.71		
	IV	1.72	0.65		
Q3	I	2.38	0.50	3.544*	III < II
	II	2.54	0.50		
	III	2.22	0.65		
	IV	2.34	0.61		
Q14	I	2.15	0.67	2.418	I < III, IV
	II	2.42	0.63		
	III	2.60	0.57		
	IV	2.48	0.78		
Q15	I	2.10	0.70	1.663	I < III
	II	2.40	0.64		
	III	2.46	0.58		
	IV	2.32	0.77		
Q17	I	2.29	0.59	2.669*	
	II	2.55	0.52		
	III	2.35	0.64		
	IV	2.23	0.59		
Q19	I	2.17	0.71	8.537***	IV < I, II, III
	II	2.47	0.64		III < II
	III	2.07	0.85		
	IV	1.69	0.68		

(continued)

Table 7.5 *(continued)*

QOL variables	Disease variables	Means	SDs	*t* or F values	Significant differences between means
Q20	I	1.86	0.73	3.304*	I < II
	II	2.23	0.62		
	III	1.90	0.76		
	IV	2.03	0.68		
Q22	I	2.52	0.68	3.233*	I < II
	II	2.86	0.35		
	III	2.66	0.66		
	IV	2.76	0.43		
Q23	I	2.52	0.68	4.279**	I < II, IV
	II	2.88	0.37		
	III	2.68	0.51		
	IV	2.86	0.44		
Q24	I	4.30	0.77	2.773*	II, III, IV < I
	II	2.75	0.51		
	III	2.70	0.54		
	IV	2.79	0.49		
Q26	I	2.60	0.68	2.771*	I, III < IV
	II	2.75	0.43		
	III	5.26	0.61		
	IV	2.86	0.35		
Q27	I	2.20	0.62	3.711**	I < II, III
	II	2.63	0.54		
	III	2.64	0.56		
	IV	2.45	0.63		
Q29	I	2.85	0.37	2.404	IV < I, II, III
	II	2.82	0.38		
	III	2.82	0.44		
	IV	2.59	0.55		
Q32	I	2.00	0.50	2.364	I < II, III, IV
	II	2.38	0.51		
	III	2.35	0.60		
	IV	2.35	0.48		
Q34	I	2.50	0.51	1.134	IV < I
	II	2.34	0.55		
	III	2.34	0.56		
	IV	2.21	0.56		
Q35	I	2.45	0.69	2.888*	I < II
	II	2.78	0.45		
	III	2.56	0.58		
	IV	2.62	0.56		

(continued)

Table 7.5 *(continued)*

QOL variables	Disease variables	Means	SDs	t or F values	Significant differences between means
Q40	I	2.60	0.50	4.070**	IV < I, II, III
	II	2.45	0.55		
	III	2.36	0.66		
	IV	2.07	0.59		
Q41	I	2.70	0.47	4.585**	IV < I, II, III
	II	2.74	0.47		
	III	2.58	0.64		
	IV	2.31	0.60		
Q44	I	2.70	0.57	4.440**	IV < I, II, III
	II	2.73	0.44		
	III	2.76	0.47		
	IV	2.38	0.56		
Q46	I	2.35	0.67	3.980**	I, IV < III
	II	2.49	0.57		
	III	2.68	0.55		
	IV	2.24	0.58		
Q47	I	2.55	0.51	3.360**	IV < II
	II	2.67	0.50		
	III	2.48	0.58		
	IV	2.32	0.55		
Q51	I	2.90	0.31	2.300	IV < II
	II	2.96	0.19		
	III	2.88	0.39		
	IV	2.79	0.42		
Q52	I	2.84	0.50	2.639*	
	II	2.54	0.73		
	III	2.71	0.54		
	IV	2.86	0.36		
Negative feelings scale	I	32.52	4.00	4.709**	IV < I, II, III
	II	33.59	3.57		
	III	32.75	4.13		
	IV	30.42	1.30		
Confusion scale	I	5.03	0.93	2.979	IV < I, II, III
	II	5.35	0.87		
	III	4.94	1.07		
	IV	4.81	0.99		

(continued)

Table 7.5 *(continued)*

QOL variables	Disease variables	Means	SDs	t or F values	Significant differences between means
Health scale	I	4.38	0.92	5.023**	I, IV < II, III
	II	5.00	0.92		
	III	4.72	1.01		
	IV	4.31	0.93		
Pain scale	I	4.90	0.89	2.648*	
	II	5.13	0.82		
	III	4.66	1.17		
	IV	4.78	1.09		
Friends scale	I	9.09	7.02	1.733	III < I, II, IV
	II	7.79	1.23		
	III	7.54	1.43		
	IV	7.79	2.69		
Stress scale	I	6.80	1.32	5.111**	IV < I, II, III
	II	7.23	1.21		
	III	6.66	1.36		
	IV	6.22	1.50		
Basic needs scale	I	15.86	1.15	3.169**	
	II	16.62	1.30		
	III	15.88	1.85		
	IV	16.34	1.51		
Recurrence of disease					
Q8	Yes	1.69	0.48	-3.418***	
	No	2.37	0.70		
Q23	Yes	3.00	0.00	6.597***	
	No	2.77	0.47		
Q49	Yes	2.88	0.33	3.204**	
	No	2.59	0.54		
Q51	Yes	3.00	0.00	4.492***	
	No	2.89	0.34		
Time since diagnosis					
Q9	Less than 5 years	2.68	0.60	-2.689**	
	More than 5 years	2.96	0.57		
Q16	Less than 5 years	2.33	0.66	3.057**	
	More than 5 years	2.00	0.70		
Q17	Less than 5 years	2.46	0.58	2.227*	
	More than 5 years	2.24	0.67		

(continued)

Table 7.5 *(continued)*

QOL variables	Disease variables	Means	SDs	t or F values	Significant differences between means
Q19	Less than 5 years	2.25	0.77	2.343*	
	More than 5 years	1.96	0.75		
Q30	Less than 5 years	2.57	0.60	−2.912**	
	More than 5 years	2.81	0.48		
Q38	Less than 5 years	2.17	0.66	2.236*	
	More than 5 years	1.92	0.70		
Q41	Less than 5 years	2.67	0.53	1.978*	
	More than 5 years	2.47	0.67		
Q45	Less than 5 years	2.28	0.66	2.088*	
	More than 5 years	2.06	0.69		
Q52	Less than 5 years	2.72	0.58	2.211*	
	More than 5 years	2.49	0.67		
Negative feelings scale	Less than 5 years	33.06	4.04	2.320*	
	More than 5 years	31.56	4.10		
Stress scale	Less than 5 years	7.02	1.36	3.672***	
	More than 5 years	6.20	1.47		
Motivation scale	Less than 5 years	8.54	0.79	2.172*	
	More than 5 years	8.25	0.91		
Time since end of treatment					
Q9	Less than 5 years	2.69	0.59	−2.656**	
	More than 5 years	2.98	0.58		
Q16	Less than 5 years	2.32	0.66	3.028**	
	More than 5 years	1.98	0.71		
Q19	Less than 5 years	2.23	0.78	2.005*	
	More than 5 years	1.98	0.74		
Q21	Less than 5 years	2.54	0.55	−2.431**	
	More than 5 years	2.74	0.44		
Q30	Less than 5 years	2.59	0.60	−2.155*	
	More than 5 years	2.78	0.51		
Q38	Less than 5 years	2.17	0.65	2.686**	
	More than 5 years	1.87	0.72		
Q41	Less than 5 years	2.67	0.54	1.990*	
	More than 5 years	2.46	0.66		

(continued)

Table 7.5 *(continued)*

QOL variables	Disease variables	Means	SDs	*t* or F values	Significant differences between means
Q45	Less than 5 years	2.28	0.65	2.049*	
	More than 5 years	2.04	0.73		
Negative feelings scale	Less than 5 years	33.01	4.07	2.238*	
	More than 5 years	31.49	4.02		
Stress scale	Less than 5 years	6.98	1.39	3.269***	
	More than 5 years	6.21	1.41		
Motivation scale	Less than 5 years	8.53	0.80	2.021*	
	More than 5 years	8.25	0.92		
Brain vs. head tumors					
Q1	Brain tumor	1.83	0.58	− 2.084*	
	Head tumor	2.40	0.70		
Q17	Brain tumor	1.83	0.58	− 3.460**	
	Head tumor	2.67	0.50		
Q20	Brain tumor	2.58	0.51	2.804**	
	Head tumor	1.80	0.79		
Q22	Brain tumor	3.00	0.00	3.973**	
	Head tumor	1.90	0.87		
Q26	Brain tumor	2.82	0.40	2.226**	
	Head tumor	2.20	0.79		
Q30	Brain tumor	3.00	0.00	2.753*	
	Head tumor	2.20	0.92		
Basic needs scale	Brain tumor	16.69	0.90	2.367*	
	Head tumor	15.00	2.11		
Head (not brain) vs. body solid tumors					
Q22	Solid body tumor	2.93	0.25	3.681**	
	Head tumor	1.90	0.88		
Q26	Solid body tumor	2.80	0.41	2.305*	
	Head tumor	2.20	0.79		
Q33	Solid body tumor	2.59	0.57	2.334*	
	Head tumor	2.10	0.57		
Q36	Solid body tumor	2.83	0.38	− 2.408*	
	Head tumor	3.00	0.00		

(continued)

Table 7.5 *(continued)*

QOL variables	Disease variables	Means	SDs	t or F values	Significant differences between means
Q37	Solid body tumor	2.73	0.45	− 3.247*	
	Head tumor	3.00	0.00		
Q44	Solid body tumor	2.57	0.57	− 2.313*	
	Head tumor	2.90	0.32		
Basic needs scale	Solid body tumor	16.73	1.44	2.419*	
	Head tumor	15.00	2.11		

Brain vs. solid tumors

Q17	Brain tumor	1.83	0.58	− 2.421*	
	Solid tumor in the body	2.37	0.67		
Q23	Brain tumor	3.00	0.00	3.247**	
	Solid tumor in the body	2.73	0.45		
Q30	Brain tumor	3.00	0.00	3.247**	
	Solid tumor in the body	2.73	0.45		
Q51	Brain tumor	3.00	0.00	2.112*	
	Solid tumor in the body	2.87	0.35		

Lymphoma vs. sarcoma

Q2	Lymphoma	2.81	0.39	2.019*	
	Sarcoma	2.63	0.61		
Q3	Lymphoma	2.49	0.53	2.331*	
	Sarcoma	2.26	0.66		
Q4	Lymphoma	2.63	0.54	2.146*	
	Sarcoma	2.39	0.68		
Q6	Lymphoma	2.86	0.45	2.143*	
	Sarcoma	2.63	0.66		
Q8	Lymphoma	2.40	0.63	2.154*	
	Sarcoma	2.13	0.63		
Q9	Lymphoma	2.86	0.46	2.817**	
	Sarcoma	2.52	0.67		

(continued)

Table 7.5 *(continued)*

QOL variables	Disease variables	Means	SDs	*t* or F values	Significant differences between means
Q10	Lymphoma	2.52	0.70	3.049**	
	Sarcoma	2.09	0.82		
Q12	Lymphoma	2.93	0.31	6.105***	
	Sarcoma	2.43	0.56		
Q13	Lymphoma	2.52	0.67	2.079*	
	Sarcoma	2.25	0.82		
Q16	Lymphoma	2.16	0.71	−2.336*	
	Sarcoma	2.44	0.57		
Q29	Lymphoma	2.87	0.33	2.644**	
	Sarcoma	2.68	0.50		
School scale	Lymphoma	13.53	1.69	2.676**	
	Sarcoma	12.68	2.12		
Pain scale	Lymphoma	5.11	0.86	2.478**	
	Sarcoma	4.66	1.19		
Play scale	Lymphoma	4.89	1.01	2.617**	
	Sarcoma	4.43	1.08		
Basic needs scale	Lymphoma	16.52	1.34	2.483**	
	Sarcoma	15.90	1.62		
Lymphoma vs. leukemia					
Q1	Lymphoma	1.95	0.69	2.301*	
	Leukemia	1.45	0.52		
Q4	Lymphoma	2.63	0.54	2.894**	
	Leukemia	2.10	0.57		
Q5	Lymphoma	2.78	0.50	2.150*	
	Leukemia	2.09	1.04		
Q27	Lymphoma	2.63	0.51	3.686***	
	Leukemia	2.00	0.63		
Q29	Lymphoma	2.87	0.33	2.466*	
	Leukemia	2.36	0.67		
Q34	Lymphoma	2.43	0.57	2.895**	
	Leukemia	2.00	0.45		

(continued)

Table 7.5 *(continued)*

QOL variables	Disease variables	Means	SDs	*t* or F values	Significant differences between means
Q35	Lymphoma	2.71	0.51	2.716**	
	Leukemia	2.27	0.47		
Q36	Lymphoma	2.73	0.50	2.235*	
	Leukemia	2.36	0.50		
Q37	Lymphoma	2.83	0.38	2.920**	
	Leukemia	2.36	0.50		
Q47	Lymphoma	2.60	0.49	2.695*	
	Leukemia	2.20	0.42		
Q48	Lymphoma	2.80	0.43	2.612**	
	Leukemia	2.38	0.52		
School scale	Lymphoma	13.53	1.69	2.927**	
	Leukemia	11.89	2.13		
Negative feelings scale	Lymphoma	32.73	3.90	1.951*	
	Leukemia	30.32	3.44		
Positive feelings scale	Lymphoma	11.11	1.27	2.826**	
	Leukemia	9.95	1.33		
Cognition scale	Lymphoma	10.98	1.17	4.094***	
	Leukemia	9.45	1.13		
Health scale	Lymphoma	4.76	0.91	2.028*	
	Leukemia	4.18	0.75		
Pain scale	Lymphoma	5.11	0.86	2.457*	
	Leukemia	4.40	1.06		
Mastery scale	Lymphoma	9.98	1.37	2.884**	
	Leukemia	8.67	1.62		
Basic needs scale	Lymphoma	16.52	1.34	3.218**	
	Leukemia	15.10	1.58		

(continued)

Table 7.5 *(continued)*

QOL variables	Disease variables	Means	SDs	t or F values	Significant differences between means
Hodgkin's lymphoma vs. non-Hodgkin's lymphoma					
Q46	Hodgkin's lymphoma	2.32	0.61	-2.186^*	
	NHL	2.63	0.56		
Q47	Hodgkin's lymphoma	2.51	0.50	-2.250^*	
	NHL	2.76	0.44		
Q50	Hodgkin's lymphoma	2.98	0.14	2.434^*	
	NHL	2.77	0.43		
Malignant vs. non-malignant tumors					
Q14	Malignant tumor	2.46	0.65	2.632^{**}	
	Non-malignant tumor	1.90	0.74		
Q45	Malignant tumor	2.23	0.65	2.456^{**}	
	Non-malignant tumor	1.73	0.79		
Q49	Malignant tumor	2.63	0.52	1.939^*	
	Non-malignant tumor	2.30	0.67		
Q51	Malignant tumor	2.89	0.33	-4.611^{***}	
	Non-malignant tumor	3.00	0.00		
Q52	Malignant tumor	2.66	0.61	-2.459^*	
	Non-malignant tumor	2.91	0.30		
Q54	Malignant tumor	2.90	0.34	-4.128^{***}	
	Non-malignant tumor	3.00	0.00		
Positive feelings scale	Malignant tumor	11.12	1.32	2.142^*	
	Non-malignant tumor	10.23	1.63		
Cognitive scale	Malignant tumor	10.87	1.29	2.166^*	
	Non-malignant tumor	10.00	1.48		

Note. The fifth column reports t values (based on t-tests) or F values (based on analyses of variance) in line with the performed comparison. The last column reports differences between pairs of means, according to the Duncan test. Because of the importance of comparing different diseases and disease stages, significant pair comparisons are reported for the 'Diagnosis' and 'Stage of disease' variables even in cases when the overall F-value was not significant. For the description of the items (Q1 to Q56) and the scales see Table 7.1.
$^*p < 0.05$, $^{**}p < 0.01$, $^{***}p < 0.001$.

functioning at home (Q14, Q15, Q22, Q26), food and other basic needs (scale of basic needs, Q23), cognitive functioning (Q35, Q27) and some indications of distress (fear and feeling successful Q32, Q46). Thus, the major QOL concerns of stage IV disease are emotional, and of stage I disease functional.

There are two important questions that are often asked concerning the QOL of children with cancer: What are the effects on QOL of duration of disease ('Time since diagnosis') and of duration of remission or survival ('Time since end of treatment'). Our data may provide answers. Concerning time since diagnosis there were significant results in 12 QOL variables, out of which 10 showed lower QOL for the longer disease duration (over 5 years as compared with less than 5 years), the only exceptions being activity in the schoolyard and external appearance. Concerning time since end of treatment, there were significant results in 11 QOL variables, out of which 9 showed lower QOL for the longer remission/survival duration (over 5 years as compared with less than 5 years), the only exceptions being activity in the schoolyard, external appearance, and ability to get things that cost money. The conclusion is that longer durations of disease or remissions are related to lower QOL. This is of particular importance because longer durations often have more positive medical connotations. Hence, QOL is not synonymous with medical state. Further, the evident implication is that in addition to treating the disease, it is also necessary to treat the QOL so that the whole child – body and soul – recover.

SOME CONCLUSIONS

The purpose of this section is to deal briefly with two issues concerning QOL. They may be presented in the form of questions: 'Where are we?' and 'Where do we go from here?'

The presentation of tools and findings in the broad domain of QOL supports several general conclusions. The first is that QOL reflects an aspect of the child's functioning and state that is neither identical with nor fully predictable from the child's medical state. It is evident, for example, that diagnoses, disease stages and being on- or off-treatment affect QOL but the effects are not pervasive across the board and mostly not trivial. Thus, not all aspects of QOL are lower in the initial stage of the disease as compared with the advanced stage, or in 'heavy' chemotherapy as compared with 'light' chemotherapy (e.g., findings based on the CQL (Kreitler and Kreitler 2003a)); some aspects of QOL are not related with estimates of disease severity by the physicians (e.g., results with MPQOLQ (Armstrong et al. 1999)); QOL of children off-treatment is not always better than that of children on-treatment (e.g., see results with the PPSC (Mulhern et al. 1990) or the generic PedsQL (Varni et al. 2002)); and the QOL of children with cancer is not lower in all respects than the QOL of healthy control children (e.g., findings with the CHQ (Bhatia *et al.* 2002)) and may even be higher (e.g., findings with CHQ (Sawyer *et al.* 1999)).

A second conclusion is that the domain of QOL in pediatric oncology samples is not a homogeneous field of functioning or experiencing. Factor analyses as well as findings comparing different subgroups suggest that it is multidimensional in its structure and contents, so that the variance of QOL is accounted for by a series of several factors or sets of items, each focused on a specific circumscribed theme (e.g., findings based on CQL (Kreitler and Kreitler 2003a), PedsQL (Varni *et al.* 2002); yet, a more global structure found with the POQOLS (Bijttebier *et al.* 2001)). This conclusion may seem to indicate the utility of broadening the scope of the domains and items represented in pediatric oncology QOL tools. Up to now, many, though by no means all, investigators seem to have followed the guidelines of the EORTC for constructing tools for assessing specific domains (i.e., school, social function-ing, cognition, physical function, and emotional state). However, it may be advisable to reconsider these guidelines in view of the following arguments: (a) the represented domains do not seem to cover all important aspects of QOL, as shown by tools that were constructed on the basis of other assumptions (e.g. Disquol (Eiser *et al.* 1999); PPSC (Mulhern *et al.* 1990)); (b) in view of children's cognitive development and style, it is possible that children's tools may need to use more concrete and specific items than the usually used ones.

A third conclusion is that QOL assessed by proxy figures, however close and informed about the child they may be, is not to be substituted for QOL based on assessments conducted with the children themselves. The reports of parents, nurses, physicians and friends may be more veridical, objective and easier to get than the children's, but they do not represent the children's QOL even when correspondences between the two kinds of reports are detected (see above section 'Difficulties in assessing QOL in children; or QOL by whom – children or parents?'). The proxy reports are to be treated as a source of information in its own right, which should be studied in order to determine what kind of information they provide and by which factors they are affected.

A fourth conclusion is that the QOL of children with cancer is the product of a matrix including multiple factors. The major factors that have been identified in research up to now are diagnosis, disease stage, current treatment (its nature and difficulty), previous treatments (e.g., whole brain radiation), as well as the child's age and gender. Since all or most of these factors play a role in regard to the child's QOL, comparing groups defined by only one of the factors yields contradictory results in different studies. For the sake of illustration, let us take diagnosis. Thus, in a study with the MPQOLQ children with leukemia or lymphoma were found to have better QOL than children with brain tumors but equal to that of children with solid tumors (Armstrong *et al.* 1999); similarly, in a study with the POQOLS children with leukemia or lymphoma had better

QOL in terms of emotional distress and discomfort due to treatment than children with solid tumors (Bijttebier *et al.* 2001); but studies with the PEDQOL (Calaminus *et al.* 2000) or CQL (Kreitler and Kreitler 2003a) showed that children with leukemia or lymphoma had lower QOL in most domains than children with brain tumors or solid tumors. Similar contradictions may be detected in the above reported findings concerning the effects of treatment (being on- or off-treatment) (e.g., CHQ, Sawyer *et al.* 1999 vs. Kreitler and Kreitler 2003a), or age (e.g., Multidimensional Fatigue Scale, Varni *et al.* 2002 vs. CQL, Kreitler and Kreitler 2003a). What these contradictions suggest is that it is probably not justified to compare groups by diagnosis without considering simultaneously at the very least whether the compared children are on- or off-treatment, and if on-treatment what kind of treatment they are getting, and how old they are.

Thus, for the time being the reported findings seem to be context- or tool-bound and do not support sweeping generalizations about the effects of particular medical or therapeutic factors on the children's QOL. One reason for this may have to do with the way children experience themselves and situations. In contrast to adults who may be better able or for whom it may make more sense to focus on one or another major factor, children may tend to experience the situation as a whole. If that is the case, then we may expect larger fluctuations in QOL of children when there is a change in some factor, such as the nature of treatment. A second possibility is that at the present stage of development of assessing QOL in pediatric oncology, still too little is known or understood about the factors operative in this domain. Hence, the findings may seem fragmentary or contradictory. The remedy for that would be to go on studying the field so as to unravel more of its components and dynamics. A third possibility is that in pediatric oncology the whole situation actually plays a larger role than in adults. If that is the case, we should beware of generalizations, not even pursue them and try instead to pose highly specific questions, exploring the QOL of groups defined precisely by a number of factors (e.g., 'What are the effects on QOL of treatment X administered to boys younger than 12 with a particular diagnosis of leukemia, in the initial phase of disease?'). Finally, a fourth possibility is that the findings are largely tool-dependent.

Finally, a fifth conclusion concerns the tools of assessing QOL in children. It may be appropriate to consider whether the commonly used tools are appropriate for children and for the studied issue of QOL in terms of contents and form. Most importantly, in view of the definition of QOL in experiential and phenomenological terms, it may not be appropriate to use pediatric QOL instruments that require children to evaluate or judge the effects of factors, such as the treatment or the disease on their QOL, as is common in health-related QOL instruments, or compare their present state with their state prior to the onset of the disease.

The five stated conclusions spell out at least two guidelines charting the way ahead in the research of QOL. One is to further explore the factors affecting the QOL of children with cancer, in an attempt to unravel the structure and dynamics of this important domain. The other is to refine and adapt the tools of assessment so that they are better adapted to the studied population and theme.

The third recommendation serves to extend the mentioned ones by suggesting that the study of QOL in children with cancer move in the direction of identifying new factors that may affect the children's QOL. Two types of such factors appear significant. One type is factors that have to do with the child's personality and coping mechanisms. This type is important because it complements the set of studied factors (e.g., disease, treatments) which are external to the children themselves. A large body of data about QOL in adult cancer patients demonstrates the importance to QOL of coping mechanisms and other resources that the patient brings into the situation. The other type of factors to be studied is those that may be expected to affect the sick child's QOL in a *positive* manner. Examples that come readily to mind would be the support of friends, family interactions, or art therapy. The study of factors of this kind is glaringly missing in the investigation of QOL in children with cancer. Studying the effects of factors with positive contributions to QOL form the bridge to the most important task of improving the sick children's QOL.

REFERENCES

Achenbach, N.K., Edelbrock, J. (Eds), (1983) *Manual for the Child Behavior Checklist and the Revised Child Behavior Profile.* Berlington, VT: University of Vermont.

Armstrong, F.D., Toledano, S.R., Miloslavich, K., Lackman-Zeman, L., Levy, J.D., Gay, C.L., Schuman, W.B., Fishkin, P. E. (1999) The Miami Pediatric Quality of Life Questionnaire: Parent scale. *International Journal of Cancer* **83**, S12, 11–17.

Bearison, D.J., Mulhern, R.K. (1994) *Pediatric Psychooncology: Psychological perspectives on children with cancer.* New York: Oxford University Press.

Bhatia, S., Meriel, E.M., Jenney, M.E.M., Bogue, M.K., Rockwood, T.H., Feusner, J.H., Friedman, D.L., Robison, L.L., Kane, R.L. (2002) The Minneapolis-Manchester Quality of Life Instrument: Reliability and validity of the adolescent form. *Journal of Clinical Oncology* **20**, 4692–4698.

Bijttebier, P., Vercruysse, T., Vertommen, H., Van Gool, S.W., Uyttebroeck, A., Brock, P. (2001) New evidence on the reliability and validity of the pediatric oncology quality of life scale. *Psychology and Health* **16**, 461–469.

Boggs, S.R., Durning, P. (1998) The Pediatric Oncology Quality of Life Scale: Development and validation of a disease-specific quality of life measure. In Drotar, D. (Ed.), *Measuring Health-related Quality of Life in Children and Adolescents: Implications for Research and Practice.* Mahwah, NJ: Erlbaum, pp. 3–24.

Bradlyn, A.S., Harris, C.V., Spieth, L.E. (1995) Quality of life assessment in pediatric oncology: A retrospective review of phase III reports. *Social Science and Medicine*, **41**, 1463–1465.

Bradlyn, A.S., Harris, C.V., Warner, J.E., Ritchey, A.K., Zaboy, K. (1993) An investigation of the validity of the Quality of Well-Being Scale with pediatric oncology patients. *Health Psychology* **12**, 246–250.

Calaminus, G., Weinspach, S., Teske, C., Gobel, U. (2000) Quality of life in children and adolescents with cancer. First results of an evaluation of 49 patients with the PEDQOL questionnaire. *Klinische Pediatrie* **212**, 211–215.

Calman, K.C. (1984) Quality of life in cancer patients – an hypothesis. *Journal of Medical Ethics* **10**, 124–127.

Canning, E.H., Canning, R.D., Boyce, W.T. (1992) Depressive symptoms and adaptive style in children with cancer. *Journal of the American Academy of Child and Adolescent Psychiatry* **31**, 1120–1124.

Challinor, J.M., Miaskowski, C.A., Franck, L.S., Slaughter, R.E., Matthay, K.K., Kramer, R.F., Veatch, J.J., Paul, S.M., Amylon, M.D., Moore, I.M. (1999) Somatisation, anxiety and depression as measures of health-related quality of life in children/adolescents with cancer. *International Journal of Cancer* **83**, S12, 52–57.

Clay, R.A. (1999) Creating the tools that measure quality of life. *APA Monitor*, **30**, 1–3.

Eder, R. (1990) Uncovering young children's psychological selves: Individual and developmental differences. *Child Development* **61**, 849–863.

Eiser, C. (1996) Choices in measuring quality of life in children with cancer: a comment. *Psycho-Oncology* **4**, 121–132.

Eiser, C., Cotter, I., Oades, P., Seamark, D., Smith, R. (1999) Health-related quality of life measures for children. *International Journal of Cancer* **83**, S12, 87–90.

Eiser, C., Jenney, M.E.M. (1996) Measuring symptomatic benefit and quality of life in paediatric oncology. *British Journal of Cancer* **73**, 1313–1316.

Eiser, C., Morse, R. (2001) Can parents rate their child's health related quality of life? Results of a systematic review. *Quality of Life Research* **10**, 347–357.

Fayers, P.M., Machin, D. (2000) *Quality of Life: Assessment, analysis and interpretation.* Chichester, UK: Wiley.

Feeny, D., Furlong, W., Barr, R.D., Torrance, G. W., Rosenbaum, P., Weitzman, S. (1992) A comprehensive multiattribute system for classifying the health status of survivors of childhood cancer. *Journal of Clinical Oncology* **10**, 923–928.

Feeny, D., Furlong, W., Boyle, M., Torrance, G.W. (1995) Multi-attribute health status classification systems: Health Utilities Index. *PharmacoEconomics* **7**, 490–502.

Feeny, D., Furlong, W., Mulhern, R.K., Barr, R.D., Hudson, M. (1999) A framework for assessing health-related quality of life among children with cancer. *International Journal of Cancer* **83**, S12, 2–9.

Goodwin, D.A.J., Boggs, S.R., Graham-Pole, J. (1994) Development and validation of the Pediatric Oncology Quality of Life Scale. *Psychological Assessment* **6**, 321–328.

Green, D.M., Zevon, M.A., Hall, B. (1991) Achievement of life goals by adult survivors of modern treatment of childhood cancer. *Cancer* **67**, 206–213.

Guyatt, G.H. (1999) Measuring health-related quality of life in childhood cancer: Lessons from the workshop (discussion). *International Journal of Cancer* **83**, S12, 143–146.

Kamphuis, R.P. (1987) The concept of quality of life in pediatric oncology. In Aronson, N.K., Beckmann, J. (Eds) *The Quality of Life in Cancer Patients.* New York: Raven Press, pp. 141–151.

Kreitler, S., Kreitler, M.M. (2003a) *The Children's Quality of Life (CQL): Instrument and manual.* Tel-Aviv, Israel: Psychooncology Unit, Tel-Aviv Medical Center.

Kreitler, S., Kreitler, M.M. (2003b) *The Adult Quality of Life (ADL): Instrument and manual.* Tel-Aviv, Israel: Psychooncology Unit, Tel-Aviv Medical Center.

Landgraf, J.M., Abetz, L., Ware, J.E. (1996) *The CHQ: The user's manual* (1st edn). Boston, MA: The Health Institute, New England Medical Center.

Landgraf, J.M., Maunsell, E., Speechley, K.N., Bullinger, M., Campbell, S., Abetz, L., Ware, J.E. (1998) Canadian-French, German and UK versions of the Child Health Questionnaire: methodology and preliminary item scaling results. *Quality of Life Research* **7**, 433–445.

Lansky, S.B., List, M.A., Lansky, L.L., Ritter-Sterr, C., Miller, D.R. (1987) The measurement of performance in childhood cancer patients. *Cancer* **60**, 1651–1656.

Lauria, M.M., Hockenberry-Eaton, M., Pawletko, T.M., Mauerer, A.M. (1996) Psychosocial protocol for childhood cancer: A conceptual model. *Cancer*, **78**, 1345–1356.

Leidy, N.K. (1994) Functional status and the forward progress of merry-go-rounds: Toward a coherent analytical framework. *Nursing Research* **43**, 196–202.

Levi, R.B., Drotar, D. (1999) Health-related quality of life in childhood cancer: Discrepancy in parent–child reports. *International Journal of Cancer* **83**, S12, 58–64.

Loonen, H.J., Derkx, B.H.H.F., Griffiths, A.M. (2002) Pediatricians overestimate importance of physical symptoms upon children's health concerns. *Medical Care* **40**, 996–1001.

Monaco, G.A. (1999) Commentary on assessing health-related quality of life in children with cancer. *International Journal of Cancer* **83**, S12, 10.

Mostow, E.N., Byrner, J., Connelly, R.R., Mulvihill, J.J. (1991) Quality of life in long term survivors of CNS tumors of childhood and adolescence. *Journal of Clinical Oncology* **9**, 592–599.

Mulhern, R.K., Horowitz, M.E., Ochs, J., Friedman, A.G., Armstrong, F.D., Copeland, D., Kun, L.E. (1989) Assessment of quality of life among pediatric patients with cancer. *Psychological Assessment* **1**, 130–138.

Mulhern, R.K., Fairclough, D.L., Friedman, A.G., Leigh, L.D. (1990) Play performance scale as an index of quality of life of children with cancer. *Psychological Assessment* **2**, 149–155.

Nayfield, S.G., Ganz, P.A., Moinpour, C.M., Cella, D.F., Hailey, B.J. (1992) Report from a National Cancer Institute (USA) workshop of quality of life assessment in cancer clinical trials. *Quality of Life Research* **1**, 203–210.

Niv, D., Kreitler, S. (2001) Pain and quality of life. *Pain Practice* **1**, 150–161.

Osoba, D.L. (1995) Measuring the effects of cancer on health-related quality of life. *PharmacoEconomics* **7**, 308–319.

Parsons, S.K., Brown, A.P. (1998) Evaluation of quality of life of childhood cancer survivors: a methodological conundrum. *Medical and Pediatric Oncology* **S1**, 46–53.

Parsons, S.K., Barlow, S.E., Levy, S.L., Supran, S.E., Kaplan, S.H. (1999) Health-related quality of lie in pediatric bone marrow transplant survivors: According to whom? *International Journal of Cancer* **83**, S12, 46–51.

Phipps, S., Hinds, P.S., Channell, S., Bell, G. (1994) Measurement of behavioral, affective and somatic responses to pediatric bone marrow transplantation: Development of the BASES scale. *Journal of Pediatric Oncology Nursing* **11**, 109–117.

Phipps, S., Dunavant, M., Jayawardene, D., Srivastiva, D.K. (1999) Assessment of health-related quality of life in acute in-patient settings: Use of the BASES instrument in children undergoing bone marrow transplantation. *International Journal of Cancer* **83**, S12, 18–24.

Phipps, S., Dunavant, M., Garvie, P.A., Lensing, S., Rai, S.N. (2002) Acute health-related quality of life in children undergoing stem cell transplant: I. Descriptive outcomes. *Bone Marrow Transplantation* **29**, 425–434.

Reynolds, C.R., Kamphaus, R.W. (1992) *BASC: Behavior Assessment System for Children manual.* Circle Pines, MN: American Guidance Service.

Sawyer, M. Antoniou, G., Toogood, I., Rice, M. (1999) A comparison of parent and adolescent reports describing the health-related quality of life of adolescents treated for cancer. *International Journal of Cancer* **83**, S12, 39–45.

Seid, M., Varni, J.W., Rode, C.A., Katz, E.R. (1999) The Pediatric Cancer Quality of Life Inventory: A modular approach to measuring health-related quality of life in children with cancer. *International Journal of Cancer* **83**, S12, 71–76.

Sprangers, M.A.G., Cull, A., Bjordal, K., Groenwold, M., Aaronson, M.K. (1993) The European Organization for Research and Treatment of Cancer Approach Quality of Life Assessment: Guidelines for Developing Questionnaire Modules. *Quality of Life Research*, **2**, 287–295.

Stephenson, R.L. (2003) Health-related quality of life in pediatric patients with brain tumors. *Dissertaton Abstracts International: Section B: The Sciences and Engineering* **62** (8-B), 3816.

Vance, Y.H., Morse, R.C., Jenney, M.E., Eiser, C. (2001) Issues in measuring quality of life in childhood cancer: measures, proxies, and parental mental health. *Journal of Child Psychology & Psychiatry & Allied Disciplines* **42**, 661–667.

Varni, J. W., Seid, M., Rode, C.A. (1999) The PedsQL™: Measurement model for the Pediatric Quality of Life Inventory™. *Medical Care* **37**, 126–139.

Varni, J.W., Katz, E.R., Seid, M., Quiggins, D.J.L., Friedman-Bender, A., Castro, C.M. (1998a) The Pediatric Cancer Quality of Life Inventory (PCQL). I. Instrument development, descriptive statistics, and cross-informant variance. *Journal of Behavioral Medicine* **21**, 179–204.

Varni, J.W., Katz, E.R., Seid, M., Quiggins, D.J.L., Friedman-Bender, A. (1998b) The Pediatric Cancer Quality of Life Inventory-32 (PCQL-32). *Cancer* **82**, 1184–1196.

Varni, J.W., Burwinkle, T.M., Katz, E.R., Meeske, K., Dickinson, P. (2002) The PedsQL™ in pediatric cancer: Reliability and validity of the Pediatric Quality of Life Inventory™ Generic Core Scales, Multidimensional Fatigue Scale, and Cancer Module. *Cancer* **94**, 2090–2106.

Ware, J.E. (1995) The status of health assessment. *Annual Review of Public Health* **16**, 327–354.

Watson, M., Edwards, L., Von Essen, L., Davidson, J., Day, R., Pinkerton, R. (1999) Development of the Royal Marsden Hospital paediatric oncology quality of life questionnaire. *International Journal of Cancer* **83**, S12, 65–70.

WHOQOL Group, the World Health Organization Quality of Life assessment (WHOQOL) (1995) Position paper from the World Health Organization. *Social Science and Medicine* **41**, 1403–1409.

Wilson, I.B., Cleary, P.D. (1995) Linking clinical variables with health related quality of life. *JAMA* **1995**, 59–65.

Worchel, F.F., Nolan, B.F., Willson, V.L., Purser, J.S., Copeland, D.R., Pfefferbaum, B. (1988) Assessment of depression in children with cancer. *Journal of Pediatric Psychology* **13**, 101–112.

Zebrack, B.J., Chesler, M.A. (2001) A psychometric analysis of the Quality of Life – Cancer Survivors (QOL-CS) in survivors of childhood cancer. *Quality of Life Research* **10**, 319–329.

Zeltzer, L.K., Dolgin, M.J., Lebaron, S., Lebaron, C. (1991) A randomized controlled study of behavioral intervention for chemotherapy distress in children with cancer. *Pediatrics* **88**, 34–42.

APPENDIX: THE CHILDREN'S QUALITY OF LIFE QUESTIONNAIRE (CQL)

Developed by the Hans Kreitler Memorial Unit of Psychooncology

Name _____ Boy/Girl _____ Age _____ Date _____

Country of birth _____ Who read the questions _____

Quality of Life

Hi. We would like to know better how you are and how you feel. For this purpose we have prepared these questions. After each question there are 3 response alternatives. In order to answer these questions, we suggest that you read each question carefully, and then check or color the answer which seems to you the most correct. This is not a test, and there are no grades. The most important thing is that you check the response that best describes your state and what is true about you.

1. **I worry about my health**

    Never   Sometimes   Often

2. **I feel healthy**

    Almost all the time   Sometimes   Almost never

3. **I feel pain**

    Never   Sometimes   Almost all the time

4. **The pain I feel is**

    Not at all strong   Not so strong   Very strong

5. **I go to school**

    Every day   Sometimes yes and sometimes not   Almost never

6. **I fulfill my duties at school**

    Like all others   Somewhat less than others   A lot less than others

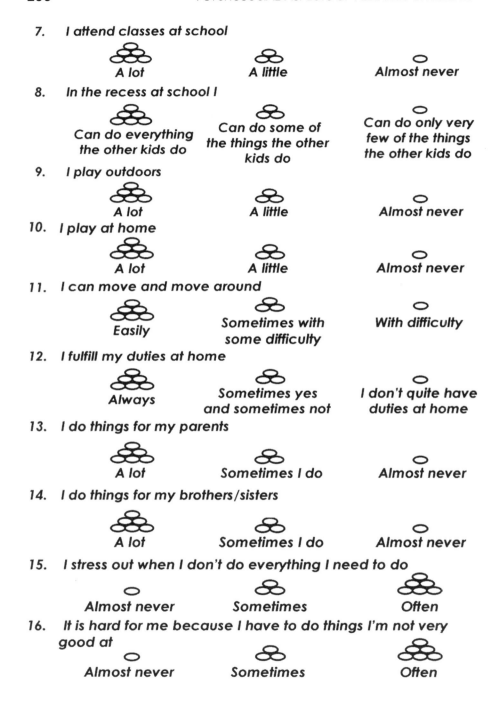

7. I attend classes at school

    A lot   A little   Almost never

8. In the recess at school I

    Can do everything   Can do some of   Can do only very
    the other kids do   the things the other   few of the things
                           kids do   the other kids do

9. I play outdoors

    A lot   A little   Almost never

10. I play at home

    A lot   A little   Almost never

11. I can move and move around

    Easily   Sometimes with   With difficulty
                           some difficulty

12. I fulfill my duties at home

    Always   Sometimes yes   I don't quite have
                           and sometimes not   duties at home

13. I do things for my parents

    A lot   Sometimes I do   Almost never

14. I do things for my brothers/sisters

    A lot   Sometimes I do   Almost never

15. I stress out when I don't do everything I need to do

    Almost never   Sometimes   Often

16. It is hard for me because I have to do things I'm not very
    good at

    Almost never   Sometimes   Often

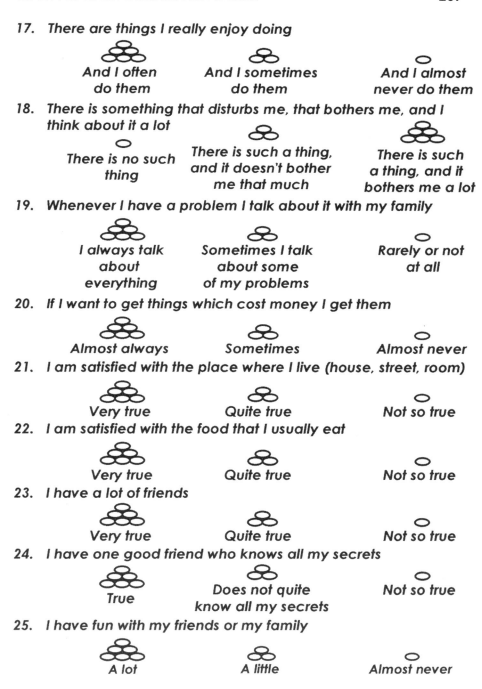

17. *There are things I really enjoy doing*

And I often
do them   And I sometimes
do them   And I almost
never do them

18. *There is something that disturbs me, that bothers me, and I think about it a lot*

There is no such
thing   There is such a thing,
and it doesn't bother
me that much   There is such
a thing, and it
bothers me a lot

19. *Whenever I have a problem I talk about it with my family*

I always talk
about
everything   Sometimes I talk
about some
of my problems   Rarely or not
at all

20. *If I want to get things which cost money I get them*

Almost always   Sometimes   Almost never

21. *I am satisfied with the place where I live (house, street, room)*

Very true   Quite true   Not so true

22. *I am satisfied with the food that I usually eat*

Very true   Quite true   Not so true

23. *I have a lot of friends*

Very true   Quite true   Not so true

24. *I have one good friend who knows all my secrets*

True   Does not quite
know all my secrets   Not so true

25. *I have fun with my friends or my family*

A lot   A little   Almost never

26. **Even when I'm alone, I can find something to do**

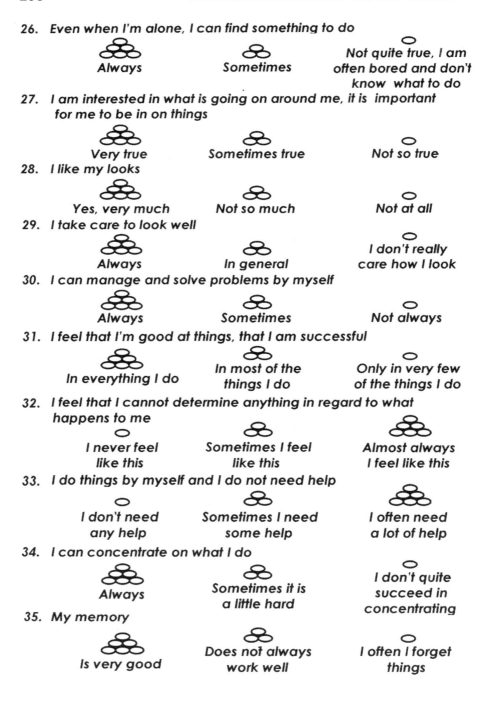

Always	Sometimes	Not quite true, I am often bored and don't know what to do

27. **I am interested in what is going on around me, it is important for me to be in on things**

Very true	Sometimes true	Not so true

28. **I like my looks**

Yes, very much	Not so much	Not at all

29. **I take care to look well**

Always	In general	I don't really care how I look

30. **I can manage and solve problems by myself**

Always	Sometimes	Not always

31. **I feel that I'm good at things, that I am successful**

In everything I do	In most of the things I do	Only in very few of the things I do

32. **I feel that I cannot determine anything in regard to what happens to me**

I never feel like this	Sometimes I feel like this	Almost always I feel like this

33. **I do things by myself and I do not need help**

I don't need any help	Sometimes I need some help	I often need a lot of help

34. **I can concentrate on what I do**

Always	Sometimes it is a little hard	I don't quite succeed in concentrating

35. **My memory**

Is very good	Does not always work well	I often I forget things

36. *I am able to think and understand things*

Always   **Sometimes it is a little hard**   **I often do not succeed**

37. *I am nervous or tense*

Almost never   Sometimes   **Often**

38. *I don't quite know what happens with me*

Almost never   Sometimes   **Often**

39. *I am sad*

Almost never   Sometimes   **Often**

40. *I feel lonely*

Never   Sometimes   **Often**

41. *Sleep is difficult for me*

Never   Sometimes   **Often**

42. *I am tired, I feel exhausted*

Almost never   Sometimes   **Often**

43. *I feel that I am guilty, that I am to blame*

Almost never   Sometimes   **Often**

44. *I am angry*

Almost never   Sometimes   **Often**

45. *I am scared*

Almost never   Sometimes   **Often**

46. *I am confused*

Almost never   Sometimes   **Often**

47. *I feel safe and protected*

Almost always   Sometimes   Almost never

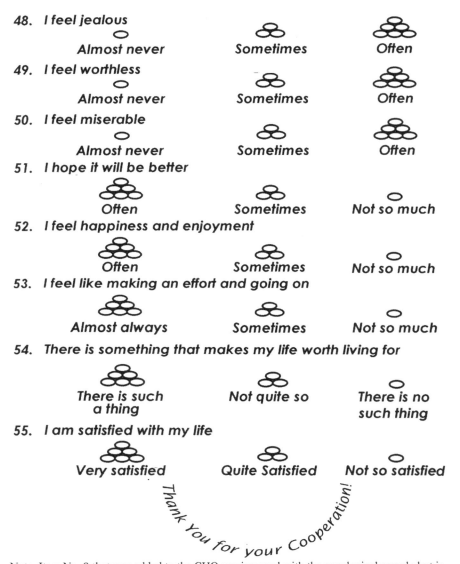

48. *I feel jealous*

    Almost never   Sometimes   Often

49. *I feel worthless*

    Almost never   Sometimes   Often

50. *I feel miserable*

    Almost never   Sometimes   Often

51. *I hope it will be better*

    Often   Sometimes   Not so much

52. *I feel happiness and enjoyment*

    Often   Sometimes   Not so much

53. *I feel like making an effort and going on*

    Almost always   Sometimes   Not so much

54. *There is something that makes my life worth living for*

    There is such   Not quite so   There is no
    a thing   such thing

55. *I am satisfied with my life*

    Very satisfied   Quite Satisfied   Not so satisfied

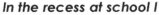

Thank You for your Cooperation!

Note. Item No. 8 that was added to the CHQ version used with the oncological sample but is not included in the CHQ standard version is as follows:

In the recess at school I

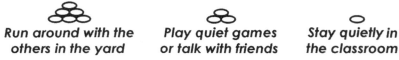

    Run around with the   Play quiet games   Stay quietly in
    others in the yard   or talk with friends   the classroom

8

Psychiatric Impact of Childhood Cancer

MARGARET L. STUBER AND DEBRA SEACORD
Neuropsychiatric Institute, University of California, Los Angeles, USA

Few would question that pediatric cancer has an emotional impact on the children and the families who deal with it. One of the challenges for clinicians is to determine what could be considered a 'normal' response to an overwhelming situation, and when the response would be considered 'pathological'. In addition, clinicians need to know how to identify children and families at risk, and to initiate appropriate preventative, as well as therapeutic, interventions. This chapter will examine what is known about these issues and outline guidelines for clinicians, based on the current (limited) database. The overview will include not only dealing with the immediate issues of diagnosis and treatment, but also the long-term concerns such as the psychiatric impact of late-effects and symptoms arising in young adulthood.

Despite the clearly overwhelming nature of the diagnosis and treatment of childhood malignancy, studies have consistently found that the majority of childhood cancer patients report minimal symptoms of long-term psycho-logical distress. In fact, there is evidence that some survivors report positive psychological effects of the cancer experience. However, clinical researchers have interpreted these data as saying more about the way that children cope with the ongoing experience of cancer treatment, which frequently goes on for years, than it does about the actual psychiatric impact. We will examine these findings, and the various interpretations.

Since no child is treated in isolation, we will also include what is known at this point about the response of the families, and the impact of their response on the children.

Psychosocial Aspects of Pediatric Oncology. Edited by S. Kreitler and M. Weyl Ben Arush
© 2004 John Wiley & Sons Ltd: ISBN 0 471 49939 0

IMMEDIATE SYMPTOMS IN PEDIATRIC ONCOLOGY PATIENTS

Chronic or life-threatening pediatric illness intensifies the challenge of the major developmental tasks of childhood and adolescence. Issues of autonomy, peer relations, and future orientation are made more complicated by the dependency of the patient role, the social isolation treatment often requires, and the potential uncertainty of chronic or relapsing conditions. The primary types of psychiatric symptoms that are of concern fall in the general categories of depression and anxiety. The mental health professional is most often consulted to assess whether the observed symptoms meet the threshold for a psychiatric diagnosis as a disorder, and if intervention is indicated. Consultations may be initiated by the treating oncologists or by the parents. Any successful assessment and intervention requires the participation of both the family and the medical team (Apter, Farbstein and Yaniv 2003, Eiser, Hill and Vance 2000).

Depression

Although depressive symptoms are not necessarily more prevalent in medically ill pediatric patients, depressive symptoms are associated with poorer medical outcome and non-adherence (Campbell and Etringer 1999). Thus depressive symptoms should not be routinely dismissed as a 'normal response to illness'. Appropriate assessment is indicated as well as intervention, if needed. Unfortunately, very few pediatric data are available that validate the use of standard depression rating scales in this patient group (Knapp and Harris 1998). There are currently several clinical investigations ongoing to develop and validate a scale for medically ill children, as has been done with adults.

One of the difficulties in evaluating symptoms of depression in children on active treatment for cancer is the differentiation of symptoms that are secondary to the cancer or treatment. Many of the somatic symptoms of depression, such as difficulty sleeping or fatigue, are common symptoms of cancer or its treatment. In a study of 454 children and adolescents, children with cancer reported fewer symptoms of depression on the Children's Depression Index than normal school children or inpatients in a psychiatric hospital. Somatic items and items concerning self-esteem did not differentiate between depressed and non-depressed children in the cancer group. They concluded that the CDI could be used with cancer patients, but must be evaluated differently for this group (Worchel et al. 1988).

It is also important to differentiate symptoms that might be interpreted as depression which are better seen as grief. Such symptoms, like those secondary to medical treatment, may still require intervention, but should be seen as a normal, rather than pathological, response to an unusual exposure to loss.

Some of the grief is a response to personal losses, such as missed opportunities or lost body functions. This is most obvious with adolescents who miss key rites of passage, such as graduation or prom. However, in addition, these children are introduced to death at an earlier age and in a more personal way than most children who have the good fortune to live in peaceful parts of the world. The typical child with cancer will come to know children his or her own age who die during the years they are on active treatment. Although this is true of most children in many parts of the world, children in the United States are commonly sheltered from such exposure, and parents often do not know how to help them with this. Appropriate assessment of the issues of concern to the child or adolescent will allow optimal intervention.

Anxiety

Anxiety is a common response to the uncertainty of cancer diagnosis and prognosis, as well as to various aspects of treatment. The recurrent body intrusions, pain, and hospitalizations, are particularly difficult for younger children, who do not have the cognitive development necessary to grasp why treatment is necessary. However, most of these anxiety symptoms do not achieve the level of psychiatric diagnosis. The most frequent clinical diagnoses during active treatment are Adjustment Disorder, Separation Disorder, or Phobias.

It is not unusual for a child to become sensitized to various items associated with pain or fear, such as needles or the procedure room. For this reason, pediatricians commonly forgo the white coat of other medical professionals, and wear bright ties or pins and attach small toys to their stethoscopes. Some clinics give small 'prizes' to children, and most give stickers, to recognize that it requires some courage to come to clinic and deal with the required procedures. However, the response can reach the level of a phobic anxiety disorder for some children and adolescents. Pre-existing generalized anxiety or other anxiety disorders appear to predispose children to phobic responses. Parental anxiety is both generated by and contributes to the anxiety response of children and adolescents. Since phobic responses can be disruptive to treatment, anxiety in both parents and children is a frequent focus of both prevention and intervention for mental health professionals working with pediatric oncology.

Conditioned responses to aversive aspects of treatment are not limited to anxiety symptoms. There have been numerous clinical reports of conditioned nausea in response to certain foods, which had become associated with chemotherapy. Children may have sufficient anticipatory anxiety that they will vomit in the car on the way to, as well as from, the clinic for treatment. These symptoms are distressing, for all concerned and require evaluation and intervention. However, they do not generally reach the level of lasting psychopathology – although certain food may be avoided for many years.

Separation anxiety, a 'developmentally inappropriate and excessive anxiety concerning separation from home or from those to whom the individual is attached' (American Psychiatric Association 1994), is most often seen in younger children and in children with prolonged hospitalizations or pre-existing anxiety. These children may experience nightmares about separation from their parents and home, be terrified that some calamity will befall them or a loved one as a result of the separation (e.g. being kidnapped), and experience physical symptoms such as headaches or nausea. These symptoms must persist for at least four weeks to meet criteria for a diagnosis, but may require intervention long before that.

Symptoms of post-traumatic stress disorder (PTSD) have been observed in some children on active treatment for cancer. Since PTSD is, by definition, only diagnosable four weeks after the traumatic event, it could be argued that children and adolescents (and their parents) who are on active treatment, with an active life-threatening illness, could only be diagnosed with Acute Stress Disorder, and not PTSD. In any case, the incidence of diagnosable PTSD in children on active treatment has been low in the studies that have assessed this. This appears to reflect the perspective of the children towards the cancer and treatment. According to the theoretical concept underlying the diagnosis of PTSD, an event must be experienced as life-threatening or a threat to physical integrity, and produce a response of intense fear, helplessness, or horror (American Psychiatric Association 1994) to generate the full complex of symptoms of PTSD. A study of 30 children, aged 3 to 18 years (mean 9.3 years) assessed them in the first week of hospitalization for bone marrow transplantation (BMT). The children were on active treatment for cancer, having had a mean duration of treatment at that point of 15.7 months (SD = 27.2 months). The families had signed a consent form indicating that they knew that the mortality of the transplant itself was approximately 15% and the overall survival after BMT was 50%. However, when the children were asked to assess the degree of life threat they were facing, 9 of the 30 reported no life threat, and 8 reported 'somewhat' of a life threat (Stuber *et al.* 1996b).

Coping and Denial

Some clinical researchers have suggested that the prevalence of anxiety and depression is under-reported in children on active treatment. A common intervention for children and families dealing with cancer is teaching the use of distraction, or the art of focused attention on something other than the cancer or treatment. This is a fundamental component of many interventions, such as guided imagery or self-hypnosis. However, there is some concern that this may lead to denial through coping or blunting of experiences. This has led to a debate among clinical researchers. Are pediatric cancer patients denying their emotional symptoms in an attempt to be positive or to live 'one day at a time'? Are they interpreting emotional symptoms as 'normal' or secondary to medical conditions, and thus not aware of psychiatric distress? Or is their coping style so effective that they are not getting depressed or anxious?

Researchers have examined the issue of denial or avoidance from a variety of perspectives. Clinical experiences suggesting that children with cancer use denial when confronted with direct questions concerning their emotional responses (Worchel *et al.* 1992) has led to recent attempts to circumvent the effects of defensiveness when assessing depression in pediatric cancer patients (Phipps and Srivastava 1999). In a study of 66 childhood cancer patients compared to 414 healthy children, the cancer patients were more likely to use an avoidant coping style than the controls. The tendency to use avoidant coping or 'blunting', defined as avoiding threat-relevant information when under stress, was positively correlated with time since diagnosis (Phipps, Fairclough and Mulhern 1995). Evaluation of self-reports from 40 adolescents and young adults found a significant association between denial of distress and higher levels of intrusive memories and avoidance, which are symptoms of PTSD (Erikson and Steiner 2000).

LONG-TERM ISSUES FOR SURVIVORS

General Psychiatric Distress

The classic study by Koocher and O'Malley (1981) found that 53% of 117 young adult survivors of pediatric cancer appeared to be well-adjusted, although 11% had severe-to-disabling problems, and problems with school, work and peer relations were common. In a large update of that study, medical and mental health status was assessed in 9535 young adult survivors of pediatric cancer who were diagnosed between 1970 and 1986, using a randomly selected cohort of the survivors' siblings ($n = 2916$) as a comparison group. Survivors were significantly more likely to report adverse general health and mental health, activity limitations, and functional impairment compared with siblings, and 44% of the survivors reported at least one adversely affected health status domain. Sociodemographic factors associated with reporting at least one adverse health status domain included being female, lower level of educational attainment, and annual income less than 20 000 dollars (Hudson *et al.* 2003). A subsample of 5736 young adults who were survivors of pediatric leukemia, Hodgkin's disease, and non-Hodgkin lymphoma were compared to 2565 sibling controls on symptoms associated with depression and somatic distress. Although, as predicted, the majority of respondents in this study did not report symptomatology indicative of depression or somatic distress, survivors were significantly more likely than sibling controls to report symptoms (Zebrack *et al.* 2002).

Despite these problems, most childhood cancer survivors do not report symptoms consistent with major psychiatric diagnoses, and are generally functioning well in school and the workplace (Madan-Swain *et al.* 2000). In a study of survivors of acute lymphoblastic leukemia, 555 young adults, ages 18 to 33 years, completed the Profile of Mood States as part of a structured telephone interview. Mood disturbance was reported by 24% of the survivors. Predictors of mood disturbance were age younger than 12.5 years at diagnosis, negative perception of current health, perception that cancer had a negative impact on employment, and status as a non-white male. High-dose cranial irradiation and intrathecal methotrexate was significantly associated with mood disturbance, but interactions between educational achievement, a history of attendance in special education classes, and sex were better predictors than treatment type or dose (Glover *et al.* 2003).

Feeling Changed or Different

Not all of the long-term impact of cancer is negative. In a study of quality of life in 176 childhood cancer survivors (age 16–28) the survivors reported that long-term effects of treatment, such as fatigue, aches, and pain negatively impact quality of life. However, the survivors reported that they were happy, feeling useful, and had high life satisfaction. Having a sense of purpose in life and perceiving positive changes as a result of cancer were associated with positive quality of life. Spiritual and religious activities appeared to be less related to quality of life in this group (Zebrack and Chesler 2002).

Similar findings were reported from an interview study of 66 childhood cancer survivors, ages 8 to 20 years. Changes in their bodies as a result of the cancer or treatment were endorsed by 42.4% of the survivors. In a more global question, 51.5% of the survivors described themselves as different as a result of the cancer experience. The vast majority (70–90%) described these differences as positive. These included improvements in the way they treat others and make friends, the way their family and others treat them, and the quality of their schoolwork and behavior, as well as their plans for the future and thoughts about life (Kazak *et al.* 1997a). Another study comparing 70 childhood leukemia survivors, aged 12 to 20 years old and at least two years off-treatment without evidence of disease to 70 matched controls in Italy found that the survivors reported a more positive and mature self-image than the controls on the Offer Self-Image Questionnaire. Included were attitude toward family, coping, and social as well as psychological aspects (Maggiolini *et al.* 2000).

Cognitive Functioning

Although the more intensive treatments introduced in the 1970s and 1980s resulted in significantly improved survival, the use of chemotherapy and radiation to eradicate disease and prevent recurrence in the central nervous system has been found to have unexpected long-term consequences. These 'cognitive late-effects' emerge over time, often not apparent until three or more years after the end of treatment. In a study comparing 100 survivors of ALL treated with chemotherapy and cranial irradiation to 50 children with a variety of malignancies treated with chemotherapy alone, and 100 healthy children, cognitive abilities were evaluated using standardized psychometric techniques. The children receiving cranial irradiation performed less well in a range of tests, with greatest differences found on verbal IQ, reading and spelling. There were no gender differences, but age less than 5 years at treatment and higher doses of radiation were correlated with lower performance in the group receiving cranial irradiation (Smibert *et al.* 1996).

As would be expected, this type of problem has an effect on education. A recent study examined the use of special education services by 12 430 young adult survivors of childhood cancer compared to 3410 full siblings. Use of special education services was reported in 23% of survivors and 8% of siblings. The greatest differences were observed among survivors who were diagnosed before age 6 years, and those who were survivors of central nervous system tumors, leukemia, and Hodgkin's disease. Treatment with intrathecal methotrexate and cranial irradiation administered alone or in combination, significantly increased the likelihood that a survivor would use special education services, as did higher doses of radiation. Survivors of leukemia central nervous system tumors, non-Hodgkin lymphoma, and neuroblastoma were significantly less likely to finish high school compared with siblings (Mitby *et al.* 2003). This suggests a need for ongoing monitoring of childhood cancer survivors, and appropriate intervention for any problems that appear.

Post-traumatic Stress

Studies of survivors of childhood cancer have shown that a subset of children and adolescents report symptoms of post-traumatic stress (Butler, Rizzi and Handwerger 1996, Stuber *et al.* 1996a). When 309 childhood cancer survivors, ages 8 to 20 years, were compared to 219 children without a significant medical history, over 10% of survivors reported moderate and approximately 3% reported severe post-traumatic stress symptoms related to the cancer and treatment experience. This severity of symptoms was not statistically significantly different from the levels of symptoms reported by healthy controls (Kazak *et al.* 1997a, Barakat *et al.* 2000).

In examining 186 survivors of childhood cancer, the two objectively quantifiable predictors of post-traumatic stress symptoms were time since end of treatment and gender. As in most studies of PTSD, girls reported more symptoms than boys, and symptoms appear to decrease over time. In addition, survivors who reported more general anxiety, and whose appraisals of life threat and treatment intensity were higher, also reported more symptoms of PTSD. Physician ratings of the intensity of the treatment protocol or severity of medical sequelae were not significant independent contributors to severity of symptoms (Stuber *et al.* 1997).

Interviews of 10 adolescents who had undergone bone marrow transplants (BMT) as part of their treatment for cancer suggest one functional consequence of both the sense of being different from peers and having been exposed to trauma. Since only approximately 50% of those who undergo BMT survive more than a year post transplant, and those who do experience a month or more of isolation and extremely intense treatment, these adolescent BMT survivors had clearly been exposed to life threat and to assaults on their body integrity. Despite this clear risk, none of the survivors reported symptoms of post-traumatic stress in the moderate or severe range. However, the control group in this study, composed of friends who had been selected by the subjects, reported more symptoms of post-traumatic stress in response to various events in their lives than the subjects. Events reported by the controls included physical injuries to themselves as well as illnesses of family members. This suggests that there may be a tendency of childhood cancer survivors to select friends who had also experienced events that would shape their perspectives and set them apart from others (Stuber and Nader 1995).

Young Adult Survivors: Symptoms

In contrast to the findings on distress in child and adolescent survivors of pediatric cancer, recent studies of survivors who are now young adults suggest that there may be more of an adverse psychiatric impact than has been apparent from previous self-report and parental report data. Seventy-eight young adults (ages 18–40) who were at least two years off-treatment for pediatric malignancy completed self-report measures assessing post-traumatic stress, anxiety, appraisal of their illness and treatment, and symptoms of psychological distress. Oncology clinicians rated treatment intensity and severity of medical late-effects based on chart review data. On the SCID, 20.5% of the participants met DSM-IV criteria for PTSD at some point since the end of their treatment. State and trait anxiety were elevated compared to norms, and clinically significant levels of intrusive (9%) and avoidant (16.7%) symptoms were reported. Participants meeting criteria for PTSD reported higher appraisal of current life threat, were rated by history as having more intense treatment histories, and reported higher (and clinically significant) levels of psychological distress than those who did not have PTSD (Hobbie *et al.* 2000). The significance of these findings is underscored by a study examining a subset of 51 of the above group. They were given self-report instruments to assess quality of life (QOL) and psychological distress (Brief Symptom Inventory (BSI)). The 20% of the survivors who met full criteria for PTSD reported clinically significant levels of psychological distress, while symptom levels for those without PTSD fell well within population norms. On all domains, QOL scores were significantly lower for the PTSD group compared to the non-PTSD group (Meeske and Stuber 2001).

Young Adult Survivors: Achievement of Life Goals

In a study of 227 young adult survivors of childhood cancer, approximately 11% reported some employment-related discrimination, and 92.4% of full-time and 90% of part-time workers were provided health insurance by their employers. The percentage who were married was significantly lower that in the general US population. Many reported that their experience with cancer had influenced their decision to have children (Green and Zevon 1991). In a more recent study of 51 childhood cancer survivors 18 to 37 years old, 22% met criteria for PTSD. None of the survivors with PTSD were married, compared to 23% of the non-PTSD group. Survivors with PTSD reported poorer quality of life across all domains, with the greatest differences reported in social functioning, emotional wellbeing, and role limitations due to emotional health and pain. Survivors without PTSD did not differ from population norms. All subscales on the psychological distress measure were higher for those with PTSD. In fact, the summative score for psychological distress was in the upper 97th percentile compared to a normative population (Meeske and Stuber 2001).

FAMILIES OF PEDIATRIC PATIENTS AND SURVIVORS

Impact on the Parents

The prevalence of post-traumatic stress symptoms appears to be significantly higher in parents of childhood cancer patients and survivors than it is in the children or adolescents. In the DSM-IV field trials, Pelcovitz and colleagues found, in a small sample, that 17% of adolescent cancer survivors and 25% of their mothers fulfilled diagnostic criteria for PTSD (Pelcovitz *et al.* 1996, 1998). A study of 65 mothers of childhood cancer survivors found that the rates of PTSD were comparable to those of adult cancer survivors (Manne *et al.* 1998). The largest study to date compared 309 mothers and 213 fathers of childhood cancer survivors to 211 mothers and 114 fathers of a healthy control group. Of the survivors' mothers, 10.1% reported severe levels of current symptoms of

PTSD and 27% reported moderate levels of symptoms. The mothers in the comparison group reported 3.0% severe and 18.2% moderate ($p = 0.001$). Of the fathers of survivors, 7.1% reported severe and 28.35% reported moderate symptoms of PTSD, compared to 0% severe and 17.3% moderate in the fathers in the comparison group ($p < 0.001$). Major predictors of symptoms were trait anxiety, perceived life threat, perceived treatment intensity, and social support. Type of treatment was not a significant contributor to symptoms (Kazak *et al.* 1998a).

Siblings

Very little formal investigation has been done with siblings of childhood cancer survivors, with the majority being qualitative studies (Murray 2002), or extremely small (Houtzager, Grootenhuis and Last 2001). A recent study examined self-report measures of anxiety, post-traumatic stress, and perceptions of the cancer experience for 78 adolescent siblings of adolescent cancer survivors. Nearly half (49%) of the participants reported mild symptoms of post-traumatic stress and 32% indicated moderate to severe levels. Over half of the siblings rated the cancer experience scary and difficult, and 25% thought their brother/sister would die during treatment. When compared to a reference group of nonaffected teens, the siblings had higher symptoms of post-traumatic stress but had similar levels of general anxiety (Alderfer, Labay and Kazak 2003).

Parental Impact on Children

The relationship between parental symptoms and psychiatric symptoms in pediatric cancer patients appears to be complex. Since anxiety is a major predictor of symptoms for both parents and survivors, it would be expected that anxiety in the family might contribute to symptoms. This might also operate at a genetic level, with pre-existing anxiety contributing to appraisal and thus to symptoms, including PTSD. For example, in the study of 186 childhood cancer survivors and their parents, mothers' perception of treatment intensity and degree of life threat contributed to anxiety and subjective appraisal for the survivor. However, neither the mothers' appraisal nor symptoms of PTSD independently contributed to the survivors' post-traumatic stress symptoms (Stuber *et al.* 1997).

THERAPEUTIC INTERVENTIONS

Family-focused Interventions

Given the interaction between the response of the parents and the pediatric patient, family-focused interventions would appear to be indicated. One of the most innovative is Kazak's use of the multiple-family group model. Adapted from use with substance abuse, this model allows parents from several families to discuss their concerns, while observed by their children, and vice versa. This facilitates open discussion of the differences between concerns of child and parents, as well as the difficulty of communicating and the impact of the other's responses. This has been used in conjunction with a cognitive behavioral model to address symptoms of PTSD in pediatric cancer survivors (Kazak *et al.* 1999).

Individual Psychotherapeutic

Hypnosis, distraction, and cognitive behavioral interventions are all well established modalities for use with children during and after active treatment for cancer (Powers 1999). The best-known treatment package was developed by Jay and colleagues. It combined filmed modeling, breathing exercises, imagery/distraction, incentives, rehearsal, and therapists coaching during medical treatments. Unlike a dose of 0.3 mg/kg of diazepam, the cognitive-behavioral package resulted in less child distress during a bone marrow aspiration than the control condition (Jay *et al.* 1987). A simpler intervention, consisting of a child blowing on a party blower, while the parent counted, and gave the child stickers for holding still, resulted in lower distress than baseline in 23 young children undergoing IV placement (Manne *et al.* 1990). Hypnosis has been found to be as effective as distraction, and in some cases has been found to be more effective than other distraction techniques in reducing children's procedural distress (Llossi and Hatira 1999).

Various approaches of complementary medicine are now being explored, including relaxation or guided imagery, massage, humor therapy, and expressive therapy for reduction of treatment-related distress. Pilot trials of massage and humor found them feasible and perceived as helpful by patients and parents. These are now being assessed in a randomized clinical trial (Phipps 2002).

Group

Various approaches have been taken to development of group approaches for pediatric cancer patients and their families. One of the main challenges of a parent group is in the composition of the members. Newly diagnosed families, who are in need of hope may find it difficult to be with a parent whose child is terminally ill or may have recently relapsed. However, experienced parents can offer help and guidance and demonstrate how to cope with the stress. Initially, most parents need to express their feelings of hopelessness, anger, fear and sadness (Kazak *et al.* 1999). A manualized group format for adult cancer patients has been successfully adapted for use with parents of adolescent oncology patients. Based on the approach of The Wellness Community, a national organization for adults dealing with cancer, participants are encouraged to become 'the patient active', and given support for maintaining a sense of humor and independence throughout treatment. Very few changes were necessary to make the format appropriate and useful to parents. Adaptation of this type of psychoeducational group for adolescents has proven more challenging. Simple adaptation of groups as usually conceptualized for adults will not meet the developmental needs of children and adolescents (Stuber *et al.* 1995).

Group approaches for pediatric cancer patients have been useful when targeted towards the impact of social isolation, dependency and the cosmetic and social effects of treatment. Groups provide opportunities for identification of common problems and reality testing about the types of problem experienced with others who have had similar experiences. Mutual problem solving and the creation of a temporary support system are the mechanisms that appear to be effective (Greenly-Adams 1989). The typical group sessions focus on the developmental tasks of adolescence and impact of the illness upon achieving separation and individuation. Groups discuss a wide variety of topics, including the impact of the illness upon social relationships, how to cope with physical appearance issues, conflicts with others, and concerns about the future.

The primary challenges to development of groups for children and adolescents on active treatment are the logistics of getting to yet another appointment, and the reluctance of the child or (especially) the adolescent to spend any more time identified with a patient role. This has sometimes been addressed by having groups during clinic time. However, the most successful groups occur within the context of a social event, such as a pizza party or camp. The uniting issue for all is cancer, but they are not brought together just to talk about cancer (which they view as unappealing), but to have fun. Cancer camps allow children who would not otherwise be able to get away from their parents to go to a safe place, and do 'normal' things such as swim. They are also among others who have had similar experiences, so it becomes easy to go without a cover on a bald head, or to remove a prosthetic limb (Briery and Rabian 1999).

Social Re-integration and Social Skills Training

Re-integration programs in schools, allowing children to re-enter the classroom and friendship groups after cancer treatment appear to have a therapeutic effect for the children. Forty-nine newly diagnosed children and their parents and teachers rated their perceptions of the utility and value of a comprehensive school re-integration intervention. The intervention included supportive counseling, educational presentations, systematic liaison between the hospital and the school, and periodic follow-ups. Overall subjective evaluations were very positive (Katz *et al.* 1992). More recently, explicit training in social skills has been used to provide coping skills to children early in the course of treatment. The hypothesis was that this might prevent later adjustment problems associated with the chronic social challenges of treatment (Katz and Varni 1993). Using a combination of social cognitive problem solving, assertiveness training, and handling teasing and name-calling, the children in the intervention evidenced less internalizing, externalizing and total behavioral problems and greater classmate and teacher social support at 9-month follow-up compared to pretreatment. The higher perceived classmate social support predicted lower depressive symptoms, lower state anxiety, lower trait anxiety, lower social anxiety, and lower internalizing and externalizing behavioral problems (Varni *et al.* 1994).

Psychopharmacology

Pharmacological approaches to preparation for procedures have been recommended for some situations and age groups by the Subcommittee on the Management of Pain Associated with Procedures in Children with Cancer (Zeltzer *et al.* 1990). The major types of medications commonly used to deal with procedural pain and anxiety are (1) topical agents such as EMLA, a 5% eutectic mixture prilocaine and lidocaine, (2) oral benzodiazepines, such as Midazolam, and (3) brief general anesthesia with agents such as propofol/fentalyl.

Advantages of topical medication are the short duration of effect and the lack of associated morbidity. However, they do take some time to become effective. EMLA is administered as a cream or patch 60 minutes prior to the procedure (Buckley and Benfield 1993). A newer agent, ELA-Max, has a more rapid onset of action (30 minutes) and has been found to be of similar efficacy for pain and anxiety in a study in which 30 well children (14 girls and 16 boys) between the ages of 7 and 13 years underwent placement of an intravenous catheter in their hands (Kleiber *et al.* 2002).

In a double-blind study Midazolam, has been shown to significantly reduce children's procedural anxiety, discomfort, and pain (Ljungman *et al.* 2000). A major advantage of Midazolam is the ability to administer the medication nasally, rectally or orally. The amnesiac effect has made it popular with anesthesiologists and intensivists. This can be an asset in use with children who have needle phobias or suffer from severe treatment anxiety. However, it can create difficulties for those who are struggling to regain a sense of control during treatment.

The need for an anesthetist and added morbidity are drawbacks to the use of anesthesia. However, there is some evidence that this is the most effective approach to painful procedures. A study of 73 children undergoing bone marrow aspirations and 105 children undergoing lumbar punctures as part of cancer treatment compared three different interventions: (1) a topical eutectic mixture of lidocaine and prilocaine (EMLA cream), (2) oral Midazolam and EMLA cream, or (3) propofol/fentanyl general anesthesia. This was not randomized, but left the choice of the intervention to patient/parent request. It was found that children receiving propofol/fentanyl general anesthesia reported significantly less procedure-related pain and distress than did those receiving either EMLA or oral Midazolam/EMLA (Holdsworth *et al.* 2003).

A combination of psychological and pharmacological interventions may be the best approach. Kazak's group used a randomized, controlled prospective design to examine the relative value of psychological only versus a combination of psychological and pharmacological intervention. They found that the addition of psychological intervention made a significant difference in decreasing the child's procedural distress (Kazak *et al.* 1998b).

Use of medication in the treatment of severe depressive and anxiety symptoms unrelated to procedures treatment is indicated when behavioral interventions are insufficient. Usual psychopharmacologic agents can be used, although care must be taken to examine potential drug interaction and to consider metabolism of the drugs, as well as the timeframe of action. For example, the mood symptoms secondary to corticosteroids may be quite disabling, but may be gone before a typical antidepressant drug has become effective (Drigen, Spirito and Gelber 1992). Steroid-induced psychosis does appear to be responsive to typical antipsychotic drugs, even in very young children (Ingram and Hagemann 2003).

Anticipatory nausea and vomiting associated with treatment is a significant concern for many children, and is not always completely addressed with behavioral interventions. A placebo-controlled trial of ondansetron has found it to be effective in reducing the incidence of post-chemotherapy vomiting for children ages 18 months to 15 years. It appeared to be even more effective when administered prior to administration of the chemotherapy (Parker *et al.* 2001). Both oral syrup and intravenous forms of ondansetron were well tolerated and almost 90% effective when administered with oral dexamethasone (White *et al.* 2000).

SUMMARY

Childhood cancer, while extremely difficult for the patient and the family, appears to cause significant psychopathology in the minority of children and their parents. A number of therapeutic approaches have been developed which are effective in preventing or treating anxiety and depression associated with painful procedures, nausea of chemotherapy, and social isolation. There remains concern about the long-term impact, both cognitively and psychologically, on survivors as they reach young adulthood. Family-based interventions, both educational and supportive, appear to be an essential aspect of good psychosocial care for all pediatric oncology patients.

REFERENCES

Alderfer, M.A., Labay, L.E., Kazak, A.E. (2003) Brief report: does posttraumatic stress apply to siblings of childhood cancer survivors? *J. Pediatr. Psychol.* **28**(4), 281–286.

American Psychiatric Association (1994) *Diagnostic and Statistical Manual.* Washington, DC: APA Press.

Apter, A., Farbstein, I., Yaniv, I. (2003) Psychiatric aspects of pediatric cancer. *Child Adolesc. Psychiatr. Clin. N. Am.* **12**(3), 473–492, vii.

Barakat, L., Kazak, A.E., Gallagher, M.A., Meeske, K., Stuber, M.L. (2000) Posttraumatic stress symptoms and stressful life events predict the long-term adjustment of survivors of childhood cancer and their mothers. *Journal of Clinical Psychology in Medical Settings* **7**(4), 189–196.

Briery, B.G., Rabian, B. (1999) Psychosocial changes associated with participation in a pediatric summer camp. *J. Pediatr. Psychol.* **24**(2), 183–190.

Buckley, M., Benfield, P. (1993) Eutectic lidocaine/prilocaine cream: a review of the topical anesthetic/analgesic efficacy of a eutectic mixture of local anesthetics (EMLA). *Drugs* **46**, 126–131.

Butler, R.W., Rizzi, L.P., Handwerger, B.A. (1996) Brief report: the assessment of posttraumatic stress disorder in pediatric cancer patients and survivors. *J. Pediatr. Psychol.* **21**(4), 499–504.

Campbell, B., Etringer, G. (1999) Posttransplant quality of life issues: depression related noncompliance in cardiac transplant patients. *Transplant. Proc.* **31**(4A), 59S–60S.

Drigan, R., Spirito, A., Gelber, R.D. (1992) Behavioral effects of corticosteriods in children with acute lymphoblastic leukemia. *Medical and Pediatric Oncology* **20**, 13–21.

Eiser, C., Hill, J.J., Vance, Y.H. (2000) Examining the psychological consequences of surviving childhood cancer: Systematic review as a research method in pediatric psychology. *Journal of Pediatric Psychology* **25**(6), 563–576.

Erickson, S.J., Steiner, H. (2000) Trauma spectrum adaptation: Somatic symptoms in long-term pediatric cancer survivors. *Psychosomatics* **41**(4), 339–346.

Glover, D.A., Byrne, J., Mills, J.L., Robison, L.L., Nicholson, H.S., Meadows, A., Zeltzer, L.K., Children's Cancer Group (2003) Impact of CNS treatment on mood in adult survivors of childhood leukemia: a report from the Children's Cancer Group. *J. Clin. Oncol.* **21**(23), 4395–4401.

Green, D.M., Zevon, M.A. (1991) Achievement of life goals by adult survivors of modern treatment for childhood cancer. *Cancer* **67**, 205–213.

Greenly-Adams, M. (1989) Psychosocial interventions in childhood cancer. In: *Handbook of Psychooncology: Psychological care of the patient with cancer.* New York: Oxford University Press, Chapter 45, pp. 562–581.

Hobbie, W., Stuber, M.L., Meeske, K., Ruccione, K., Kazak, A.E. (2000) PTSD in young adult survivors of childhood cancer. *Journal of Clinical Oncology* **18**, 4060–4066.

Holdsworth, M.T., Raisch, D.W., Winter, S.S., Frost, J.D., Moro, M.A., Doran, N.H., Phillips, J., Pankey, J.M., Mathew, P. (2003) Pain and distress from bone marrow aspirations and lumbar punctures. *Ann. Pharmacother.* **37**(1), 17–22.

Houtzager, B.A., Grootenhuis, M.A., Last, B.F. (2001) Supportive groups for siblings of pediatric oncology patients: impact on anxiety. *Psychooncology* **10**(4), 315–324.

Hudson, M.M., Mertens, A.C., Yasui, Y., Hobbie, W., Chen, H., Gurney, J.G., Yeazel, M., Recklitis, C.J., Marina, N., Robison, L.R., Oeffinger, K.C., Childhood Cancer Survivor Study Investigators (2003) Health status of adult long-term survivors of childhood cancer: a report from the Childhood Cancer Survivor Study. *JAMA* **290**(12), 1583–1592.

Ingram, D.G., Hagemann, T.M. (2003) Promethazine treatment of steroid-induced psychosis in a child. *Ann. Pharmacother.* **37**(7–8), 1036–1039.

Jay, S.M., Elliott, C., Katz, E., Siegel, S. (1987) Cognitive-behavioral and pharmacologic interventions for children's distress during painful medical procedures. *Journal of Consulting and Clinical Psychology* **55**, 860–865.

Katz, E.R., Varni, J.W. (1993) Social support and social cognitive problem solving in children with newly diagnosed cancer. *Cancer* **71**, 3314–3319.

Katz, E.R., Varni, J.W., Rubenstein, C.L., Blew, A., Hubert, N. (1992) Teacher, parent, and child evaluative ratings of a school reintegration intervention for children with newly diagnosed cancer. *Child Health Care* **21**(2), 69–75.

Kazak, A.E., Stuber, M.L., Barakat, L.P., Meeske, K. (1997a) Assessing posttraumatic stress related to medical illness and treatment: The Impact of Traumatic Stressors Interview Schedule (ITSIS). *Families, Systems and Health* **14**(3), 365–380.

Kazak, A.E., Barakat, L.P., Meeske, K., Christakis, D., Meadows, A.T., Casey, R., Penati, B., Stuber, M.L. (1997b) Posttraumatic stress symptoms, family functioning, and social support in survivors of childhood leukemia and their mothers and fathers. *Journal of Consulting and Clinical Psychology* **65**(1), 120–129.

Kazak, A.E., Stuber, M.L., Barakat, L.P., Meeske, K., Guthrie, D., Meadows, A.T. (1998a) Predicting posttraumatic stress symptoms in mothers and fathers of survivors of childhood cancer. *Journal of the American Academy of Child and Adolescent Psychiatry* **37**(8), 823–831.

Kazak, A.E., Penati, B., Brophy, P., Himelstein, B. (1998b) Pharmacologic and psychologic interventions for procedural pain. *Pediatrics* **102**, 59–66.

Kazak, A.E., Simms, S., Barakat, L., Hobbie, W., Foley, B., Golomb, V., Best, M. (1999) Surviving cancer competently intervention program (SCCIP): a cognitive–behavioral and family therapy intervention for adolescent survivors of childhood cancer and their families. *Family Process* **38**(2), 175–191.

Kleiber, C., Sorenson, M., Whiteside, K., Gronstal, B.A., Tannous, R. (2002) Topical anesthetics for intravenous insertion in children: a randomized equivalency study. *Pediatrics* **110**(4), 758–761.

Knapp, P.K., Harris, E.S. (1998) Consultation-liaison in child psychiatry: a review of the past 10 years. Part II: Research on treatment approaches and outcomes. *J. Am. Acad. Child Adolesc. Psychiatry* **37**(2), 139–146.

Koocher, G., O'Malley, J. (1981) *The Damocles Syndrome: Psychosocial consequences of surviving childhood cancer.* New York: McGraw-Hill.

Ljungman, G., Kreuger, A., Andréasson, S., Gordh, T., Sörensen, S. (2000) Midazolam nasal spray reduces anxiety in children. *Pediatrics* **105**(1), 73–78.

Llossi, C., Hatira, P. (1999) Clinical hypnosis versus cognitive behavioral training for pain management with pediatric cancer patients undergoing bone marrow aspirations. *The International Journal of Clinical and Experimental Hypnosis* **47**(2), 104–116.

Madan-Swain, A., Brown, R.T., Foster, M.A., Vega, R., Byars, K., Rodenberger, W., Bell, B., Lambert, R. (2000) Identity in adolescent survivors of childhood cancer. *Journal of Pediatric Psychology* **25**(2), 105–115.

Maggiolini, A., Grassi, R., Adamoli, L., Corbetta, A., Charmet, G.P., Provantini, K., Fraschini, D., Jankovic, M., Lia, R., Spinetta, J., Masera, G. (2000) Self-image of adolescent survivors of long-term childhood leukemia. *J. Pediatr. Hematol. Oncol.* **22**(5), 417–421.

Manne, S., Redd, W.H., Jacobsen, P., Gorfunkle, K., Schorr, O., Rapkin, B. (1990) Behavioral intervention to reduce child and parent distress during venipuncture. *Journal of Clinical and Consulting Psychology* **58**, 565–572.

Manne, S.L., Du Hamel, K., Gallelli, K., Sorgen, K., Redd, W.H. (1998) Posttraumatic stress disorder among mothers of pediatric cancer survivors: diagnosis, comorbidity, and utility of the PTSD checklist as a screening instrument. *Journal of Pediatric Psychology* **23**, 357–366.

Meeske, K., Stuber, M.L. (2001) PTSD, Quality of life and psychological outcome in young adult survivors of pediatric cancer. *Oncology Nursing Forum* **28**(3), 481–489.

Mitby, P.A., Robison, L.L., Whitton, J.A., Zevon, M.A., Gibbs, I.C., Tersak, J.M., Meadows, A.T., Stovall, M., Zeltzer, L.K., Mertens, A.C., Childhood Cancer Survivor Study Steering Committee (2003) Utilization of special education services and educational attainment among long-term survivors of childhood cancer: a report from the Childhood Cancer Survivor Study. *Cancer* **97**(4), 1115–1126.

Murray, J.S. (2002) A qualitative exploration of psychosocial support for siblings of children with cancer. *J. Pediatr. Nurs.* **17**(5), 327–337.

Parker, R.I., Prakash, D., Mahan, R.A., Giugliano, D.M., Atlas, M.P. (2001) Randomized, double-blind, crossover, placebo-controlled trial of intravenous ondansetron for the prevention of intrathecal chemotherapy-induced vomiting in children. *J. Pediatr. Hematol. Oncol.* **23**(9), 578–581.

Pelcovitz, D., Goldenberg, B., Kaplan, S., Weinblatt, M., Mandel, F., Meyers, B., Vinciguerra, V. (1996) Posttraumatic stress disorder in mothers of pediatric cancer survivors. *Psychosomatics* **37**(2), 116–126.

Pelcovitz, D., Libov, B.G., Mandel, F., Kaplan, S., Weinblatt, M., Septimus, A. (1998) Posttraumatic stress disorder and family functioning in adolescent cancer. *Journal of Traumatic Stress* **11**(2), 205–221.

Phipps, S. (2002) Reduction of distress associated with paediatric bone marrow transplant: complementary health promotion interventions. *Pediatr. Rehabil.* **5**(4), 223–234.

Phipps, S., Fairclough, D., Mulhern, R.K. (1995) Avoidant coping in children with cancer. *J. Pediatr. Psychol.* **20**(2), 217–232.

Phipps, S., Srivastava, D.K. (1999) Approaches to the measurement of depressive symptomatology in children with cancer: Attempting to circumvent the effects of defensiveness. *Development and Behavioral Pediatrics* **20**(3), 150–156.

Powers, S.W. (1999) Empirically supported treatments in pediatric psychology: Procedure-related pain. *Journal of Pediatric Psychology* **24**(2), 131–145.

Smibert, E., Anderson, V., Godber, T., Ekert, H. (1996) Risk factors for intellectual and educational sequelae of cranial irradiation in childhood acute lymphoblastic leukaemia. *Br. J. Cancer* **73**(6), 825–830.

Stuber, M.L., Nader, K. (1995) Psychiatric sequelae in adolescent bone marrow transplant survivors: Implications for psychotherapy. *The Journal of Psychotherapy Practice and Research* **4**(1), 30–42.

Stuber, M.L., Meeske, K., Gonzalez, S., Houskamp, B., Pynoos, R. (1994) Traumatic stress after childhood cancer I: Response to treatment. *Psycho-Oncology* **3**, 305–312.

Stuber, M., Gonzalez, S., Benjamin, H., Golant, M. (1995) Fighting for recovery: Group interventions for adolescent with cancer patients and their parents. *The Journal of Psychotherapy Practice and Research* **4**, 286–296.

Stuber, M.L., Christakis, D., Houskamp, B.M., Kazak, A.E. (1996a) Post trauma symptoms in childhood leukemia survivors and their parents. *Psychosomatics* **37**, 254–261.

Stuber, M.L., Nader, K.O., Houskamp, B.M., Pynoos, R.S. (1996b) Appraisal of life threat and acute trauma responses in pediatric bone marrow transplant patients. *Journal of Traumatic Stress* **9**(4), 673–686.

Stuber, M.L., Kazak, A.E., Meeske, K., Barakat, L., Guthrie, D., Garnier, H., Pynoos, R.S., Meadows, A. (1997) Predictors of posttraumatic stress symptoms in childhood cancer survivors. *Pediatrics* **100**(6), 958–964.

Varni, J.W., Katz, E.R., Colegrove, R., Dolgin, M. (1994) Perceived social support and adjustment of children with newly diagnosed cancer. *Journal of Developmental and Behavioral Pediatrics* **15**, 20–26.

White, L., Daly, S.A., McKenna, C.J., Zhestkova, N., Leal, C., Breatnach, F., Smelhaus, V., Hung, I.J., Kowalczyk, J., Ninane, J., Mitchell, T., Haigh, C. (2000) A comparison of oral ondansetron syrup or intravenous ondansetron loading dose regimens given in combination with dexamethasone for the prevention of nausea and emesis in pediatric and adolescent patients receiving moderately/highly emetogenic chemotherapy. *Pediatr. Hematol. Oncol.* **17**(6), 445–455.

Worchel, F.F., Nolan, B.F., Wilson, V.L., Purser, J.S., Copeland, D.R., Pfefferbuam, B. (1988) Assessment of depression in children with cancer. *Journal of Pediatric Psychology* **13**, 101–112.

Worchel, F.F., Rae, W.A., Olson, T.K., Crowley, S.L. (1992) Selective responsiveness of chronically ill children to assessments of depression. *J. Pers. Assess.* **59**(3), 605–615.

Zebrack, B.J., Chesler, M.A. (2002) Quality of life in childhood cancer survivors. *Psychooncology* **11**(2), 132–141.

Zebrack, B.J., Zeltzer, L.K., Whitton, J., Mertens, A.C., Odom, L., Berkow, R., Robison, L.L. (2002) Psychological outcomes in long-term survivors of childhood leukemia, Hodgkin's disease, and non-Hodgkin's lymphoma: a report from the Childhood Cancer Survivor Study. *Pediatrics* **110**(1, Pt 1), 42–52.

Zeltzer, L.K., Altman, A., Cohen, D., LeBaron, S., Munuksela, E.L., Schechter, N.L. (1990) Report of the subcommittee on the management of pain associated with procedures in children with cancer. *Pediatrics* **86**, 826–833.

Zevon, M.A., Neubauer, N.A., Green, D.M. (1990) Adjustment and vocational satisfaction of patients treated during childhood or adolescence for acute lymphoblastic leukemia. *The American Journal of Pediatric Hematology/Oncology* **12**(4), 454–461.

9

The Family of the Child with Cancer

DAFNA MEITAR

Department of Behavioral Science, Sackler School of Medicine, Tel-Aviv University, Israel

Most families are not ready or prepared for a cancer diagnosis of their child; thus the diagnosis of cancer in a child is a crisis for the child and the family (Martinson and Cohen 1988, Binger *et al.* 1969). The family as a unit is shaken, as each individual is facing a new reality and has to relocate in the unit and re-examine self and relationships to the other family members – the parents to their sick child, to their other children to one another and to their own parents; the siblings to the sick child and other siblings, to their parents and grandparents; the sick child to his parents, siblings and grandparents. The grandparents have to face a new 'world order' with their children, the sick grandchild and the other grandchildren.

They all have to refer to the wider circle of their relationships including extended family members, friends, relatives, neighbors, school and others.

Despite recent advances in treatment of childhood malignancies that have dramatically altered survival rates, the 'word' cancer is associated with death, and for most people cancer cannot be associated with children (Grootenhuis and Last 1997). The life-threatening nature of the disease and its invasive treatment present both practical and emotional stresses for family members.

Dealing with fear becomes an inseparable part of life. Fear of death, of the unknown, of self-abilities and limitations. Family members have to deal with other's prejudice, ignorance and interference. Mostly they have to deal with the change in everyday life.

Being confronted with a diagnosis of childhood cancer in the family causes various emotional reactions. Those reactions change concomitantly with the different stages of treatment of the sick child.

Psychosocial Aspects of Pediatric Oncology. Edited by S. Kreitler and M. Weyl Ben Arush
© 2004 John Wiley & Sons Ltd: ISBN 0 471 49939 0

PARENTS

Receiving the Bad News

At first the parents are usually stunned and disbelieving at the outset, and there is an initial period of shock, confusion and numbness. There may be denial of the diagnosis, or intellectual acceptance without any emotional release (Binger *et al.* 1969).

Most parents experience uncertainty and helplessness due to loss of parental control and they initially relinquish control over the management of the disease. They do not want to be in control – but they need to know that someone is (doctors, God). They simply want to provide food, comfort and social experiences for their children (Martinson and Cohen, 1988). Trying to retrieve control, some parents get carried away trying to get as much information as possible. Being flooded with information – their feelings are blocked, bringing up feelings of guilt when they later deal with them. This stage is characterized by being overwhelmed with thoughts, fears and the need to *do* something.

Reorganization

During the period *after their child's diagnosis* of cancer, parents face a number of new demands. They must adapt not only to the threat of the death of their child and the need to provide him emotional support, but also to day-to-day disruptions that accompany an intensive, uncomfortable medical treatment regimen that is likely to involve inpatient hospitalization. They have to help their child cope with unpleasant and painful treatments and at the same time arrange medical or hospital appointments. As well, they must help maintain their own employment despite considerable disruption to personal and family routines. It is hardly surprising that many parents experience considerable distress during this period of time (Martinson and Cohen 1988, Sloper 2000). However, they are reluctant to acknowledge their distress because of concern that they may upset their sick child or because they feel guilty about the onset of their child's illness and their inability to shield their child from distressing and uncomfortable treatments (Sawyer *et al.* 1998). There is often guilt over a perceived delay in diagnosis and fear, for the siblings and themselves, that they will develop the same illness. Feelings of anger, sadness, depression, anxiety and inability to function are common, as well as insomnia and somatic and social dysfunctioning (Binger *et al.* 1969, Grootenhuis and Last 1997, Grossman 1998, Dahlquist *et al.* 1993, Magni *et al.* 1986, Manne *et al.* 1995).

Parents at this stage are confused regarding their relationships with the sick child. They question their own 'parenting' abilities and tend to develop a dual discipline for the other children and the ill child, becoming overprotective for the latter (Grossman 1998, Kübler-Ross 1983). This often worsens their relationships with their children, more so when they are teenagers.

Stabilization

During the following time of curative attempts for the sick child, family life stabilizes, as a new routine and reality is taking over.

Gradually parents reclaim control over the management of the disease – they know more about the disease and its effects and become more assertive advocates on the child's behalf (Martinson and Cohen 1988).

Different parents use various coping strategies. Some use a more 'practical' or 'doing' type of coping strategies – they keep seeking information and help and they look for problems to solve. Acquisition of information provides a sense of control because it allows an individual to assess the event and take action, such as participation in decision-making (Averill 1973). Others use a more 'emotional' type of coping – they are trying to maintain emotional balance, rely on religion, be optimistic and accepting, or use denial (Grootenhuis and Last 1997).

Some parents, although not religious, rely on praying and wishful thinking. They attribute special positive characteristics to the child as a proof that he is one of the survivors and are hoping for a miracle (Grootenhuis and Last 1997).

Women are reported to more often use religion and information-seeking, whereas men more often use denial (Grootenhuis and Last 1997). While some studies indicate that parents eventually cope well and can carry out daily tasks adequately (Grootenhuis and Last 1997, Sawyer *et al.* 2000, Hoekstra-Weebers *et al.* 1999, 2001, Brown *et al.* 1992, Kupst and Schulman 1988, Dahlquist, Czyzewski and Jones 1996), others find that parents continue to suffer from somatic and psychological symptoms and even psychiatric disturbances (Sloper 2000, Hoekstra-Weebers *et al.* 1999, Brown *et al.* 1992, 1993). Several demographic risk factors are mentioned: younger parents, parents of younger children, parents with lower occupational level, parents with less education, parents with lower socioeconomic status and low income, and those with religious affiliation (Grootenhuis and Last 1997, Hoekstra-Weebers *et al.* 1999, Sawyer *et al.* 2000, Kupst and Schulman 1988, Morrow, Carpenter and Hoagland 1984). Evidence on differences between mothers and fathers is inconclusive. Some studies report mothers are in higher risk of negative outcome than fathers (Sloper 2000, Dahlquist, Czyzewski and Jones 1996); but other find no difference (Speechley and Noh 1992). Trait anxiety is a risk factor for both mothers and fathers (Kazak *et al.* 1998).

In mothers a strong predictor of both the long term and the short-term psychological adjustment appears to be a personality characteristic. Mothers who use assertive behaviors less frequently with time are at risk (Hoekstra-Weebers *et al.* 1999).

End of Treatment

Upon *end of treatment* the parents have to face the difficulties of living with uncertainty and the possibility of recurrence over the longer term – most feel that life will never get back to normal (Martinson and Cohen 1988, Sloper 2000, Hoekstra-Weebers *et al.* 1999, 2001). Some show symptoms of post-traumatic stress disorder (Sloper 2000, Kazak *et al.* 1998). Parents may feel very dependent on the medical caregivers and question again their own parental abilities.

THE COUPLE

Adjustment is variable between individuals; thus each parent separately tries to cope with the situation. Cooperation between spouses is critical to manage the intense demands of this period and thus puts an enormous pressure on the couple as such. A considerable number of studies found an increased incidence of marital distress (Grootenhuis and Last 1997, Dahlquist *et al.* 1993, Lansky *et al.* 1978) and impaired sexual relationships after diagnosis (Grootenhuis and Last 1997, Hughes and Lieberman 1990).

The greater the difference in anxiety level between parents, the greater the reported marital distress (Dahlquist *et al.* 1993).

Overall adequate family coping is reflected in stable marital status (Sawyer *et al.* 2000).

Families with strong relationships are more likely to become stronger as a result of the illness, in contrast to families with a previously disputable marriage that report worsening in relationships (Grootenhuis and Last 1997, Sloper 2000). Despite the pressure no higher divorce rates are reported (Grootenhuis and Last 1997, Lansky *et al.* 1978).

SINGLE-PARENT FAMILIES

For a single-parent family the burden of care is much heavier. Loneliness is accentuated and previous choices are re-contemplated. There is no one to share responsibility, despair and change in life routine with. Immediate need for help is raised, especially if there is more than one child in the family. This burden usually falls on grandparents, if they are available, and the extended family is much more involved. This often brings up again old controversy regarding life-style choices. There are no controlled studies looking at the mechanisms single parents use in dealing with this crisis, nor at the outcome.

SIBLINGS

Siblings have been described as the most emotionally forgotten and afflicted of all family members during severe childhood illness (Murray 1995, 1999a, 2000).

Objective

During the course of their brother or sister's illness, siblings feel left out and suffer. Their stress is similar to or even more intense than the sick child's (Spinetta *et al*. 1999, Kramer and Moore 1983). Without any ill-intention on the part of already overburdened and concerned parents, siblings are often inadvertently ignored. Siblings have feelings of isolation because their parents perforce are frequently at the hospital and gone from home and they are left in the care of others with the immediate family not there. The preoccupation with the sick child limits the parent's ability to attend to and support the needs of the healthy children in the family (Spinetta *et al*. 1999, Kramer and Moore 1983).

Studies have found that the healthy children experience drastic changes in their relationship with parents, the ill sibling, extended family members, and friends. They complain about diminished parental physical and emotional availability (Murray 1999a, Kramer and Moore 1983). Also the ill child receives preferential treatment, with parents tending to be more lenient in discipline as well as overindulgent and overprotective (Kübler-Ross 1983, Kramer and Moore 1983, Hilden, Watterson and Chrastek 2000). Sometimes this is interpreted as rejection of themselves (Binger *et al*. 1969).

Consequently, sibling rivalry intensifies with the healthy siblings feeling jealous and resentful of this inequitable treatment. The healthy siblings are reticent about confronting their parents. They fear that complaining will worsen the situation (Kramer and Moore 1983). Siblings are reported to be ashamed of these negative feelings, expressing guilt for being the 'healthy one' and maybe causing the illness, which in itself denies them the right to complain (Kübler-Ross 1983, Kramer and Moore 1983). These internalized feelings of shame and guilt can be tormenting, especially when intensified by fears of the ill child's possible death.

Although the disease and therapy directly involves the ill child, it also has a significant impact on the well child. Dramatic physical changes such as amputation or hair loss are extremely frightening to witness.

Having a sibling with cancer labels the family as being 'different', causing the healthy siblings embarrassment and frustration over answering endless questions about the ill child's condition.

Siblings Response at Time of Illness

Siblings of children with cancer feel jealousy, anger and confusion. They wonder if their family will be the same again. They sometimes hate and resent their sick sib and feel everybody is not sensitive to their need (Kübler-Ross 1983, Murray 1995). Siblings have to adapt to the change in the family's routines. Sometimes because of income changes the financial situation changes which demands further adaptation (Spinetta *et al.* 1999).

Studies show variably that one-quarter to one-half of siblings of children with cancer had experienced problems in behavioral adjustment and had negative changes in their behavior, either at home or at school, since the diagnosis (Binger *et al.* 1969, Sloper and While 1996). They often have somatic complaints and symptoms (eye-blinking, head-tilting tics), significant anxiety, periods of depression and acting-out behavior (Murray 1999a, Hilden, Watterson and Chrastek 2000). Problems described also include an onset of enuresis, headaches, poor school performance, school phobia, severe separation anxiety, and persistent abdominal pains (Binger *et al.* 1969).

School experiences can change both ways. Academic functioning can decline because of illness-related distractions and a general state of anxiety. Conversely, performance can improve. The healthy children may immerse themselves in their schoolwork to fill the void left by a decrease in family involvement. They experience changes in their relationships with their classmates. Initially friends, not knowing what to say or fearing that cancer is contagious, often make themselves scarce. Out of fear and ignorance, insensitive teasing can occur, which intensifies feelings of isolation (Kramer and Moore, 1983).

Communication

Siblings tend to fear the worst, even for their own health. They sometimes believe the medical staff is trying to kill their sib (Binger *et al.* 1969, Hilden, Watterson and Chrastek 2000). When parents and members of the healthcare team attempt in good faith to shield the siblings from knowledge about the illness, such well-intentioned hiding of the truth often drives the siblings to fear even worse possibilities, and can lead to feelings of isolation, guilt and resentment. Their fears will never be addressed if they are not included in discussions of, for example, why a certain procedure is being done.

This is even more pertinent when siblings are to be tested for potential bone marrow donation. They should have the reasons explained in detail, including the option for rejection of the graft regardless of its 'quality'.

GRANDPARENTS

Grandparents are expected to take an active role in the life of their son/daughter/in-law's families when a grandchild becomes sick. They are the 'natural' supporters. It is much a matter of culture and geography how much a grandparent was involved in the life of the sick child's family until the moment of illness; however, when a grandchild has a cancer a grandparent is expected and usually wishes to be involved. The new situation brings turmoil for the 'older parents'.

They might not have been in good terms with their own child/in-law, but this is not foreseen to matter. They are maybe very busy with their own life – work, business, and social commitments. They might be preoccupied with their own health problems or their spouse's – but are expected to be available for assistance.

Physical changes are much harder in advanced age. Helping often means relocating – to their grandchild's house or to another nearby relative, or even staying in the hospital overnight.

Grandparents are expected to find the delicate balance between helping and not being 'too much', not being another burden for the little reorganizing family. How much is enough and how much is too much?

Grandparents are expected to support and not bring their own additional worries. They feel they have the right to know, but since they are not the primary guardians they are not getting direct information unless the parents of the child consent. They are trying to replace the absent parents at home, and in doing it are confronted with the anger and despair of the siblings of the sick child. They are often blamed by the other grandchildren for not being as good as the parent at anything – cooking, making beds, reading stories, driving.

They feel very lonely and are expected to be the strongest, the wisest and the advice-givers.

FAMILY-ORIENTED TREATMENT PLAN

The challenge of treating a child with cancer is far beyond cure of the disease. The treatment plan has to be holistic in approach, consider the individual family, and include comprehensive support for the family. This approach is important, not only for the sick child who trusts his parents first and will benefit from a strong, cohesive and united family, but also for the family members themselves. Each one of them is facing a crisis, and relating to their mental, physical and spiritual needs is an acute as well as preventive medical care.

Parents

Often, in the pediatric setting, the primary focus is on reducing the child's anxiety and on providing parents with information to function collaboratively in their child's care. It is also important to address parents' anxiety during treatment and, given the long-term impact of anxiety, parents may benefit from specific interventions after treatment ends (Kazak *et al.* 1998).

The initial consultation has a significantly important role in the way the family will further cope with the new crisis. One of the most important goals is establishing effective communication with the parents – it is crucial for the effective care and, even more so, later on if and when palliative care becomes necessary (Stevens 1998). A team approach at the initial conference provides an opportunity for the family to know the care-takers and for health professionals to know the family.

One has to remember that on receiving the diagnosis the child's parents sometimes assume the worst: that their child is certainly going to die soon. Clear explanation can help reduce confusion and help the parents to readjust expectations to a more hopeful level in keeping with the child's actual prognosis (Stevens 1998).

The parent's emotional state at time of initial consultation does not allow a full taking in and comprehension of the information given, so facts should be provided on a continuous basis (Chesler and Barbarin 1984). While the way information is being delivered is very much dependent on an individual's style, the content of what is said needs to consider that some parents are reluctant to discuss certain issues. Among the more sensitive topics are: side effects, statistics of success and failure, relapse, research, testicular biopsies, emotional effects of cancer on the patient and parents, discipline, family stress, and coping with painful procedures (Wells *et al.* 1990).

Aiming to minimize distress, a clear layout at the treatment center and the availability of friendly, non-clinical areas for children and parents are important to emphasize. The availability of 24-hour telephone support by staff who are familiar with the children and the provision of accommodation for the children and parents who must live away from home are helpful as well (Sawyer *et al.* 2000).

An important component of the initial consultation is making a conscious effort to encourage parents to continue to be the primary caregiver for their child. Through the active treatment period parents should be consulted about the best way to make the child comfortable for procedures and treatments. They also should be given the opportunity to have a special, specific role in preparing the child for procedures and in supporting the child during and after these procedures. It helps when the hospital staff is honest with the parents about what the child is going to experience and gives them some choices about how they can be involved (Grossman 1998). Decisions during all stages of treatment are best made collaboratively; thus information delivered needs to be clear, accurate and current (Pyke-Grimm *et al.* 1999). Information giving must be individualized to the needs of the family, probably as determined by ongoing evaluation and assessment of the family's needs.

While communicating with the parents, caregivers need to be aware of the changing needs at different stages of disease. Parents become less patient as time goes by. They feel tired and are very sensitive to resentment. They may become very demanding and caregivers have to be prepared accordingly (Martinson and Cohen 1988).

During the highly stressful initial diagnostic and treatment period it is important to consider their personal needs as well as the marital unit when assessing parental adjustment (Dahlquist *et al.* 1993). A failure to identify parents in distress and to provide them with adequate support may, in the long term, significantly disadvantage the sick child as well as the whole family (Sawyer *et al.* 1998). The continuation of high levels of distress over time for a number of parents points to the importance of interventions to identify those at risk in the early treatment stages and of the provision of ongoing support. Such support could usefully focus on the important resources that can help parents withstand the stresses of the illness: family relationships and appraisal, that is, their feelings about the demands of the illness and their ability to deal with these demands.

It is worth recalling that fathers in particular are reporting difficulties in accessing support at all stages (Sloper 2000).

THE VALUE OF SUPPORT – RESOURCES AND PLANNING

Sources for support varies for different individuals – parents turn to each other, to the physician, sometimes to clergy, social workers, parents of other sick children.

One variable that may help explain why some parents adjust well whereas others are more at risk is social support. Studies supporting the stress-moderating role of social support show that a higher level of perceived support is related to lower levels of psychological distress for parents of children after diagnosis and during treatment (Grootenhuis and Last 1997, Sloper 2000, Magni *et al.* 1986, Kupst and Schulman 1988, Morrow, Carpenter and Hoagland 1984). However the relationship between perceived family and extra-familial support and post-traumatic stress disorders for parents of childhood cancer survivors is unclear (Hoekstra-Weebers *et al.* 2001, Speechley and Noh 1992).

In planning support we need to recall that parents receive the most support around the time of diagnosis. This support may be considered a crisis support. They get less support during the time they are coping with the more chronic stress (Hoekstra-Weebers *et al.* 2001).

Parents groups are a very useful means of helping parents in sharing and expressing their feelings, fears and hopes. It enables 'legitimization' of bad and unspoken feelings.

Supporting Siblings

Clearly the healthy siblings of cancer patients have a unique set of problems with which they have to cope. However, research has shown that there are barriers to providing support to siblings of children with cancer such as staff issues, access to siblings, institutional constraints, and the role boundary issues (Murray 1999b).

Supportive therapy for siblings should be considered an essential aspect of total care of the family. Members of the healthcare team and parents should involve the siblings from the beginning, keep them informed – taking into account the sibling's social, emotional, and cognitive capacity – with written, audio, and/or video material through the different phases of the disease. It should be explained to them that they were in no way responsible for causing the cancer.

Parents should be encouraged to participate more in their 'other' children activities, include them in the discussions of the diagnosis and keep them informed thereafter. Siblings should be offered the opportunity to actively participate in the patient's care. They should be brought to the hospital to see their sib. Emphasizing the positive and optimistic sides of treatment should be encouraged (Binger *et al.* 1969, Spinetta *et al.* 1999, Kramer and Moore 1983).

Siblings should have opportunities to talk about implications of the disease, especially worries about death.

Parents should be encouraged to take turns staying at the hospital or at home with the patient.

Siblings groups can effect an exceptionally high level of understanding and support.

Supporting Grandparents

Grandparents benefit considerably from an early consultation with the child's physician, undertaken under the parents' consent. This allows clarifying and dealing with questions and misconceptions such as irrational guilt.

Acknowledging their important role and suggesting modes of help alleviates conflicts. Grandparents as well can benefit from group support.

SHARING INFORMATION WITH THE SICK CHILD

This important issue has a tremendous influence over family's dynamics. The subject should be raised as part of the family's planning. Parents have to decide whether and how much they should share information with the ill child. There are two different approaches: the 'protective' and the 'open'. The first one is trying to shield the young child from full knowledge of the disease. It talks about unnecessarily elevating the child's anxieties and fears. It is based on the assumption that young children are very concrete thinkers, without conceptual schemas for processing abstract notions about extended illness. Therefore a disclosure of the diagnosis and prognosis is not necessary. Supporters of this approach also argue that the frightening reality of the diagnosis/prognosis should not be allowed to interfere with a calm and normal family life (Chesler, Paris and Barbarin 1986). Also it is claimed that by protecting children from knowledge of their illness parents could delay their own loss of authority, continue to play the role of responsible parent, and preserve family integrity and privacy.

The open approach suggests that shielding the children does not necessarily alleviate anxiety or fear but may even heighten these emotions (Waechter 1971). When the children know but their parents do not want them to, they experience isolation and loneliness which is complicated by the lack of meaningful communication and candor (Binger 1969, Chesler, Paris and Barbarin 1986, Spinetta, Rigler and Karon 1973). Moreover parents cannot control what the child hears once he leaves the hospital to meet with friends and in school. The presence of older siblings is another cause for 'telling the child' because of the possibility that something will leak out (Chesler, Paris and Barbarin 1986). Many practitioners argue that the family's energy and time can be spent better in dealing honestly with the illness and related feelings than in maintaining an unreal facade of normality. As Issner (1973) points out: 'In denying the child an honest relationship, we deny him the opportunity for hope. An air of mystery implies reason for despair'.

There is data to suggest that open communication may be related to better psychological and emotional adjustment for the ill child and siblings (Chesler, Paris and Barbarin 1986). The 'open' approach is usually used more by older parents and by parents with more children (Chesler, Paris and Barbarin 1986).

Sharing information is a family process and is developing with time and events (Chesler, Paris and Barbarin 1986). Whatever approach the family chooses it should be honored by caregivers and delivered to the sick child.

WHEN THE CHILD IS DYING

As the children's cancer advances, parents' understanding that the child no longer has a realistic chance for cure is usually delayed. Although nearly all parents report having a discussion at some point with a medical caregiver about their child having no realistic chance for cure, only 49% report that they have come to understand that their child was terminally ill through the discussion (Wolfe *et al.* 2000).

As the terminal phase of the illness progresses, parents are faced with the inevitable death of their child. Parents are confronted with the decision of whether to continue treatment with investigational drugs to treat the disease, to continue extraordinary life-support measures, or to choose the cessation of treatment (Ross-Alaolmolki 1985). The stresses created by these decisions on an already strained family system may lead to major physical and psychosocial difficulties for various family members. Some families do not want to 'give up' and see it as an obligation to the child to fight off death at all costs. Some, although not choosing to go on, need reassurance that everything possible has been done, to enable them to live with the decision they have made (Vickers and Carlisle 2000).

Living with a dying child impacts on each family member and can have long-term disruptive effects on the family system, such as divorce, separation, depression, and an increased incidence of alcoholism (Ross-Alaolmolki 1985, Heller and Schnider 1978). A series of interrelated and interdependent processes takes place during anticipatory mourning in parents of children with a life-threatening illness. Parents of children with cancer have been observed to experience the following processes: (1) Acknowledgement, in which parents are struggling between hope and despair with an intensifying awareness as they realize the death of the child is inevitable. (2) Grieving, which fluctuates in intensity throughout the child's illness. Parents manifest all aspects of 'anticipatory' grief reactions: intellectualization, irritability, depression, somatization, denial and frenzied activity. (3) Reconciliation, which involves reconstructing the child's past and present life and helps the parents reaffirm the value of the child's life. (4) Detachment, which, depending on the parent's concept of the child's life expectancy, may include gradual withdrawal or becoming involved in other relationships. (5) Memorialization, a process by which memories of the ill child become fixed and idealized (Futterman and Hoffman 1973).

Parents protect themselves and others in an attempt to maintain normal family functioning and relationships. They will avoid crying in front of their children, or expressing anger to the care-takers. They will even avoid expressing their doubts, fears or anxieties to each other in a fruitless effort to shield the other from pain and feelings of loss (Ross-Alaolmolki 1985). These same responses may be the cause of misunderstanding and pain in the partner, the ill child, and the siblings (Ross-Alaolmolki 1985, Bluebond-Langner 1978).

The terminal nature of the illness confronts the parents with decisions relating to whether the child is to be kept in the hospital or taken home to die in the comfort of the family environment. Home care for dying children is reported to be both a feasible and desirable alternative to hospitalization during the final days (Vickers and Carlisle 2000, Martinson 1978, Mulhern, Lauer and Hoffmann 1983, Lauer *et al.* 1985).

Home keeps the family together. For most families, palliative home care facilitates the 'deprofessionalization' of dying, with the family providing the main source of care for the child (Vickers and Carlisle 2000).

Home care has a major impact upon parental adaptation following a child's death. Parents providing home care for their dying child indicate a reduction in guilt and content for being able to treat their child (Lauer *et al.* 1983).

Caregivers, who can provide alternative decisions for families, facilitate the maintenance of control. The process of selecting alternatives provides families with an opportunity to develop and enhance their sense of mastery during a time when they feel they have a very little control.

Parents raise questions and concerns surrounding the actual death of the child. Questions are often related to how the child will die, whether or not the child will be alert or in pain. At this stage parents become increasingly dissatisfied with the quality and quantity of the information they are given (Martinson and Cohen 1988).

Caregivers can facilitate the family's capacity to ask questions and can encourage open communication between family members and caregivers.

Parents frequently ask whether the child is aware or knows of his impending death. Research has shown that children with a life-threatening illness are aware that theirs is no ordinary illness (Bluebond-Langner 1978, Waechter 1971, Spinetta, Rigler and Karon 1973, Ross-Alaolmolki 1985, Vickers and Carlisle 2000). They can sense the extraordinary stress of their parents and doctors when death is imminent. They may feel tremendous isolation if they are not given permission to talk openly about their illness and impending death (Hilden, Watterson and Chrastek 2000, Faulkner 1997, Whittam 1993). When given the opportunity to communicate, children can conquer their fears as well as express their love (Hilden, Watterson and Chrastek 2000). Families that speak about the disease and prognosis feel a more meaningful relation with the child.

Parents may indicate an intense need to talk about the child, including his physical appearance (this is not the child I know – due to steroids, progressive disabilities etc.). The caregiver must be accepting and make the parents feel free to speak in a safe environment.

At the dying phase, mothers have reported a greater degree of difficulty with the problems of helplessness, loss of confidence in the ability to be a good parent, financial difficulties. Also being avoided by others, growing apart from their spouse, and fear of being unable to cope if the child should die. Fathers report significantly greater difficulty with two problems: feeling left out of the ill child's life and being worried that their spouse was too preoccupied with the dead child (Black 1998).

AFTER THE DEATH OF A CHILD

A child who is dying shapes the texture of the family in many different ways. Thus, each person's response to a potential or impending loss is an expression of one's own coping style, as that person tries to make meaning out of the loss.

Parents

Parents of children that have died suffer general malaise, an inability to return to normal functioning, continued apathy and feelings of sadness and an inability to confront reminders of the child and to plan for the future. They demonstrate significantly poorer adjustment in their extended family relationships and domestic environment, as well as in their overall psychosocial adjustment (Morrow, Carpenter and Hoagland 1984, Heller and Schnider 1978). Sometimes, serious medical problems arise: hypertension, ulcers, somatic complaints, colitis and obesity. Many parents manifest morbid grief reactions that can include daily visits to the cemetery, refusing to refer to the dead child, depression. There are work-related problems – although most stay in the same job – school difficulties and marital discord. An increased divorce rate is reported (Ross-Alaolmolki 1985, Heller and Schnider 1978, Lauer *et al.* 1983).

Three factors were found to be predictive of good post-death adjustment: (1) The availability of ongoing support from a 'significant other'. (2) The adherence to a philosophy of life within which the diagnosis and its implications could be accepted. (3) An awareness that the deceased child had received information and emotional support at a level consistent with its questions, age and stage of development (Pettle and Lansdown 1986). Social support is not found beneficial (Morrow, Carpenter and Hoagland 1984).

Parents may feel that they can never recover fully from the loss of a child. For some parents, the new identity is a stronger one – they feel they have been through 'the fire' and that nothing can affect them so profoundly again. The cost may be a reduction in their sensitivity to their other children or partner that may threaten the marriage or even disrupt it (Black 1998).

Siblings

An array of emotional and behavioral sequels have been reported in siblings of a child that has died. These children are at increased risk for developing severe psychological and behavioral problems. These include disturbed ego functioning and identity problems, poor self-concept while idealizing the dead sibling, guilt-laden reactions, death phobias, and character distortions. Other major symptoms are feelings of loneliness, sadness, sleep disturbances, increased physical demands, and loss of parental availability (Murray 1999a, Pettle and Lansdown 1986, Cobb 1956).

Teachers report that these siblings are often worried, have poor concentration, tend to do things alone, are very restless, and are not liked by other children. This leads to poor school performance (Binger *et al.* 1969, Murray 1999a, Pettle and Lansdown 1986).

In psychiatric patients that have lost a sibling, reported reactions had a heavy emphasis on guilt including depression, withdrawal, and accident-prone and constant acting-out behaviors (Murray 1999a).

Research indicates the importance of preparing children for a sibling's death. Siblings have the ability to comprehend such information; and the fact is that the bereavement period is eased if siblings receive such preparation (Lauer *et al.* 1985, Spinetta *et al.* 1999, Hilden, Watterson and Chrastek 2000). Many parents choose not to inform children about their brother or sister's terminal status. Preparation for the death is a crucial factor in facilitating children's adjustment (Murray 1999a, Lauer *et al.* 1985, Hilden, Watterson and Chrastek 2000).

Children who have participated in home care describe a significantly different experience than those whose sibling died in hospital. The majority of home care children reported that they were prepared for the impending death, received consistent information and support from their parents, were involved in most activities concerning the dying child, were present for the death, and viewed their own involvement as the most important aspect of the experience. Non-home care children generally described themselves as having been inadequately prepared for the death, isolated from the dying child and their parents, unable to use their parents for support or information, unclear as to the circumstances of death, and useless in terms of their own involvement (Kübler-Ross 1983, Lauer *et al.* 1985).

Grandparents

Grandparents expect to predecease their grandchildren even more than parents expect to predecease their children. Since grandparents are also parents, many of the issues pertinent to bereaved parents are conspicuous for bereaved grandparents. However, grandparents' grief is threefold in that they must grieve for their deceased grandchild, their son or daughter who parented the child, and themselves (Reed 2000, Ponzetti 1992). Grandparent's hopes and dreams are often being fulfilled through the grandchildren. Death of a grandchild kills the hope for immortality through continuity.

The time after the death of the grandchild can be a source for tension between grandparents and their children. They may feel not important because they are not considered with the funeral arrangements, they do not know many of the visiting friends and neighbors and they feel their sadness is not important. Grandparents express guilt over being unable to help their child. They feel isolation and, often resentment (Reed 2000). During the bereavement period grandparents can become a burden but in many families they offer considerable support (Binger 1969).

Similar to parents, grandparents too experience physical symptoms following the child's death. Insomnia or some other sleep disturbance are mentioned most often (Ponzetti 1992).

Those grandparents who have coped well during the child's illness will also cope more successfully with bereavement after the child's death (Stevens 1998). Therefore it is very important to include grandparents in the family's plan of support during and after the bereavement period.

REFERENCES

Averill, J. (1973) Personal control over aversive stimuli and its relationship to stress. *Psychological Bulletin* **80**, 286–303.

Binger, C.M., Ablin, A.R., Feurstein, R.C., Kushner, J.H., Zoger, S., Mikklesen, C. (1969) Childhood leukemia. *New Engl. J. Med.* **280**, 414–418.

Black, D. (1998) The dying child. *BMJ* **316**(7141), 1376–1378.

Bluebond-Langner, M. (1978) *The Private Worlds of Dying Children.* Princeton, NJ: Princeton University Press.

Brown, R.T., Kaslow, N.J., Hazzard, P., Madan-Swain, A., Sexson, S.B., Lambert, R., Baldwin, K. (1992) Psychiatric and family functioning in children with leukemia and their parents. *J. Am. Acad. Child Adolesc. Psychiatry* **31**, 495–502.

Brown, R.T., Kaslow, N.J., Madan-Swain, A., Doepke, K.J., Sexon, S.B., Hill, L.J. (1993) Parental psychopathology and children's adjustment to leukemia. *J. Am. Acad. Child Psychiatry* **32**, 554–561.

Chesler, M.A., Barbarin, O.A. (1984) Difficulties of providing help in a crisis: relationships between parents and children with cancer and their friends. *Journal of Social Issues* **40**, 113–134.

Chesler, M.A., Paris, J., Barbarin, O.A. (1986) 'Telling' the child with cancer: Parents choices to share information with ill children. *J. Pediatr. Psychol.* **11**, 497–515.

Cobb, B. (1956) Psychological impact of long illness and death of a child on the family circle. *Journal of Pediatrics* **49**, 746–751.

Dahlquist, L.M., Czyzewski, D.I., Copeland, K.G., Jones, C.L., Taub, E., Vaughan, J.K. (1993) Parents of children newly diagnosed with cancer: anxiety, coping and marital stress. *Journal of Pediatric Psychology* **18**, 365–376.

Dahlquist, L.M., Czyzewski, D.I., Jones, C.L. (1996) Parents of children with cancer: a longitudinal study of emotional distress, coping style, and marital adjustment two and twenty months after diagnosis. *J. Pediatr. Psychol.* **21**, 541–554.

Faulkner, K.W. (1997) Talking about death with a dying child. *Am. J. Nurs.* **97**, 64–69.

Futterman, E.H., Hoffman, I. (1973) Crisis and adaptation in the families of fatally ill children. In Anthony, E. and Koupernick, C. (Eds) *The Child in his Family: the impact of disease and death.* New York: John Wiley.

Grootenhuis, M.A., Last, B.F. (1997) Adjustment and coping by parents of children with cancer: a review of the literature. *Support Care Cancer* **5**, 466–484.

Grossman, L.S. (1998) Understanding anger in parents of dying children. *Am. Fam. Physician* **58**(5), 1211–1212.

Heller, D.B., Schnider, C.D. (1978) Interpersonal methods for coping with stress: helping families of dying children. *Omega* **8**, 319–330.

Hilden, J.M., Watterson, J., Chrastek, J. (2000) Tell the children. *JCO* **18**(17), 3193–3195.

Hoekstra-Weebers, J.E., Jaspers, J.P., Kamps, W.A., Klip, E.C. (1999) Risk factors for psychological maladjustment of parents of children with cancer. *J. Am. Acad. Child Adolesc. Psychiatry* **38**(12), 1526–1535.

Hoekstra-Weebers, J.E., Jaspers, J.P., Kamps, W.A., Klip, E.C. (2001) Psychological adaptation and social support of parents of pediatric cancer patients: a prospective longitudinal study. *J. Pediatr. Psychol.* **26**(4), 225–235.

Hughes, P.M., Lieberman, S. (1990) Troubled parents: vulnerability and stress in childhood cancer. *Br. J. Med. Psychol.* **63**, 53–64.

Issner, N. (1973) Can the child be distracted from his disease? *Journal of School Health* **43**, 468–471.

Kazak, A.E., Stuber, M.L., Barakat, L.P., Meeske, K., Guthrie, D., Meadows, A.T. (1998) Predicting post traumatic stress symptoms in mothers and fathers of survivors of childhood cancers. *J. Am. Acad. Child Adolesc. Psychiatry* **37**(8), 823–831.

Kramer, R.F., Moore, I.M. (1983) Childhood cancer: meeting the special needs of healthy siblings. *Cancer Nurs.* **6**, 213–217.

Kübler-Ross, E. (1983) *On Children and Death*. New York: Touchstone.

Kupst, M., Schulman, J. (1988) Long-term coping with pediatric leukemia: a six year follow-up study. *Journal of Pediatric Psychology* **13** 7–22.

Lansky, S.B., Cairns, N.U., Hassanein, R., Wehr, J., Owman, J.T. (1978) Childhood cancer: Parental discord and divorce. *Pediatrics* **62**, 184–188.

Lauer, M.E., Mulhern, R.K., Bohne, J.B., Camitta, B.M. (1985) Children's perception of their sibling's death at home or hospital: The precursors of differential adjustment. *Cancer Nurs.* **8**, 21–27.

Lauer, M.E., Mulhern, R.K., Wallskog, J.M., Camitta, B.M. (1983) A comparison study of parental adaptation following a child's death at home or in the hospital. *Pediatrics* **71**, 107–112.

Magni, G., Silvestro, A., Carli, M., De Leo, D. (1986) Social support and psychological distress of parents of children with acute lymphocytic leukaemia. *Br. J. Med. Psychol.* **59**, 383–385.

Manne, S.L., Lesanics, D., Meyers, P., Wollner, N., Steinhertz, P., Redd, W. (1995) Predictors of depressive symptomatology among parents of newly diagnosed children with cancer. *J. Pediatr. Psychol.* **20** 491–510.

Martinson, I.M. (1978) Home care for children dying of cancer. *Pediatrics* **62**, 106–113.

Martinson, I.M., Cohen, M.H. (1988) Themes from a longitudinal study of family reactions to childhood cancer. *J. Psychosoc. Oncol.* **6**, 81–98.

Mulhern, R.K., Lauer, M.E., Hoffmann, R.G. (1983) Death of a child at home or in the hospital: subsequent psychological adjustment of the family. *Pediatrics* **71**(5), 743–747.

Morrow, G.R., Carpenter, P.J., Hoagland, A.C. (1984) The role of social support in parental adjustment to pediatric cancer. *Journal of Pediatric Psychology* **9**, 317–329.

Murray, J.S. (1995) Social support for siblings of children with cancer. *J. Pediatr. Oncol. Nurs.* **12**(2), 62–70.

Murray, J.S. (1999a) Siblings of children with cancer: a review of the literature. *J. Pediatr. Oncol. Nurs.* **16**(1), 25–34.

Murray, J.S. (1999b) Methodological triangulation in a study of social support for siblings of children with cancer. *J. Pediatr. Oncol. Nurs.* **16**(4), 194–200.

Murray, J.S. (2000) Development of two instruments measuring social support for siblings of children with cancer. *J. Pediatr. Oncol. Nurs.* **17**(4), 229–238.

Pettle Michael, S.A., Lansdown, R.G. (1986) Adjusment to the death of sibling. *Arch. Dis. Child* **61**, 278–283.

Ponzetti, J.J. (1992) Bereaved families: a comparison of parent's and grandparent's reactions to the death of a child. *Omega* **25**(1), 63–71.

Pyke-Grimm, K.A., Degner, L., Small, A., Mueller, B. (1999) Preferences for participation in treatment decision making and information needs of parents of children with cancer: a pilot study. *J. Pediatric Oncology Nursing* **16**(1), 13–24.

Reed, Mary Lou (2000) *Grandparents Cry Twice*. Baywood Publishing Company, Inc., Amityville, NY.

Ross-Alaolmolki, K. (1985) Supportive care for families of dying children. *Nurs. Clin. North America* **20**, 457–467.

Sawyer, M., Antoniou, G., Toogood, I., Rice, M., Baghurst, P. (2000) Childhood cancer: a 4-year prospective study of the psychological adjustment of children and parents. *J. Pediatr. Hematol. Oncol.* **22**(3), 214–220.

Sawyer, M.G., Streiner, D.L., Antoniou, G., Toogood, I., Rice, M. (1998) Influence of parental and family adjustment on the later psychological adjustment of children treated for cancer. *J. Am. Acad. Child. Adolesc. Psychiatry* **37**(8), 815–822.

Sloper, P. (2000) Predictors of distress in parents of children with cancer: a prospective study. *J. Pediatr. Psychol.* **25**(2), 79–91.

Sloper, P., While, D. (1996) Risk factors in the adjustment of siblings of children with cancer. *J. Child Psychol. Psychiatry* **37**(5), 597–607.

Speechley, K.N., Noh, S. (1992) Surviving childhood cancer, social support, and parents' psychological adjustment. *Journal of Pediatric Psychology* **17**, 15–31.

Spinetta, J.J., Jancovic, M., Eden T., Green, D., Martins, A.G., Wandzura, C., Wilbur, J., Masera, G. (1999) Guidelines for assistance to siblings of children with cancer: report of the SIOP working committee on psychosocial issues in pediatric oncology. *Medical and Pediatric Oncology* **33**, 395–398.

Spinetta, J.J., Rigler, D., Karon, M. (1973) Anxiety in the dying child. *Pediatrics* **52**, 841–845.

Stevens, M.M. (1998) Care of the dying child and adolescent: family adjustment and support. In Doyle, D., Hanks, G.W.C., MacDonald, N. (Eds) *Oxford Textbook of Palliative Medicine*. New York: Oxford University Press, pp. 1057–1075.

Vickers, J.L., Carlisle, C. (2000) Choices and control: parental experiences in pediatric terminal home care. *Journal of Pediatric Oncology Nursing* **17**(1), 12–21.

Waechter, E.H. (1971) Children's awareness of fatal illness. *Am. J. Nurs.* **71**, 1168–1172.

Wells, L.M., Heiney, S.P., Swygert, F., Troficanto, G., Stokes, C., Ettinger, R.S. (1990) Psychosocial stressors, coping resources and informational needs of parents of adolescent cancer patients. *J. Pediatr. Oncol. Nurs.* **7**, 145–148.

Whittam, E.H. (1993) Terminal care of the dying child. *Cancer* **71**, 3450–3462.

Wolfe, J., Klar, N., Grier, H.E., Duncan, J., Salem-Schatz, S., Emanuel, E.J., Weeks, J.C. (2000) Understanding of prognosis among parents of children who died of cancer. *JAMA* **284**, 2469–2475.

10

Psychosocial Effects of Hematopoietic Cell Transplantation in Children

RONIT ELHASID

Pediatric Hematology Oncology Department, Meyer Children's Hospital, Rambam Medical Center, Haifa, Israel

MICHAL M. KREITLER

Psychooncology Unit, Tel Aviv Medical Center, Tel Aviv, Israel

SHULAMITH KREITLER

Pychooncology Unit, Tel Aviv Medical Center, and Psychology Department, Tel Aviv University, Tel Aviv, Israel

MYRIAM WEIL BEN ARUSH

Pediatric Hematology Oncology Department, Meyer Children's Hospital, Rambam Medical Center, Technion Faculty of Medicine, Haifa, Israel

INTRODUCTION: OUTLINES OF THE PROCEDURE

Stem cell transplantation (SCT) is an established treatment of many malignant and non-malignant hematological, hereditary and immunological diseases. The widespread use of SCT in the treatment of a steadily increasing number of life-threatening disorders is the culmination of over four decades of research by a great number of investigators. The first successful allogeneic transplants (i.e., SCT from a donor) of hematopoietic stem cells were done in 1968 in three children with congenital immunodeficiency diseases (Bach *et al.* 1968). Since

Psychosocial Aspects of Pediatric Oncology. Edited by S. Kreitler and M. Weyl Ben Arush
© 2004 John Wiley & Sons Ltd: ISBN 0 471 49939 0

then, thousands of patients have received SCT to treat life-threatening malignant and non-malignant diseases.

Hematopoietic stem cells are the most important stem cells needed for successful transplantation. These cells can be harvested from the bone marrow and more recently from peripheral blood. Rapid hematopoietic recovery was shown after peripheral blood stem cell transplantation as compared with bone marrow transplantation (BMT) (Bensinger *et al.* 2001). Stem cells are taken from the patient, in the case of autologous peripheral blood stem cell transplantation (PBSCT), or from a donor, in the case of allogeneic PBSCT. A donor may be found in the patient's close family, usually a matched sibling, and if not, through a search designed to identify an unrelated donor matched in HLA (human leukocyte antigens) system. Genes of the HLA system encode a complex array of histocompatibility molecules that play a central role in immune responsiveness and in determining the outcome of tissue transplantation (Bodmer, 1972). Umbilical cord blood stem cells are another alternative source of hematopoietic stem cells in patients lacking a suitable sibling donor. Advances in histocompatibility testing and development of marrow donor registries, such as the National Marrow Donor Program in the USA, as well as the establishment of cord blood banks have facilitated the use of unrelated donors and thus enabled the expansion of the number of patients who could receive transplants.

The transplant process is often described as consisting of five phases: (a) conditioning, which typically lasts for 7–10 days and in which chemotherapy and/or radiation are administered for eliminating malignancy, preventing rejection of new stem cells and creating space for the new cells; (b) stem cell infusion, which usually lasts about an hour, whereby the period varies with the volume infused and procedure of stem cell processing; (c) the neutropenic phase, which lasts 2–4 weeks, and in which the patient is highly susceptible to infections, such as mucositis, herpes simplex virus, and various skin and gut pathogens, and is treated mainly by antibiotics, antifungal agents and supportive care; (d) the engraftment phase, which may last for several weeks, and in which the infections start slowly to clear, whereby the greatest challenge becomes the management of graft versus host disease (GVHD) and prevention of viral infections; (e) the post-engraftment phase, which may last for months to years, and is marked by the gradual development of tolerance, weaning off of immunosuppression, management of chronic GVHD, and immune reconstitution.

There are multiple and diverse indications for each type of transplant. Autologous SCT is usually performed in recurrent solid tumors, such as brain tumors or Ewing sarcoma as well as in advanced stage neuroblastoma. Allogeneic SCT is done in recurrent or high-risk hematological malignancies, immunodeficiency states, metabolic diseases, and hematological diseases, such as thalassemia major or stem cell disorders, such as aplastic anemia.

Diverse complications can arise during and after SCT. Infections remain a major problem due to the myelosuppression caused by the conditioning regimen. Gram-negative as well as gram-positive bacteria are responsible for much of the morbidity (Meyers, 1985). Isolation, use of high-efficiency particulate air filtration systems and hand washing are used to minimize contact of these compromised hosts with infectious agents. In patients undergoing allogeneic SCT the depressed immunity continues after transplant due to the use of immunosuppression given post-transplant to prevent GVHD. Viral and fungal infections predominate during this period (Peterson et al. 1983).

Veno-occlusive disease of the liver is a common and often fatal complication of high dose chemo-radiotherapy. It consists of the triad of weight gain, platelet transfusion refractoriness and hyper-bilirubinemia. It is now the most common life-threatening complication of preparative regimen-related toxicity of BMT (Shulman and Hinterberger 1992).

GVHD results from HLA disparity between the hematopoietic stem cell donor and the transplant recipient. In GVHD the new transplanted immune system attacks, as it were, the whole body. It generally involves the skin, the gastrointestinal tract and the liver, causing rash and blistering, diarrhea and hyper-bilirubinemia, respectively. Acute GVHD is usually observed within 30–40 days of marrow infusion, but with the advent of more potent immunosuppressive agents such as cyclosporine, its onset may now be delayed by several months. Chronic GVHD usually occurs more than 100 days after allogeneic stem cell infusion, and the clinical pattern differs somewhat from that observed in acute GVHD. The most commonly involved organs are skin, liver, salivary glands, mucous membranes and muscles (Rowe et al. 1994). Acute and chronic GVHD can cause high morbidity and mortality. Immunosuppression administered as prophylaxis treatment for GVHD decreases further the immune status. However, since it involves a delay in immune reconstitution, it may bring about more morbidity. Chronic GVHD remains one of the prime determinants of late transplant-related morbidity and impaired quality of life (QOL). It includes abnormalities of growth and development in children, and problems of employment and functional performance status in the survivors as adults (Duell et al. 1997).

ISOLATION AND OTHER STRESSORS

Length of hospitalization for stem cell transplantation is about one month. To minimize complications the child is isolated in a room with a high-efficiency particulate air filtration system, and is not allowed to leave the room for the whole period of the transplantation. An early study reported on the psychological responses of children to isolation in a protected environment

(Kellerman, Rigler and Siegel, 1979). The participants in the study were cancer patients with advanced stage solid tumors, treated in a laminar airflow unit. Behavioral observations of 14 children were carried out over a period of 2 years, whereby the total number of available observations was 3629. The results referred to perception, sleep, intellectual functioning, physical discomfort, mood, management problems, activity patterns, social-communicative behavior, and sedation. No changes were observed in intellectual functioning as measured by standard psychometric tools. In general, no debilitating or long-term psychological effects related to prolonged treatment in a protected environment were noted. No child had to be removed from isolation because of psychological factors. The investigators concluded that children adapt more easily than adults to protected environments. Nevertheless, and despite a strong program of psychosocial support, some of the children had hallucinatory experiences and regressive symptoms in mood and communication, mostly after 6 weeks or more in isolation. Notably, the average isolation period of the patients in that study was 90 days, which is longer than nowadays.

Another study described factors that affect the coping processes of adolescents with aplastic anemia and infants with severe combined immuno-deficiency disease treated in laminar flow isolation rooms (Kutsanellou-Meyer and Christ 1978). The children in the study stayed in rooms devoid of windows. An intercom system was the only means of communication between the patient, the family, and the staff. This study was descriptive, presenting examples of coping with the isolation experience, relying on informal observations, without the use of any standard psychological tests. The findings indicate clearly that isolation, with its concomitant drastic reduction in normal emotional supports, enhances appreciably the stress of being ill and of having to undergo BMT.

Nowadays laminar airflow isolation is no longer a must and the protected environments are achieved by using rooms with hepafiltration. There is only one study that examined stress reactions and psychic adaptation of 15 children aged 8–12 years after SCT in single-room treatment under such isolation conditions. This prospective longitudinal study was based on free diagnostic interviews, projective tests and self-report questionnaires as well as intelligence tests administered in order to evaluate different adaptation processes in the children (Gunter et al. 1999). The responses to the self-report questionnaires revealed predominantly the conscious levels of emotional organization. This perspective highlighted the children's strong tendencies to adapt to the situation and to normalize their behavior under the isolation conditions. A comparison of pre- and post-transplant responses showed an 'overnormalization' of the scores for anxiety, depression, neuroticism, and extraversion and a relatively undifferentiated perception of one's own body. In contrast, the psychoanalytic interview, and the projective tests (e.g.,

Rorschach) tapped deeper levels of emotional responsiveness and exposed a completely different angle of the children's change in emotional adjustment from before to after the transplantation. Of the 15 children, nine dealt much more intensely than before with fears of death, feelings of depression, loneliness, and rage and had fantasies of guilt and punishment. Only two children showed a decreased intensity of their emotions and a more rigid organization of defenses than prior to transplantation. The limitations of this study are mainly the small number of studied children and their restricted age range.

In the Oncology/Hematology Department at the Rambam hospital the transplant rooms are equipped with a high-efficiency particulate air filtration system. The child is not allowed to leave the room but is not alone. Usually, one of the parents stays with the child in the same room for the whole transplant period. Other people who enter the room are the nurse, the physician in charge, and the teacher of the department. Thus, the physical isolation is not as extreme as it used to be when the laminar airflow system was used. However, in the course of transplantation the patient cannot leave the room or meet other family members or friends for a long period. It seems that changes in isolation practices have reduced the difficulties of isolation in general and the emotional burden in particular. Thus, a prevalent impression of health professionals is that isolation per se is less of a problem than it used to be. However, this impression still remains to be tested empirically.

Yet, even nowadays prolonged hospitalization in a protected environment and the enforced isolation both during and subsequent to hospitalization remain serious stressors for the patients. Further BMT-related stressors include the life-threatening nature of the BMT procedure, the disruption and dislocation of the family, the acute toxicity of the high-dose chemotherapy and radiotherapy used in conditioning regimens, the intense physical discomfort involved in the treatment, the required compliance with aversive daily routines, and the generally high levels of transient treatment-related morbidity (Patenaude, 1990). It is important to note also the stressful impact of the pain that most children undergoing BMT experience. A study with 20 children, aged 5–17, undergoing BMT, showed that despite getting continuous-infusion opioid therapy with additional boluses as needed for pain, all children reported pain after one month of treatment (Pederson, Parran and Harbaugh, 2000). The impact of the stressors is enhanced by the extended period of the treatment, which is long per se and may be further prolonged through the frequent complications. Studies show that the parents of children undergoing BMT also experience high levels of stress (Manne *et al.* 2002, Streisand *et al.* 2000). This may further enhance the children's distress.

The magnitude of the children's stress is such that the responses of some pediatric BMT patients have been described as representing a variant of post-traumatic stress disorder, with symptoms similar to those observed in children who have been traumatized by violence (Pot-Mees 1989, Stuber *et al.* 1991). All those stressors could affect the children's QOL post-transplant.

One indication of the extremity of the stress involved in BMT is the high incidence of non-compliance noted in pediatric BMT patients. It was found that almost all of these patients had at some point difficulties with ingesting oral medication (due to the unpalatable mouth rinses they were required to do), and all but the youngest group had compliance problems which in over 50% of the cases required intervention (Phipps and DeCuir-Whalley 1990).

EFFECTS ON QUALITY OF LIFE

During the past decades better use of high-dose chemotherapy and improved management of supportive care have resulted in higher survival rates for children with cancer in general and of patients who have undergone BMT in particular. These advances have highlighted the importance of the issue of maintaining a good QOL. Health, as defined by the World Health Organization as early as 1948, is not only the absence of disease, but also the presence of physical, mental, and social wellbeing (World Health Organization 1952). The terms 'quality of life' and more specifically, 'health-related quality of life' refer to the effects of health on the physical, psychological and social domains of life, considered as distinct areas that are influenced by a person's perceptions, experiences, expectations, and beliefs (see Chapter 7 on quality of life).

The impact of health on each of these domains can be measured in terms of two dimensions: objective assessments of functioning or health status, and more subjective perceptions of health. The two dimensions are distinct, since two people with the same health status may have different levels of QOL (Testa and Simonson 1996).

Understanding the impact of the BMT on QOL can assist in counseling children and their families who are considering BMT as a treatment option, and may lead to changes in the current medical and nursing protocols across phases of the transplant process to long-term rehabilitation (Grant 1999).

Two models were proposed for analyzing the relations of SCT to the patient's QOL. Ferrell *et al.* (1992a, 1992b) proposed a model that focuses on four dimensions of QOL they have identified: physical wellbeing, psychological wellbeing, social wellbeing, and spiritual wellbeing. Each dimension was analyzed according to the patients' responses in interviews conducted with them. Ford *et al.* (1996) presented another model that focuses on examining separately each of the following four specific phases: pre-SCT, day of SCT up to 100 days, post-SCT from 100 days to 1 year, and 1 or more years since SCT.

The four-dimensional model and the four-phase model provide jointly a theoretical framework for assessing QOL after SCT. Notably, each dimension may differ in each phase, for example, physical wellbeing between the day of SCT up to 100 days is not the same as it is one or more years following SCT. Thus, applying the two models together makes it possible to identify ways for intervention in regard to each dimension at each phase, covering the whole period.

Parsons et al. (1999) have raised the following important question: Health-related QOL in pediatric BMT survivors: according to whom?[1] In the past, QOL assessments of BMT survivors have been based on proxy reports, provided primarily by the parents. Several studies have shown that maternal distress and depression, marital adjustment and health locus of control influence parents' assessment of the child's functioning and behavior (Mulhern et al. 1992, Renouf and Kovacs 1994, Sanger et al. 1992). Parsons et al. (1999) studied 82 patients in the age range of 5 to 12 years. Forty-seven patients (57%) had received an allogeneic transplant, and thirty-five patients (43%) received an autologous transplant. The majority (96%) of patients had an underlying malignancy. The time interval between BMT and the assessment of QOL ranged from 24 days to 8.4 years. The perceptions of parents and children's health status following BMT were compared, using the Child Health Rating Inventories (CHRIs) and its companion measure the Disease Impairment Inventory – BMT (DSII-BMT). The findings showed good agreement between parental reports and child self-assessment in regard to 'objective' issues, such as missed school days and utilization of resources (e.g., emergency room visits). Children's scores were correlated highly with physicians' ratings of clinical disease severity and varied within each functional status domain both by transplant type and by time after BMT, in predictable ways. In contrast, parental ratings for disease-specific problems and pain were not significantly correlated with disease severity ratings. Further, little agreement was found between parental and child ratings in regard to the dimensions of mental health or QOL, regardless of the time after BMT, the type of transplant or the presence vs. absence of chronic GVHD. Children who had undergone BMT within the previous 6 months reported doing better in all areas of functioning than their parents reported about them. In the later time periods, the pattern was reversed, with the parents reporting higher scores than the children in regard to physical functioning, role function and energy. It is evident that children and parents base their reports on different considerations, for example, in the first period after SCT parents could be considering the toxicity of the transplant, whereas the children could be focusing on the recent isolation and the fate of other children on the unit. Be that as it may, the results of Parsons et al. (1999) suggest that children are capable of providing valid and

---

[1] See also Chapter 7 concerning the issue of measuring QOL on the basis of proxy reports, and for the description of the QOL measures mentioned in this chapter.

reliable information about their health-related QOL, information that varies predictably among clinical subgroups.

Phipps *et al.* (1999) used the Behavioral, Affective and Somatic Experiences Scale (BASES) to assess aspects of health-related QOL in children undergoing BMT. There were separate versions for parent, nurse and patient reports. In regard to patients at least 5 years old, BASES data were obtained weekly from parent, patient and nurse. For patients less than 5 years of age data were obtained only from the parent and nurse. Once-weekly observations were obtained through week + 6, followed by once-monthly observations through month + 6. Nurse observations were stopped when the patient was discharged from the initial BMT hospitalization. For patients at least 5 years old, BASES data were obtained weekly from the patient, a parent and the nurse. Longitudinal data were obtained from a cohort of 105 children (61 had allogeneic BMT and 44 autologous). Yet, only 45 children were older than 5 years and completed the patient version of the BASES. Clear patterns of change from one phase to another were found on measures from all respondents. The parental reports showed significant effects over time for all scales. The children's reports showed significant changes on all BASES subscales except Quality of Interaction. The nurses' reports showed significant changes on all subscales except Quality of Interaction and Compliance. All separately checked items of the Somatic Distress Scale (viz. nausea/vomiting, mucositis) and the Mood Disturbance Scale (viz., cheerful/friendly, sad/subdued, fearful anxious, and angry/irritable) showed significant declines according to the parents' and nurses' reports. Again, in line with parents' and nurses' reports, most somatic distress items showed a high peak in the week after BMT conditioning, followed by a decline to baseline or lower by week + 4 or + 5. Both parents' and nurses' reports show a difference in line with the type of transplantation: the patients undergoing allogeneic BMT experienced significantly higher effects on the subscales of Somatic Distress and Activity, but not on the subscales of Compliance, Mood Disturbance and Quality of Interaction. According to parents and nurses, the lowest degrees of somatic distress were experienced by the youngest children, the highest degrees by adolescents and intermediate degrees by children in the 6–12 year group. In all subscales of the BASES, younger patients had scores indicating better QOL than adolescents. There were no differences between the genders in any of the subscales, except one (Compliance subscale, in which males were reported by the nurses as having greater difficulties).

A recent study by Phipps *et al.* (2002) focused on assessing the acute effects of BMT on 153 children (age range <1 year to 20), especially in regard to somatic distress and mood disturbances. The instruments (the BASES, parent version and child version for children above 5 years of age) and the observation schedule were similar to those used in a previously reported study (Phipps *et al.* 1999). The findings showed that when the children enter the hospital for BMT their QOL is already compromised: they have high levels of somatic and mood disturbance symptoms, and low levels of activity. The situation exacerbates during the BMT procedure and peaks about one week after the transplant. But by the fourth to fifth week post-transplant there is a decline in distress back to the levels at admission, and a further decline in the 4–6 months after the transplant.

QUALITY OF LIFE OF BMT SURVIVORS

Several studies focused on QOL assessments in cancer survivors who have undergone BMT. One of the early studies reported observations on 43 children with normal cognitive abilities, 26 of whom were 5–16:8 years old, and 17 were younger than 5 years (Pot-Mees 1989). They were followed for 12 months post-transplant. Most of the children had leukemia. Three kinds of comparisons were undertaken: first, the status of the BMT children 6 and 12 months post-transplant were compared; secondly, the BMT children were compared to children who had undergone another kind of serious medical procedure (cardiac surgery); and thirdly, the BMT children were compared to healthy children who had not undergone any stressful procedure. The findings indicated an increase in behavior problems from pre-BMT (15%) to 6 months post-transplant (about 3 months after discharge from the hospital) (40%). The observed rate was higher than in the normal population (15%). The characteristic pattern for the children over 5 years included depressive symptoms, decreased interest in enjoyable activities, fear of disease recurrence, emotional detachment from parents and friends and difficulties in concentration, as well as eating difficulties and temper tantrums. No effects were observed on general cognitive functioning but there were significant declines in scholastic achievement (viz. arithmetic) and difficulties in dealing with academic pressures in general. The characteristic pattern for children under 5 included lethargy, eating problems, and social difficulties, with a tendency for regression in self-help skills. Twelve months after BMT, most of the children (80.8%), regardless of their age, improved in their psychological state and were already on their way to reintegration into normal life. Yet, comparisons with the healthy children showed that the BMT survivors manifested more disturbed behavior in the academic, social and emotional domains even 12 months after transplant (35% as compared with 15% in the controls). However, the BMT survivors resembled greatly in their behavior symptoms and rate of disturbance (though not in the deficit in cognitive functioning) another group of children who had undergone cardiac surgery, which also qualifies as a life-threatening stressful medical procedure. It is possible that the serious effects noted in this study are due to the stringent conditions of BMT and the absence of psychosocial awareness of the risks and difficulties for the pediatric patients almost 20 years ago.

Another early study of BMT survivors (Alby 1986) also noted their psychological difficulties, in particular in the social field in the framework of the school. A more recent study was done specifically in order to evaluate the behavioral reputation and social acceptance of pediatric BMT survivors (Vannatta et al. 1998). The comparison of peer, teacher and self-report data was done between a group of 48 BMT survivors, aged 8–16, and 48 healthy children in the same classroom, with a similar gender distribution. The study showed that BMT survivors had fewer friends and were described by their peers (though not by the teachers or by themselves) as more socially isolated. The peers also described them as physically less attractive and less skilled in sports, that is to say, as being deficient in properties that are commonly considered as socially desirable. It is possible that prolonged absenteeism from the school coupled with deficiency in socially desirable characteristics may lay the groundwork for social difficulties that could impair the children's social and emotional QOL.

However, not all studies of BMT survivors report difficulties. A study based on 39 patients, who had at least 2 years of follow-up after they had undergone allogeneic BMT (with a median follow-up of 5.7 years), did not reveal any evident impairment in QOL as assessed in terms of psychosocial functioning (Uderzo et al. 2000). Further, another study (Schmidt et al. 1993) used a mixed sample of 162 adults and 50 pediatric survivors, who had all been allogeneic marrow recipients. The data was obtained by means of interviews during clinic visits (5%), or over the telephone (95%). The interview referred to three domains of QOL: (1) productive activity and functioning; (2) health status and treatment-related physical symptoms; and (3) qualitative aspects of daily life. The patients graded their overall QOL on a 1–10 scale. The Karnofsky score was determined thereafter. The patients were contacted at least one year following their BMT. The majority (90%) of the 40 pediatric transplant recipients, who had attended school full-time before diagnosis, had been able to return to full-time attendance or employment when surveyed. Also those who had not been enrolled in school pre-diagnosis were all enrolled in school or employed full-time when surveyed. All pediatric patients were rated with Karnofsky performance status of 90 or 100 at the time of the survey. A subjective rating of their overall QOL, on a scale running from 0 to 10 (i.e., low to high, respectively), showed that the median score was 9.5. The authors concluded that the younger patients might overcome the treatment-related toxicity more completely than older (adult) persons.

Another study (Nespoli et al. 1995) focused on 36 children and adolescents, who had been in the age range of 2 to 16 years when transplantation took place. Patients who had undergone BMT at least 6 months before were included. This survey consisted of self-rating questionnaires, for the recipients and for the parents according to the patients' age. The investigators used a self-devised questionnaire for parents, the Busnelli anxiety scale for 17 patients aged 8–15 years, the Children's Depression Scale for 17 patients aged 9–16 years, the Parent Symptoms questionnaire for 13 parents of patients aged 4–9 years, and the Offer self image questionnaire for 11 adolescent patients. According to the parents, most of the children did not think back about BMT with anxiety, although many preferred not to talk about it with their parents (41%) or friends (50%). Only 16% of the interviewed patients complained about physical problems. Return to school figured as the cause of most difficulties. Tests that evaluate affective status indicated normal levels of anxiety, while in adolescents a slight depression state was reported, causing a sense of inadequacy. Self-image was substantially normal. Anxiety levels appeared to be higher in pre-school children. The investigators concluded that in their respondents QOL was good. Nevertheless, homogeneous instruments would be more appropriate for identifying those at risk for having future difficulties in coping with the BMT procedure.

Notteghem *et al.* (2003) evaluated the neuropsychological and adaptive functioning of children who have undergone autologous BMT without previous cranial irradiation. The major goal of the study was to determine whether high-dose chemotherapy alone might cause cognitive deficits. There were 76 children in the sample. They had all undergone BMT as treatment for an extracranial solid tumor. The BMT conditioning regimen consisted of high-dose chemotherapy without either total body irradiation or supratentorial cranial irradiation. The inclusion criteria were continuous complete remission 5 years or more after BMT, no sign of mental retardation, no developmental delay, and no psychosis prior to diagnosis. Median age at the time of the transplant was 4.5 years, and at neuropsychological examination, 15.7 years. The median interval between transplantation and neuropsychological examination was 9.1 years. Overall, the performance and skills of the participants were in the normal range and their professional and academic outcomes were satisfactory. A deleterious effect of deafness on verbal IQ associated with the previous administration of cisplatin was observed. In addition, reading difficulties had arisen that could be related to absence from kindergarten or primary school during hospitalization. Finally, in the younger subgroup, visual–perceptual skills were found to be more fragile.

Further aspects of the QOL of BMT survivors were highlighted in another study of 73 survivors after allogeneic BMT with an observation time of 1 to 15 years (median: 5.6 years) (Matthes-Martin *et al.* 1999). The Karnofsky–Orlansky scale was used for assessing functional status. Lack of a more specific tool for assessing in a comprehensive way the QOL of children induced the investigators to design a questionnaire focusing on the practical aspects of daily life. The first part included questions concerning frequency of medical consultation in the last 4 months prior to the study, school attendance after transplantation and professional career. The second part included 12 items referring to physical and psychological aspects. All but one patient (with severe neurological impairment) had Karnofsky–Orlansky scores over 80. In the case of children younger than 12 years, the QOL questionnaires were completed by the parents. Responses to the questionnaire of QOL revealed that 75% of the patients reported non-physical or psychological impairment. QOL was related inversely with the diagnosis of chronic GVHD. The findings of the study are, however, to be interpreted with caution, first, because its design was cross-sectional with a variable time interval between BMT and self-assessment; and second, because no age-adjusted control group of healthy individuals was used.

An innovative approach to assessing QOL in pediatric patients who have undergone BMT was adopted by Kreitler, Kreitler and Ben Arush (in press). In contrast to most studies that focus either on comparing BMT patients with themselves in different periods or sometimes with healthy controls, Kreitler, Kreitler and Ben Arush compared BMT patients ($n = 18$) with other pediatric cancer patients, matched to the BMT patients in diagnoses and the various demographic variables ($n = 56$). All patients have terminated their treatment (mean time since end of treatment 3.88 years, SD = 2.27). The major difference between the groups was undergoing BMT or not. There were no significant differences between the groups in disease stage, recurrence, time since diagnosis, time since end of treatment, age (9–17 years), gender distribution, and country of origin. They were administered the CQL questionnaire. Significant differences between the groups were not found in any of the scales or the total QOL score but only on the five following items (out of 56 items): those who received BMT scored higher on feeling healthy, doing things one likes to do, taking care of the way one looks, and motivation for coping, and lower on jealousy (see items Q2, Q18, Q30, Q54 and Q49, respectively in Table 7.1, Chapter 7). In this study, data is still being collected. In view of the small sample size the reported findings are to be considered as preliminary. However, the trend of the findings is suggestive of the possibility that precisely because of the severe stressfulness of BMT, psychosocial efforts are invested by the patients, their families and the staff to alleviate and remedy the situation, with the result that the overall QOL of BMT survivors is better than that of 'regular' pediatric cancer patients.

PSYCHOSOCIAL FACTORS OF CHILDREN'S ADJUSTMENT

As may be expected, there are individual differences in the responses of children undergoing BMT (Pot-Mees 1989). The study of these differences and of the determining factors is of great importance, both in order to identify as early as possible children who may be at risk for enhanced psychological distress and later psychological difficulties, and for providing all children the preparation prior to the treatment that may help them cope as best as possible. Pot-Mees (1989) focused on two kinds of determinants: coping styles and social environment. He found that the most effective attitude on the part of the children was a coping style of inner-directedness, withdrawal, waiting, 'holding back impulses', seeking distraction even if only temporary, rather than attempting to get an active solution. Further, the children who were better adjusted post-transplant were those with a resilient personality who responded to the stressful situation with denial and self-protectiveness. Insofar as the social environment is concerned, Pot-Mees noted that the best-adjusted children were those whose parents were emotionally adjusted, experienced marital satisfaction and were able to provide the children social support.

Some further studies focused specifically on identifying psychological factors that could contribute to differential adjustment of children undergoing BMT. Thus, Phipps and Mulhern (1995) used a prospective longitudinal design in order to examine the psychological adjustment of survivors of pediatric BMT, and to determine predictors of adjustment, particularly by identifying variables that confer protection from, or indicate vulnerability to, the stresses of BMT. Measures of patients' social competence, behavior problems, and self-esteem, as well as perceived family conflict, cohesion and expressiveness, were obtained before hospital admission for BMT and again 6 to 12 months following BMT. There were significant declines in social competence and overall self-concept after BMT. Before BMT, perceptions of family conflict had a moderate negative correlation with patient adjustment, whereas family cohesion and expressiveness were unrelated or only weakly related with adjustment measures. But all variables of family environment obtained pre-BMT were highly predictive of adjustment post-BMT. By means of a cross-lagged correlation it was shown that perceived family cohesion and expressiveness act as protective factors, enabling resilience to the stresses of BMT. The findings provide clues for designing programs to improve the QOL of pediatric patients undergoing BMT.

Barrera *et al.* (2000) examined children's QOL and behavioral adjustment pre-BMT and 6 months post-BMT. Their measure was specifically developed for children with cancer and it assesses physical wellbeing, role restriction and emotional wellbeing. They compared the pre- and 6 months post-BMT QOL (assessed only by parents' reports), behavioral adjustment and severity of medical symptoms of pediatric BMT patients as well as maternal psychological adjustment and family functioning. The participants were 26 children (mean age 8.5 years) and their mothers, 18 with allogeneic transplant and 8 with autologous transplant. The children undergoing BMT improved in their overall QOL at 6 months after BMT and did not present with symptoms of serious psychological maladjustment at either pre- or 6 months post-BMT, as measured by the Child Behavior Checklist behavioral scores. On the bases of the mothers' reports, there was an increase in the children's overall QOL by 6 months post-BMT, as well as specific decrease in the extent of physical discomfort and role restriction, as measured by the Pediatric Oncology Quality of Life. They emphasized that these interpretations need to be put to further empirical tests using children' self-reports in addition to parental reports of the children's psychological wellbeing. Of all the child, parent, family, and medical variables assessed at pre-BMT only family cohesion and child adaptive functioning were significantly related to children's QOL and behavioral adjustment 6 months following BMT. Higher levels of family cohesion were related with better QOL in survivors. Thus, family connectedness pre-BMT appeared to play the role of a protective factor against the stresses characteristic of the post-BMT period.

PSYCHOSOCIAL EFFECTS ON DISEASE COURSE AND OUTCOME

In view of studies with adult patients that showed effects of psychosocial factors on disease course in cancer (Fox, 1998), interest arose in studying the effects of psychological variables on medical outcomes after BMT. A retrospective cross-sectional study (McConville et al. 1990) with 32 pediatric BMT patients found four factors that contributed to so-called 'unexpected' severe physical complications (i.e., they accounted for 55% of the variance): the child's functional impairment, family dysfunction, paternal psychopathology and geographical dislocation. The same study showed that four similar factors contributed to predicting 'unexpected' deaths in the patients' sample (accounting for 36% of the variance): the child's functional impairment, parental psychopathology, family dysfunction and the child's personality. The major limitations of this study are the small size and poor medical state of the sample, and the retrospective nature of the design. A more recent study investigated the hypothesis that in addition to clinical factors, family characteristics would contribute to predicting the physical outcomes of BMT in pediatric patients (Dobkin et al. 2000). This prospective study was done over a 6.5-year period, with 68 pediatric patients who underwent BMT (29.4% autologous, 70.6% allogeneic). At transplant, their mean age was 7.5 years (range 4 months to 18 years). Their initial prognosis was rated by physicians, on the basis of the child's diagnosis, known risk factors, and donor type. Both parents completed two questionnaires assessing family wellbeing and marital satisfaction. Nurses also rated the children's' QOL 120 and 365 days following the BMT on the Play Performance Status scale. The two outcome measures used were medical complications and death of the child. The study found no effect of family stress or marital satisfaction on the child's survival. There were no predictors in the data for medical complications or the Play Performance score. The best predictor of deaths was the initial prognosis. The authors emphasize that in order to get proof for the effect of social support on survival it would have been necessary to check directly the children's perceptions rather than rely only on the parents' reports.

SOME CONCLUSIONS

In his excellent review paper of BMT, Phipps (1994) noted a certain lagging of psychological studies of BMT behind the rapid medical advances in BMT. Although well-designed studies designed to shed light on the psychological effects of BMT have been published in the meantime, there is still a gap between the levels of psychological and medical information in regard to the effects of BMT. Basically, the studies showed that the BMT procedure has a marked psychosocial impact on the pediatric patient, which may last beyond the medical procedure itself, and which is largely dependent on the physical sequelae of the treatment. However, the studies also show that the effects seem to be reversible and are remediable by proper psychosocial interventions. The social and emotional support the child gets, particularly from the family, seems to be an important beneficial factor in regard to the child's QOL. At present the pronounced deficit in psychosocial research consists in regard to intervention procedures designed to improve the coping of the children and raise the level of their QOL during and after the treatment.

ACKNOWLEDGEMENTS

Thanks are due to Jawdat Eid and Rivka Rosenkranz for their help and contributions.

REFERENCES

Alby, N. (1986) Difficultés psychologiques de la période post-greffe de moelle osseuse [Psychological problems in the period after bone marrow transplantation]. *Soins. Chirurgie* **38–40**, 483–484.

Bach, F.H., Albertini, R.J., Joo, P., Anderson, J.L., Bortin, M.M. (1968) Bone marrow transplantation in a patient with the Wiskott–Aldrich syndrome. *Lancet* **2**, 1364–1366.

Barrera, M., Boyd Pringle, L.-A., Sumbler, K., Saunders, F. (2000) Quality of life and behavioral adjustment after pediatric bone marrow transplantation. *Bone Marrow Transplantation* **26**, 427–435.

Bensinger, W.I., Martin, P.J., Storer, B., Clift, R., Forman, S.J., Negrin, R., Kashyap, A., Flowers, M.E., Lilleby, K., Chauncey, T.R., Storb, R., Appelbaum, F.R. (2001) Transplantation of bone marrow as compared with peripheral-blood cells from HLA-identical relatives in patients with hematologic cancers. *New England Journal of Medicine* **344**, 175–181.

Bodmer, W.F. (1972) Evolutionary significance of the HLA system. *Nature* **237**, 139–145.

Dobkin, P.L., Poirier, R.-M., Robaey, P., Bonny, Y., Champagne, M., Joseph, L. (2000) Predictors of physical outcomes in pediatric bone marrow transplantation. *Bone Marrow Transplantation* **26**, 553–558.

Duell, T., van Lint, M.T., Ljungman, P., *et al.* (1997) Health and functional status of long-term survivors of bone marrow transplantation. EBMT Working Party on Late Effects and EULEP Study Group on Late Effects. European Group for Blood and Marrow Transplantation. *Annals of Internal Medicine* **126**, 184–192.

Ferrell, B., Grant, M., Schmidt, G. M., *et al.* (1992a) The meaning of quality of life for bone marrow transplant survivors. Part 1: The impact of bone marrow transplant on quality of life. *Cancer Nursing* **15**, 153–160.

Ferrell, B., Grant, M., Schmidt, G.M., *et al.* (1992b) The meaning of quality of life for bone marrow transplant survivors. Part 2: Improving quality of life for bone marrow transplant survivors. *Cancer Nursing* **15**, 247–253.

Ford, R., McDonald, J., Mitchell-Supplee, K.J., Jagles, B.A. (1996). Marrow transplant and peripheral blood stem cell transplantation. In McCorkle, R., Grant, M., Frank-Stromborg, M., Baird, S.B. (Eds). *Cancer Nursing: A comprehensive textbook* (2nd edn). Philadelphia, PA: W.B. Saunders, pp. 504–530.

Fox, B.H. (1998) Psychosocial factors in cancer incidence and prognosis. In Holland, J.C. (Ed.), *Psycho-oncology*. New York: Oxford University Press, pp. 110–124.

Grant, M. (1999) Assessment of quality of life following hematopoietic cell transplantation. In Thomas, E.D., Forman, S.J., Blume, K.G. *Hematopoietic Cell Transplantation* (2nd edn). Oxford, England: Blackwell, pp. 407–413.

Gunter, M., Karle, M., Werning, A., Klingebiel, T. (1999) Emotional adaptation of children undergoing bone marrow transplantation. *Canadian Journal of Psychiatry* **44**, 77–81.

Kellerman, J., Rigler, D., Siegel, S.E. (1979) Psychological response of children to isolation in a protected environment. *Journal of Behavioral Medicine* **2**, 263–274.

Kreitler, S., Kreitler, M M., Ben Arush, M. (in press). The quality of life of children with cancer: a retrospective and prospective study.

Kutsanellou-Meyer, M., Christ, G.H. (1978) Factors affecting coping of adolescents and infants on a reverse isolation unit. *Social Work in Health Care* **4**, 125–137.

Manne, S., DuHamel, K., Nereo, N., Ostroff, J., Parsons, S., Martini, R., Williams, S., Mee, L., Sexson, S., Wu, L., Difede, J., Redd, W.H. (2002) Predictors of PTSD in mothers of children undergoing bone marrow transplantation: the role of cognitive and social processes. *J. Pediatr. Psychol.* **27**, 607–617.

Matthes-Martin, S., Lamche, M., Ladenstein, R., Emminger, W., Felsberger, C., Topf, R., Gadner, H., Peters, C. (1999) Organ toxicity and quality of life after allogeneic bone marrow transplantation in pediatric patients: a single center retrospective analysis. *Bone Marrow Transplantation* **23**, 1049–1053.

McConville, B.J., Steichen-Asch, P., Harris, R., Neudorf, S., Sambrano, J., Lampkin, B., Bailey, D., Fredrick, B., Hoffman, C., Woodman, D. (1990) Pediatric bone marrow transplants: Psychological aspects. *Canadian Journal of Psychiatry* **35**, 769–775.

Meyers, J.D. (1985) Infections in marrow recipients. In Mandell, G.L., Douglas, R.G., Bennett, J.E. (Eds). *Principles and Practice of Infectious Diseases*. New York: Wiley, pp. 1674–1676.

Mulhern, R.K., Fairclough, D.L., Smith, B., Douglas, S.M. (1992) Maternal depression, assessment methods, and physical symptoms affect estimates of depressive symptomatology among children with cancer. *Journal of Pediatric Psychology* 17, 313–326.

Nespoli, L., Verri, A.P., Locatelli, F. *et al.* (1995) The impact of pediatric bone marrow transplantation on quality of life. *Quality of Life Research* 4, 233–240.

Notteghem, P., Soler, C., Dellatolas, G., Kieffer-Renaux, V., Valteau-Couanet, D., Raimondo, G., Hartmann, O. (2003) Neuropsychological outcome in long-term survivors of a childhood extracranial solid tumor who have undergone autologous bone marrow transplantation. *Bone Marrow Transplantation* 31, 599–606.

Parsons, S.K., Barlow, S.E., Levy, S.L., Supran, S.E., Kaplan, S.H. (1999) Health-related quality of life in pediatric bone marrow transplant survivors; according to whom? *International Journal of Cancer, Supplement* 12, 46–51.

Patenaude, A.F. (1990) Psychologic impact of bone marrow transplantation: Current perspective. *Yale Journal of Biological Medicine* 63, 515–519.

Pederson, C., Parran, L., Harbaugh, B. (2000) Children's perceptions of pain during 3 weeks of bone marrow transplant experience. *Journal of Pediatric Oncology Nursing* 17, 22–32.

Peterson, P.K., Mcglave, P., Ramsay, N.K.C., *et al.* (1983) A prospective study of infectious diseases following bone marrow transplantation: Emergence of aspergillus and cytomegalovirus as the major causes of mortality. *Infection Control* 4, 81–89.

Phipps, S. (1994) Bone marrow transplantation. In Bearison, D.J., Mulhern, R.K. (Eds), *Pediatric Psychooncology: Psychological perspectives on children with cancer.* New York: Oxford University Press, pp. 143–170.

Phipps, S., DeCuir-Whalley, S. (1990) Adherence issues in pediatric bone marrow transplantation. *Journal of Pediatric Psychology* 15, 459–475.

Phipps, S., Mulhern, R.K. (1995) Family cohesion and expressiveness promote resilience to the stress of pediatric bone marrow transplant: a preliminary report. *Journal of Development and Behavior in Pediatrics* 16, 257–263.

Phipps, S., Dunavant, M., Jayawardene, D., Srivastava, D.K. (1999) Assessment of health-related quality of life in acute in-patients settings use of the BASES instrument in children undergoing bone marrow tyransplantation. *International Journal of Cancer, Supplement 12* 18–24.

Phipps, S., Dunavant, M., Garvie, P.A., Lensing, S., Raj, S.N. (2002) Acute health-related quality of life in children undergoing stem cell transplant: I. Descriptive outcomes. *Bone Marrow Transplantation* 29, 425–434.

Pot-Mees, C.C. (1989) *The Psychological Effects of Bone Marrow Transplantation in Children.* Delft, The Netherlands: Eburon.

Renouf, A.G., Kovacs, M. (1994) Concordance between mothers' reports and children's self-reports of depressive symptoms: a longitudinal study. *Journal of the American Academy of Child and Adolescent Psychiatry* 33, 208–216.

Rowe, J.M., Ciobanu, N., Ascensao, J., *et al.* (1994) Recommended guidelines for the management of autologous and allogeneic bone marrow transplantation. A report from the Eastern Cooperative Oncology Group (ECOG). *Annals of Internal Medicine* 120, 143–158.

Sanger, M.S., Maclean, W.E. Jr., Van Slyke, D.A. (1992) Relation between maternal characteristics and child behavior ratings. *Clinical Pediatrics* 31, 461–466.

Schmidt, G.M., Niland, J.C., Forman, S.J., Fonbuena, P.P., Dagis, A.C., Grant, M.M., *et al.* (1993) Extended follow-up in 212 long-term allogeneic bone marrow transplant survivors. Issues of quality of life. *Transplantation* 55, 551–557.

Shulman, H.M., Hinterberger, W. (1992) Hepatic venoocclusive disease–liver toxicity syndrome after bone marrow transplantation. *Bone Marrow Transplantation* **10**, 197–214.

Streisand, R., Rodrigue, J.R., Houck, C., Graham-Pole, J., Berlant, N. (2000) Brief report. Parents of children undergoing bone marrow transplantation: documenting stresss and piloting a psychological intervention program. *Journal of Pediatric Psychology* **25**, 331–337.

Stuber, M.L., Nader, K., Yasuda, P., Pynoos, R. S., Cohen, S. (1991) Stress response after pediatric bone marrow transplantation: Preliminary results of the prospective longitudinal study. *Journal of the American Academy of Child and Adolescent Psychiatry* **30**, 952–957.

Testa, M.A., Simonson, D.C. (1996) Assessment of quality of life outcomes. *New England Journal of Medicine* **334**, 835–840.

Vannatta, K., Zeller, M., Noll, R.B., Koontz, K. (1998) Social functioning of children surviving bone marrrow transplantation. *Journal of Pediatric Psychology* **23**, 169–178.

Uderzo, C., Biagi, E., Rovelli, A., Balduzzi, A., Schiro, R., Longoni, D., Arrigo, C., Nicolini, B., Placa, L., Da-Prada, A., Mascaretti, L., Giltri, G., Galimberti, S., Valsecchi, M.G., Locasciulli, A., Masera, G. (2000) Bone marrow transplantation for childhood hematological disorders: a global pediatric approach in a twelve year single center experience. *Medical and Surgical Pediatrics* **21**, 157–163.

World Health Organization (1952) Constitution of the World Health Organization. In *Handbook of Basic Documents* (5th edn). Geneva Palais des Nations: UN Publications, pp. 3–20.

11

The Survivors of Childhood Cancer

AMITA MAHAJAN AND MERIEL E.M. JENNEY

Department of Paediatric Oncology, Llandough Hospital, Penarth, Wales, UK

INTRODUCTION

Dramatic improvements in childhood cancer over the last three decades have resulted in a rapidly growing number of long-term survivors. A successful outcome for these survivors is largely dependent on the underlying diagnosis and the therapy they have received. With overall cure rates currently exceeding 65% in the developed world, it is estimated that 1 in 900 adults is a survivor of childhood malignancy (Bleyer 1993). This population is at an increased risk of a number of medical problems such as specific organ toxicities, delayed growth and other endocrinological problems, reduced fertility, neurocognitive impairment and second malignancies (Green 1993, Meadows and Hobbie 1986, Green *et al.* 2001) with over half of the patients experiencing at least one chronic medical problem. Does this population also have a higher incidence of disturbances in psychosocial adjustment given their frequency of chronic medical complications, their 'at-risk' status of disease recurrence and the psychological trauma of their earlier illness experiences? The aim of this review is to explore these issues – in particular, whether there are specific treatment experiences that lead to well-defined long-term problems and whether age at the time of treatment influences outcome? Finally, what do we know about the coping mechanisms of these survivors in the long-term?

There are large differences in reporting of maladjustment amongst survivors which is as high as 50% (Greenberg, Kazak and Meadows 1989) in some settings. Yet, other studies have shown a very low incidence of psychopathology. These differences almost certainly relate to differences in the populations

Psychosocial Aspects of Pediatric Oncology. Edited by S. Kreitler and M. Weyl Ben Arush
© 2004 John Wiley & Sons Ltd: ISBN 0 471 49939 0

studied (e.g. the inclusion of brain tumor survivors with significant neurocognitive problems), different treatment regimens (e.g. the inclusion of patients with significant physical sequelae) and variations in the methods of assessment used to determine psychopathology (e.g. measures used self-report vs. parent/teacher reports). Strategies that are currently used to influence and improve psychological function in the long term will also be discussed.

FOLLOWING COMPLETION OF TREATMENT: THE TRANSITION

At first sight, completion of therapy would appear to be a positive experience for families. However, it is frequently a time of distress, anxiety and uncertainty. The significance of this transition phase for families can be underestimated by their carers. Patients and families are often ambivalent about terminating the use of chemotherapeutic agents known to be responsible for cancer remission (Lewis and LaBarbera 1983). Consequently, they often report heightened anxiety, fears and feeling of vulnerability as active treatment ends (Haase and Rostad 1994). The protocols and treatment modalities, which have provided structure and reassurance, are replaced by a 'wait and watch' period during which recurrence is still a possibility.

A formal conference at the end of treatment is appropriate to address these issues and prepare the family for the future. This provides a sense of closure to the active treatment. It also provides an opportunity to move from active treatment to a focus on a healthy lifestyle and a perspective that reflects an understanding of the disease, and potential late-effects.

PHYSICAL SEQUELAE OF SUCCESSFUL THERAPY

Successful therapy can be associated with a number of potential long-term physical sequelae. The functional status of individual patients in adolescence and adulthood largely depends on the severity of these effects and how effectively they develop coping strategies. The presence or absence of long-term physical toxicity may be one of the major determinants of psychological well-being in adulthood. The physical sequelae of successful treatment have been extensively reported elsewhere (Green 1993, Meadows and Hobbie 1986, Green et al. 2001, Hawkins, Draper and Kingston 1987). They include physical disfigurement (e.g. radiotherapy to face, chronic hair loss or amputation) or limitation of function, e.g. following limb salvage procedures, chronic bladder and bowel dysfunction. Growth impairment and other endocrine abnormalities are reported in a number of patients, particularly following cranial radiotherapy or BMT.

The *central nervous system* (CNS) late-effects include a range of neuropsychological disorders varying from subtle learning difficulties to overt neurological deterioration depending on the modality of treatment given. Common problems include deficiencies in mental processing speed, verbal and non-verbal memory, freedom from distractibility, attention and arithmetic.

Studies of mortality of long-term survivors suggest that there is an increased risk of early death (Robertson, Hawkins and Kingston 1994, Mertens *et al.* 2001). The patients at most risk of increased late mortality are those who survived relapse of their primary tumor. Second malignant neoplasm is probably the most devastating consequence of childhood cancer therapy. It has been estimated that within 25 years of diagnosis, 4% of survivors develop a second primary cancer (Hawkins, Draper and Kingston 1987).

The presence or absence of these late-effects may have a significant effect on the subsequent psychological adjustment of the survivors.

PSYCHOLOGICAL ADJUSTMENT OF CHILD AND ADOLESCENT CANCER SURVIVORS AND IMPACT ON SOCIAL SKILLS

General Issues

The psychological impact of having had childhood cancer can continue long after treatment ends for survivors and their families. However, reassuringly most survivors appear to have a reasonable level of psychosocial adjustment. This adjustment in the years after completion of therapy depends on a number of variables. The age at diagnosis, level of academic functioning and family cohesiveness are major determinants in childhood and adolescence. In adulthood, the presence or absence of physical sequelae and economic status (specifically successful employment) are important factors influencing adequate psychosocial adjustment.

The diagnosis of cancer and subsequent treatment may challenge the child's normal development by limiting opportunities, restricting play and activities, delaying the attainment of autonomy and potentially compromising family and peer relationships. These effects may differ specifically as a function of the child's age. For infants, cancer is most likely to affect parent–child relationships, restrict mobility, or limit opportunities to socialize with peers. For older children, the impact of cancer can lead to reduced schooling, compromised peer relationships, more time with adults, concern about body image and awareness of vulnerability and possible death. Cancer in adolescence may extend the period of dependency on parents and may reduce opportunities to establish close interpersonal relationships for example with the opposite sex.

We will explore these issues for children with cancer at different ages and stages of maturity.

Psychological Adjustment in Childhood in the First Few Years Following Completion of Therapy

A number of issues are of particular importance for the intellectual and psychological well-being of the pre-pubertal child. These include freedom from symptoms, growth, spontaneous progression through puberty and normal physical development. Adjusting to normal family life rather than being the centre of attention may also be challenging for some. A number of studies have investigated peer relationships, interactions and perceptions during the critical period of reintegration into school during the late-treatment phase and immediately following completion of therapy. For example, in a study evaluating teacher ratings of children who were either on treatment or had ceased therapy within the last year (Noll *et al.* 1990), 24 patients (ages 8–18 years) were compared with matched classroom controls. A wide variety of malignancies were represented, although children with brain tumors were not included. The teachers completed a modified version of 'Revised Class Play'. This instrument was modified to obtain teachers' impressions of three fundamental dimensions of interpersonal style: 'sociability–leadership', 'aggressive–disruptive', 'sensitive–isolated'. When compared to matched controls, children with cancer were perceived by teachers as being (a) less sociable and prone towards leadership and (b) more socially isolated and withdrawn. The same cohort was also evaluated for peer and self-perceptions of sociability, social isolation, overall popularity, mutual friendships and feelings of loneliness. The reports from peers suggested that children with cancer were perceived as being more socially isolated. However, no significant differences were found in their popularity, number of friends or self-worth (Noll *et al.* 1991).

In contrast Spirito *et al.* (1990) examined the social adjustment of 56 children aged 5–12 years who had been off-treatment for at least 6 months. In comparison with their healthy peers, teachers rated the survivors as being better adjusted socially. Specifically the children were rated as being teased less and arguing less frequently with classmates. The survivors themselves, however, reported fewer friends of the same age and greater loneliness and isolation.

In other settings the impact of chronic illness itself has been shown to influence psychological adjustment but the influence is variable. Spirito *et al.* (1990) noted that chronic illness frequently disrupts peer interactions because of observed physical limitations and differences. Other reported studies specifically examining the social competency of children with chronic illnesses, however, show generally good adjustment.

The degree of psychosocial adjustment and social competence among survivors of childhood cancer appears to be most closely associated with the functional status of the child, parental education and family functioning (Wallander *et al.* 1989). Newby *et al.* (2000) reported that social skills, in one cohort, as rated by both parents and teachers, are best predicted by academic functioning. They demonstrated a significant association between fewer school-related difficulties with better psychological adjustment. Greenberg and Meadows also reported a significant association between academic function-ing, physical impairments and lower levels of distress in a group of cancer survivors in the first few years following completion of treatment.

Adequacy of family support and adaptability are strongly associated with good psychological adjustment. The family represents the primary system that influences adjustment. Following completion of therapy, the interactions of child and family assume an important role. Kupst *et al.* (1995) reported that coping and perceived adjustment in survivors were positively associated with mothers' coping and adjustment particularly in the younger age group (those less than 7 years at diagnosis).

Psychological Adjustment during Adolescence

Adolescence is a time of change and normal psychological progression through adolescence is well described in a number of models. Havinghurst (1972) and Newman and Newman (1987) have identified five tasks related to adolescence: relationship with peers, emotional independence, preparation for career, sense of morality and development of sex-role identity. The adolescent survivor from cancer also has to cope with fear of relapse, insecurity of the future, damage to self-esteem, loss of autonomy and, for some, distorted appearance and body image. It is therefore not surprising that in a number of individuals, normal progression through adolescence may be compromised. Despite this, most research suggests that the majority of adolescent survivors show positive psychosocial functioning.

Meadows, McKee and Kazak (1989) compared a cohort of 95 long-term survivors to their healthy siblings. There was no significant difference in social competence, frequency of adverse behaviors, or school achievement compared to siblings. In another study (Noll *et al.* 1993) adolescent survivors were rated by peers as being more socially isolated although friendships and popularity were not affected. Again most studies highlight that the most important determinants of the level of psychological adjustment are the survivors' functional status (degree of physical/cognitive impairment) and adaptability.

A number of studies emphasize the importance of family functioning in predicting overall adjustment during this period. One surprising finding is that the survivors from families who report significant cohesiveness exhibit poorer adjustment (Newby *et al.* 2000). Specifically, a higher frequency of behavioral problems in the survivors as reported by the teachers was associated with reports of greater cohesiveness within families. Family cohesiveness, which is generally considered to be a positive attribute of family life for healthy children, appears to be associated with more adjustment difficulties in young people who have survived cancer (Kazak 1994). A possible explanation for this is that adolescents who have survived cancer have a greater need for autonomy than their healthy peers. Thus any perceptions of intrusion from the family system may be associated with symptoms of adjustment difficulties among survivors. Additional research is needed to determine the veracity of these findings.

Finally, length of time following completion of treatment also appears to significantly affect overall psychological adjustment; children and adolescents who had completed therapy longer ago were rated by parents and teachers as being better adjusted than those who had only recently completed therapy (Newby 2000). Adolescents appear to experience significant initial anxiety and emotional turbulence following cessation of therapy, perhaps because of fear of possible recurrence. It appears that the psychological adjustment improves with the passage of time since therapy.

PSYCHOSOCIAL ADJUSTMENT DURING ADULTHOOD

The ability to establish identity and functional independence and to form intimate relationships are hallmarks of a successful transition from adolescence to adulthood. A number of studies have attempted to look at adult psychosocial functioning after childhood cancer. Again variability in methods used and deficits in design have contributed to conflicting findings. Discrepancies have arisen from small sample sizes, the inclusion largely of chronic attendees where follow-up is not universal (a self-selected cohort) and the use of siblings as controls despite the documented emotional and behavioral difficulties amongst siblings of survivors (Sahler et al. 1994). Most studies of adult psychosocial outcome have relied on questionnaires that assess current function but are dependent on the respondent's understanding of the issues explored.

Irrespective of the incidence of psychological problems reported in the various studies, once again the key determinants appear to be functional status, specifically freedom from symptoms, and the individuals' or the families' resilience and adaptability. Even if there are no long-term medical or psychological problems there is still the issue of the continuing stigma of having had cancer earlier in life that may restrict employment and career choices. In a study assessing the eligibility for compulsory military service of childhood cancer survivors, it was reported that childhood cancer survivors were less likely to meet the requirements set for military service. Furthermore

30% were rejected merely on the basis of a former diagnosis of cancer (Paivi *et al.* 1999).

In a large study exploring psychosocial adjustment of long-term survivors, Koocher and O'Malley (1981) utilized both patient and parent self-reports as well as interview data from 117 survivors. They reported that, although most long-term survivors were able to lead relatively normal lives in terms of academic, vocational and social functioning, nearly half showed some evidence of significant psychological problems, primarily in the form of anxiety and difficulties in interpersonal relationships. A similar study limited to survivors of childhood Hodgkin's disease (Cella *et al.* 1988), utilizing interview data and study staff ratings, documented maladjustment defined by social incompetence, and poor interpersonal relationships in nearly a third of their sample. A more recent study of 102 adult survivors of childhood acute leukemia and Wilms' tumor did not find increased incidence of psychiatric disorder in this population or a significant difference in current social functioning but did report significant long-term problems with interpersonal functioning and day-to-day coping (Mackie *et al.* 2000). A number of other studies report generally low levels of psychological distress with an absence of significant psycho-pathology (Elkin *et al.* 1997, Spirito *et al.* 1990). Elkin *et al.* 1990 studied a cohort of 161 patients at a median age of 19 years at the time of evaluation. A symptom inventory (self-report) that had been designed to reflect the psychological symptom patterns of psychiatric and medical patients (SCL-90-R) was used. Comparisons were made with the normative standardization and the relationship of selected demographic and medical variables with psychological distress was explored. The results showed very low levels of psychological distress in this population. Only three factors were identified which were associated with an increased risk of maladjustment: older patient age at follow-up, greater number of relapses and presence of severe functional impairment.

In general there is a suggestion that those studies relying primarily on self-report to demonstrate a better outcome (Fritz, Williams and Amylon 1988, Fritz and Williams 1988, Greenberg, Kazak and Meadows 1989), compared to those utilizing parent, teacher or staff reports which appear to show higher levels of maladjustment (Koocher and O'Malley 1981, Cella *et al.* 1988). It may well be that self-reports are biased towards minimization of affective distress and a propensity to present themselves in a more favorable light, or it may simply reflect successful coping mechanisms (Worchel 1989, Canning, Canning and Boyce 1992, Phipps and Srivastava 1996). These studies have demon-strated a high incidence of a repressive adaptive style in cancer survivors, which may account for their lower scores on self-report measures of affective distress. Individuals identified as repressors have lower scores on measures of anxiety, depression and anger expression i.e. are better functioning. It has been hypothesized that repressive defenses may decrease the self-report of negative psychological outcomes for this population. This highlights the difficulties in the interpretation of self-reporting. Whether patients repress symptoms or demonstrate self-denial, the identification of a lack of adjustment is difficult and requires careful assessment. These may be the patients at greatest risk of later problems and interventions may be particularly important for this cohort.

Successful relationships in survivors depend both on achieving a biological cure and a positive psychological adaptation as well as the successful negotiation of adolescent developmental milestones. Marriage can be viewed as a surrogate marker of positive psychological functioning among adult survivors. In a study looking at self-reported data from 10 425 cancer survivors in North America (Rauck et al. 1999) 32% reported being married or living as married, 6% being divorced or separated and 62% having never been married. These figures are significantly lower than those of the general population. Survivors of the central nervous system (CNS) tumors were even less likely to be married.

In summary, it would appear that while severe psychopathology is relatively rare, mild to moderate adjustment difficulties may be present in a significant proportion of adult survivors. The majority of individuals seem to overcome these difficulties reasonably well and appear to have adequate social functioning. The available evidence also suggests that repressive adaptation is a stable personality trait that might be expected to endure after completion of therapy. However, a significant proportion of survivors continue to have problems with interpersonal relationships.

SURVIVORS OF BRAIN TUMORS DURING CHILDHOOD

The survivors of brain tumors during childhood have additional problems that warrant further discussion. It is in this group of patients that the physical and psychological sequelae of successful therapy are the most profound.

Brain tumors are the second commonest malignancy in childhood after acute lymphocytic leukemia and account for nearly 20% of all malignancies in childhood. This subgroup represents a major cause of acquired neurological disability. A number of studies attest to the physical, cognitive, linguistic and behavioral problems experienced by children with primary brain tumors.

Psychological testing reveals that between 40% and 100% of long-term survivors of CNS tumors have some form of cognitive dysfunction (Glauser and Packer 1991), the variation being attributable to the type of tumor and use of radiotherapy. Impaired intelligence as evidenced by a reduction in full-scale IQ is seen in the majority of patients with medulloblastoma treated conventionally with localized radiotherapy (Dennis et al. 1996). There is also increasing evidence that cognitive and academic abilities may deteriorate progressively over time (Anderson et al. 2000). Two neuropsychological processes contribute to this progressive decline. Children may lose previously acquired information and skills but more importantly the acquisition of new skills and information happens at a much slower rate than healthy age-related peers (Hopewell 1998, Twaddle *et al.* 1986). The dose of radiotherapy and the age at which it was administered correlate significantly with the neurocognitive outcome (the higher the dose and the younger the age, the greater the impairment).

In addition to the reduction in full-scale IQ, children with intracranial tumors show evidence of impairment across a range of cognitive function, including visual attention and memory, verbal fluency, perceptual abilities, freedom from distraction and social problem solving (Kazak *et al.* 1999, Garcia-Perez *et al.* 1994, Butler *et al.* 1994). Such cognitive impairments can create serious problems in a classroom setting. It is important to establish whether early intervention can limit this progressive decline and this is currently under investigation. A recent study looking at various aspects of cognitive impairment demonstrated that nonverbal and information processing skills continued to decline progressively while other deficits remained relatively stable over time. Literacy skills, however, increased with time, with educational intervention assisting progress, emphasizing the gains that can occur with remediation (Anderson *et al.* 2000).

POST-TRAUMATIC STRESS DISORDER

A cluster of anxiety and avoidance symptoms has been identified in pediatric cancer survivors and their parents. These symptoms are consistent with a trauma response and have led researchers to propose that the long-term psychosocial impact of cancer may best be understood by using the framework of post-traumatic stress disorder (PTSD) (Butler, Rizzi and Handwerger 1996, Kazak *et al.* 1997). There are many aspects of cancer diagnosis and treatment that evoke intense fear and helplessness. Treatment can be visualized as a chronic process of traumatic stress, including painful invasive procedures, repeated hospitalizations, separation from family members, and painful complications following treatment. In addition, late-effects of treatment such as infertility and growth problems, physical changes such as amputation and cardiac and pulmonary dysfunction; and cognitive changes can serve as lifelong reminders. For individuals who are treated during childhood, these long-term effects are understood and recognized in new ways at each level of development and provide lifelong opportunities for retraumatization. However, despite research documenting psychological symptoms in children that are consistent with PTSD in the months and years following cancer treatment, recent work has found that pediatric cancer survivors actually report fewer PTSD symptoms than do their parents (Butler, Rizzi and Handwerger 1996) and on formal measures tend to respond in a manner similar to children who have never been ill.

CURRENT STRATEGIES TO MINIMIZE LONG-TERM MEDICAL AND COGNITIVE PROBLEMS

It is important to recognize that to minimize the incidence of psychological maladjustment in the long term, constant efforts must be made to reduce the incidence of medical and cognitive problems. For a number of childhood cancers, the survival rates have improved to a level where the intensity and duration of therapy, particularly radiotherapy and mutilating surgery, can be reduced. Effective systemic chemotherapy has allowed the use of lower doses and volumes of radiotherapy with a profound improvement in quality of life for the survivor with no reduction in the survival rates (D'Angio *et al.* 1989, Donaldson and Link 1987). Additionally, modifications in the delivery of radiation, e.g. the use of conformal radiotherapy and more accurate imaging with field reduction, have also diminished the musculoskeletal and other complications associated with the use of this modality (Donaldson and Kaplan 1982).

It is now well known that cranial radiation used to treat children with ALL has significant long-term sequelae in terms of poorer academic achievement and psychosocial functioning (Hill *et al.* 1998). The most important clinical intervention in recent years has been to abandon the routine use of this modality in the treatment of childhood acute lymphoblastic leukemia preserving its use only in those with disease in the CNS or undergoing total body irradiation as part of conditioning for BMT (at a significantly lower dose).

Infertility following cancer therapy is a major issue for cancer survivors. However, recent advances in the field of reproduction have potentially opened opportunities for the preservation of the reproductive potential of young cancer patients with good long-term prognosis for survival.

The management of bone tumors involving the extremities requires surgical resection, historically an amputation. Although effective in tumor control, it leads to cosmetic deformities, functional abnormalities, and potential psychological sequelae in cancer survivors. Limb-salvage surgery, with endoprosthetic replacement is now being increasingly performed when feasible to overcome these problems. However, the long-term outcome of patients undergoing these procedures is under evaluation and improved psychological outcome has not yet been proven.

STRATEGIES TO COPE WITH LONG-TERM SEQUELAE

The majority of pediatric oncology centres have evolved a mechanism to follow up survivors of childhood cancer well into adult life. 'Long-term follow-up' or 'after completion of therapy' (ACT) clinics have been set up in most centres to counsel patients and their parents about late-effects and to detect subtle late-effects as early as possible. These clinics are usually multidisciplinary and involve input from a number of specialists such as endocrinologists, neurologists and cardiologists. Most units would have access to the services of a clinical psychologist and family therapy unit. If there is a perceived need for intervention, particularly psychological support or counselling, this should be provided.

It has been suggested that continued monitoring of cancer survivors in specialty clinics might increase anxiety and potentially stigmatize a group who are without disease and only at minimal risk of new complications. One way to minimize this would be to formulate individualized follow-up plans that are based on an individual's risk. An increasing literature base is becoming available to underpin decisions about the clinical follow-up of long-term survivors largely based on retrospective studies, and prospective evaluation of new treatments is needed. Information to guide the follow-up of survivors will come from national population-based cohort studies, large multicentre clinical studies, and randomized clinical trials designed to evaluate both survival and long-term toxicities associated with different strategies. As this information accumulates, the level of clinical surveillance can be developed to match the clinical need. An evidence base is clearly required (Wallace *et al.* 2001).

Some centers have tried novel approaches to reduce symptoms of distress and improve family functioning and development. Intervention programs combining cognitive-behavioral and family therapy are well received and appear to be effective in reducing the symptoms of post-traumatic stress and anxiety (Kazak *et al.* 1999). Other programs have been directed more specifically at helping the child with cancer acquire the social skills to cope with school life. Clearly, return to school can be a difficult time for children with cancer but there are early indications (Haase and Rostad 1994) that this can be eased with intervention. Whether or not these interventions have an impact on later functioning remains to be established.

A proportion of survivors are likely to have some neurocognitive impairment. Special strategies may be needed to optimize their education. Even those who do not have obvious learning difficulties may have subtle problems such as short-term memory loss and problems with mental arithmetic and abstract conceptualization. It is essential these are recognized and addressed within both the medical and educational systems for the child.

CONCLUSION

It appears that most children have an impressive ability to come to terms with the cancer experience and develop adequate psychosocial adjustment in later life. At the same time, it is important to recognize that a proportion of survivors experience genuine difficulties in adjustment which may be aggravated by physical sequelae or adverse social or family circumstances. As future studies of survivorship issues are undertaken, attempts to understand physical and psychological effects of childhood cancer must be made in parallel. It is only by adopting equal emphasis in both mental and physical health that young adults will have the best chance to attain their full potential.

REFERENCES

Anderson, V.A., Godber, T., Smibert, E., Weiskop, S., Ekert, H. (2000) Cognitive and academic outcome following cranial irradiation and chemotherapy in children: a longitudinal study. *Br. J. Cancer* **82**(2), 255–262.

Bleyer, W.A. (1993) What can be learned about childhood cancer from 'Cancer Statistics Review 1973–1988'. *Cancer* **71**, 3229–3236.

Butler, R.W., Hill, J.M., Steinherz, P.G., Meyers, P.A., Finlay, J.L. (1994) Neuropsychologic effects of cranial irradiation, intrathecal methotrexate, and systemic methotrexate in childhood cancer. *J. Clin. Oncol.* **12**(12), 2621–2629.

Butler, R., Rizzi, L.l., Handwerger, B. (1996) The assessment of posttraumatic stress disorder in pediatric cancer patients and survivors. *Journal of Pediatric Psychology* **21**, 499–504.

Canning, E.H., Canning, R.D., Boyce, T.B. (1992) Depressive symptoms and adaptive style in children with cancer. *J. Amer. Acad. Child Adolesc. Psychiatry* **31**, 1120–1124.

Cella, D., Tan, C., Sullivan, M., Weinstock, L., Alter, R., Jow, D. (1988) Identifying survivors of pediatric Hodgkin's disease who need psychologic interventions. *J. Psychosoc. Oncol.* **5**, 83–96.

D'Angio, G.J., Breslow, N., Beckwith, B., *et al.* (1989) Treatment of Wilms' tumor: Results of the Third National Wilms' Tumor Study. *Cancer* **64**, 349.

Dennis, M., Spiegler, B.J., Hethrington, C.R., *et al.* (1996) Neuropsychological sequelae of the treatment of children with medulloblastoma. *J. Neurooncol.* **29**, 91–101.

Donaldson, S.S., Kaplan, H.S. (1982) Complications of treatment of Hodgkin's disease in children. *Cancer Treatment Rep.* **66**, 977.

Donaldson, S.S., Link, M.P. (1987) Combined modality treatment with low-dose radiation and MOPP chemotherapy for children with Hodgkin's disease. *J. Clin. Oncol.* **5**, 742.

Elkin, T.D., Phipps, S., Mulhern, R.D., Fairclough, D. (1997) Psychological functioning of adolescent and young adult survivors of pediatric malignancy. *Med. Pediatr. Oncol.* **29**, 582–588.

Fritz, G.K., Williams, J.R. (1988) Issues of adolescent development for survivors of childhood cancer. *J. Am. Acad. Child. Adolesc. Psychiatry* **27**, 712–715.

Fritz, G.K., Williams, J.R., Amylon, M. (1988) After treatment ends: psychosocial sequelae in pediatric cancer survivors. *Am. J. Orthopsychiatry* **58**, 552–561.

Garcia-Perez, A., Sierrasesumaga, L., Narbona-Garcia, J., Calvo-Manuel, F., Aguirre-Ventallo, M. (1994) Neuropsychological evaluation of children with intracranial tumors: impact of treatment modalities. *Med. Pediatr. Oncol.* **23**(2), 116–123.

Glauser, T.A., Packer, R.J. (1991) Cognitive deficits in long-term survivors of childhood brain tumors. *Childs Nerv. Syst.* **7**, 2–12.

Green D.M. (1993) Effects of treatment for childhood cancer on vital organ systems. *Cancer* **71**, 3299–3306.

Green, D.M., Grigoriev, Y.A., Nan, B., Takashima, J.R., *et al.* (2001) Congestive cardiac failure after treatment for Wilms' tumor: A report from the National Wilms' Tumor Study Group. *J. Clin. Oncol.* **19**(7), 1926–1934.

Greenberg, H.S., Kazak, A.E., Meadows, A.T. (1989) Psychological functioning in 8–16-year-old cancer survivors and their parents. *J. Peds.* **114**, 488–4893.

Haase, J.E., Rostad, M. (1994) Experiences of completing cancer therapy: children's perspectives. *Oncol. Nurs. Forum* **21**(9), 1483–1492.

Havinghurst, R. (1992) *Developmental Tasks and Education.* New York: David McKay.

Hawkins, M.M., Draper, G.J., Kingston, J.E. (1987) Incidence of second primary tumors among childhood cancer survivors. *Br. J. Cancer* **56**, 339–347.

Hill, J.M., Kornblith, A.B., Jones, D., *et al.* (1998) A comparative study of the long term psychosocial functioning of childhood acute lymphoblastic leukemia survivors treated by intrathecal methotrexate with or without cranial irradiation. *Cancer* **82**(1), 208–218.

Hopewell, J.W. (1998) Radiation injury to the central nervous system. *Med. Ped. Oncol. Suppl.* **1**, 1–9.

Kazak, A. (1994) Implications of survival: pediatric oncology patients and their families. In D.J. Bearison, R.K. Mulhern (Eds), *Pediatric Psycho-Oncology: Psychological perspectives on children with cancer*, pp. 171–192.

Kazak, A.E., Barakat, L.P., Meeske, E., *et al.* (1997) Posttraumatic stress, family functioning, and social support in survivors of childhood leukemia and their mothers and fathers. *Journal of Consulting and Clinical Psychology* **65**, 120–129.

Kazak, A.E., Simms, S., Barakat, L., Hobbie, W., Foley, B., Golomb, V., Best, M. (1999) Surviving cancer completely intervention program (SSCIP): a cognitive-behavioral and family therapy intervention for adolescent survivors of childhood cancer and heir families. *Family Process* **38**(2), 175–191.

Koocher, G., O'Malley, J. (1981) *The Damocles Syndrome.* New York: McGraw-Hill.

Kupst, M.J., Natta, M.B., Richardson, C.C., *et al.* (1995) Family coping with paediatric leukaemia: ten years after treatment. *J. Pediatr. Psychol.* **20**, 601–617.

Lewis, S., LaBarbera, J.D. (1983) Terminating chemotherapy: another stage in coping with childhood leukemia. *Am. J. Pediatr. Hematol. Oncol.* **5**, 33–37.

Mackie, E., Hill, J., Kondryn, H., McNally, R. (2000) Adult psychosocial outcomes in long-term survivors of acute lymphoblastic leukaemia and Wilms' tumour: a controlled study. *Lancet* **355**(9212), 1310–1314.

Meadows, A.T., Hobbie, W.L. (1986) The medical consequences of cure. *Cancer* **58**, 524–528.

Meadows, A.T., McKee, K., Kazak, A.E. (1989) Psychosocial status of young adult survivors of childhood cancer: a survey. *Med. Pediatr. Oncol.* **17**, 466–470.

Mertens, A.C., Yasui, Y., Neglia, J.P., Potter, J.D., Nesbit, M.E. Jr, Ruccione, K., Smithson, W.A., Robison, L.L. (2001) Late mortality experience in five-year survivors of childhood and adolescent cancer: the childhood cancer survivor study. *J. Clin. Oncol.* **19**, 3163–3172.

Newby, W.L., Brown, R.T., Pawletko, T.M., Gold, S.H., Whitt, J.K. (2000) Social skills and psychosocial adjustment of child and adolescent cancer survivors. *Psycho-Oncology* **9**, 113–126.

Newman, B., Newman, P. (1987) *Development Through Life: A Psychosocial Approach.* Chicago: The Dorsey Press.

Noll, R., Bukowski, W., LeRoy, S., Kulkarni, R. (1990) Social interaction between children and their peers: teacher ratings. *J. Pediatr. Psychol.* **7**, 75–84.

Noll, R., LeRoy, S., Bukowski, W., Rogosch, F.A., Kulkarni, R. (1991) Peer relationships and adjustment in children with cancer. *J. Pediatr. Psychol.* **6**, 307–326.

Noll, R.B., Bukowski, W.M., Davies, W.H., *et al.* (1993) Adjustment in the peer system of adolescents with cancer: a two year study. *J. Pediatr. Psychol.* **18**, 351–364.

Paivi, M.L., Heikki, A.S., Toivo, T.S., Hans, H., *et al.* (1999) Military service of male survivors of childhood malignancies. *Cancer* **85**(3), 732–740.

Phipps, S., Srivastava, D.K. (1997) The repressor personality in children with cancer. *Health Psychol.* **16**, 521–528.

Rauck, A., Green, D.M., Yasui, Y., *et al.* (1999) Marriage in survivors of childhood cancer: A preliminary description from the childhood cancer survivor study. *Med. Pediatr. Oncol.* **33**, 60–63.

Robertson, C.M., Hawkins, M.M., Kingston, J.E. (1994) Late deaths and survival after childhood cancer: implications for cure. *British Medical Journal* **309**, 162–167.

Sahler, O.J.Z., Mulhern, R., Dolgin, M.J., *et al.* (1994) Sibling adaptation to childhood cancer collaborative study: prevalence of sibling distress and definition of adoptions levels. *J. Dev. Behav. Pediatr.* **15**, 353–366.

Spirito, A., Stark, L., Cobiella, C., Drigan, R., Androkites, A., Hewitt, K. (1990) Social adjustment of children successfully treated for cancer. *J. Pediatr. Psychol.* **15**, 359–371.

Twaddle, V., Britton, P.G., Kernahan, J., Craft, A.W. (1986) Intellect after malignancy. *Arch. Dis. Child.* **61**, 700–702.

Wallace, H.W.B., Blacklay, A., Eiser, C., Davies, H., Hawkins, M., Levitt, G.A., Jenney, M.E.M. (2001) Developing strategies for long term follow up of survivors of childhood cancer. *British Medical Journal* **232**, 271–274.

Wallander, J., Varni, J., Babani, L., Banis, H., Wilcox, K. (1989) Family resources as resistance factors for psychologically ill and handicapped children. *J. Pediatr. Psychol.* **14**, 157–174.

Worchel, F.F. (1989) Denial of depression: adaptive coping in pediatric cancer patients? *Newslet. Soc. Ped. Psychol.* **13**, 8–11.

PART THREE
PSYCHOSOCIAL INTERVENTIONS

12

Speaking to Children about Serious Matters

JANE E. SKEEN AND M. LOUISE WEBSTER

Starship Children's Hospital, Auckland, New Zealand

INTRODUCTION

Communication with seriously ill children about their disease, treatment and prognosis, is an area that in the past was often overlooked or neglected. Prior to the 1970s the majority of both paediatric and adult patients with cancer were not told their diagnosis in the belief that this would spare them anxiety and distress. While there has been a significant change in standard medical practice with respect to adult patients, studies within the past 10 years still report that as many as a third of children with cancer aged 8–12 and a fifth of those aged 13–15 have not been told that they have cancer (Last and van Veldhuizen 1996). In keeping with this only 19% of families of terminally ill children were found to have acknowledged with their child, the child's impending death (Goldman and Christie 1993). The majority of the families either actively blocked discussion (6%), felt the child had died unaware of the situation (29%), or did not know what their child knew or felt (23%). There remains for many adults the mistaken belief that children are not able to understand the seriousness of their condition and are best spared the burden of such knowledge. A further factor that inhibits adults from talking to children about their illness is the grief and feeling of impotence that many health professionals and parents experience when having to acknowledge the unthinkable and deal with life-threatening or terminal illness in children.

Psychosocial Aspects of Pediatric Oncology. Edited by S. Kreitler and M. Weyl Ben Arush
© 2004 John Wiley & Sons Ltd: ISBN 0 471 49939 0

There are many serious issues that arise for the child or young person who develops cancer. Diagnosis, prognosis, treatment regimes and side effects, invasive procedures, body image alteration, amputation, major surgery, bone-marrow transplantation, fertility loss, and loss of a sense of invulnerability are all issues that may be encountered during and after treatment and therefore require explanation and discussion with children and their families. Even with the best treatments currently available, 20% of children and adolescents diagnosed with cancer will die from their malignancy. These young people will need to know that further curative treatment is not possible, but that palliative care and support will continue. They need the opportunity to talk about death and about their own death, and to be involved, where possible, in decisions about how they will live the life they still have. Although the past 30 years have seen a growing awareness of these issues in published research, clinical case forums, national body guidelines, popular press articles, and paediatric oncology service policies regarding children's rights to information, many parents and health professionals still find it difficult to speak with children about serious matters.

This chapter will first review the evidence base for a practice of being open and honest with children about cancer, the factors that make it hard for parents to talk to their children about serious matters, children's understanding of illness and of death, and child and family preference regarding how information is given. In the second part of the chapter we present practical strategies in speaking with children. In our consideration of all of these matters it is important to remember, throughout this, that children and adolescents cannot be considered in isolation, but must always be seen in the context of their family, the family's cultural affiliation and spiritual beliefs, and the wider societal systems. In approaching communication about serious illness with children we need to include the important people in the child's world – their parents, siblings, extended family, and often friends and classmates.

LITERATURE REVIEW

Information Given to Children and Psychological Outcomes

In the 1970s when the majority of children with cancer died from their disease and standard practice was to 'protect' children from full knowledge of the disease, observational studies of such children revealed that most did nevertheless find out about their disease and prognosis from other children (Bluebond-Langner 1978). However the isolation and distrust that resulted from the secrecy surrounding them, left many children unable to communicate with family or hospital staff about their fears or their situation (Chesler, Paris and Barbarin 1986). A small number of subsequent studies involving direct interview or assessment of children and adolescents with cancer have explored the relationship between information given to the child about diagnosis and prognosis, and subsequent psychological adjustment. Claflin and Barbarin (1990) conducted structured interviews with children and adolescents with cancer as part of a longitudinal study of family coping in childhood cancer. Children aged less than 9 years at diagnosis were significantly less likely to have been given any specific information by their parents about diagnosis, compared to those aged 9–18 years (11% vs. 60%). The younger children were also less likely to have been given information about prognosis, or specific explanations and rationalisation for treatments and procedures. Despite being 'protected' from such information, the younger children experienced the same levels of distress and of side effects as did the older children and adolescents, and had the same levels of awareness of parental distress.

Slavin *et al.* (1982) studied a random sample of 116 long-term survivors of childhood cancer to examine the relationship between long-term psychosocial adjustment (based on a composite of standardised psychiatric examination and standardised psychological measures of symptoms and adjustment) and early communication of the cancer diagnosis to the child. Those patients who had been told by a parent or physician that they had cancer within one year of initial diagnosis (or before the sixth birthday for those who were infants at diagnosis) showed significantly better psychosocial adjustment than did patients who had either not been told about their cancer within a year of diagnosis or who had found out by themselves about their diagnosis from peers or by reading the medical chart. Interviews with the parents and siblings of the patients revealed that the vast majority of parents now believed that children should be told early about their diagnosis. Many parents who had not told their children the diagnosis early identified this 'lack of candor as a source of stress or other difficulty both during and after the treatment period'.

A more recent study of 56 children aged 8–16 years attending an oncology clinic (Last and van Veldhuizen 1996) used structured interviews with parents to determine the amount and depth of information given to children about their diagnosis, prognosis and the possibility of dying from the cancer. The children, who were either receiving active treatment or follow-up, completed standardised measures of anxiety and depression. Children who received open information about their diagnosis and prognosis early in their illness showed significantly less anxiety and depression and identified greater availability of sources of information. Type of cancer and disease prognosis had no effect on depression and anxiety scores or on parent communication, but parents were less likely to give information to younger children.

These findings are consistent with those from studies of communication between parents who themselves have cancer and their children. Children and adolescents who are not informed openly about their parents' disease report more anxiety and psychological distress than those who are well informed (Kroll *et al.* 1998). While some have questioned whether such findings reflect general family functioning and mental health, of which open communication is just one of many markers (Slavin *et al*. 1982), in families in which some children have been told and some have not been told, the children who are better informed are less anxious than their siblings (Rosenheim and Reicher 1985).

In summary, studies looking at the relationship between timing and specificity of information given to children with cancer by their parents or physicians and the emotional wellbeing of such children have not demonstrated any 'protective effect' of withholding information from children. Instead the studies have shown that children who are not given information about their diagnosis and treatments early in the course of their illness are more vulnerable to anxiety and depression during cancer treatment, and to long-term psychosocial adjustment problems following treatment. Moreover it seems to be important that such information is given openly by trusted adults in the child's life such as parents and physicians, rather than being covertly acquired from peers or other sources.

Information Given to Children and Physical Health Outcomes

Treatment outcome and long-term physical health may also be jeopardised when a young person is not adequately informed about their cancer, or does not have an open and trusting relationship with their parents and medical team. Treatment adherence in adolescents with cancer is generally reported to be poor, with figures for non-adherence to medication as high as 59% being found in adolescent outpatients. While there are many factors that influence treatment adherence, adolescents and parents who are in agreement about chemotherapy dosage and timing, and about information given by the medical team regarding the cancer and treatments, are more likely to achieve good adherence to chemotherapy (Tebbi 1993, Tebbi *et al*. 1986). Long-term survivors of childhood cancer are at risk of physical late-effects of treatment including growth and hormonal deficiencies, cardiac complications, infertility, and second malignancies. As adults they need to be able to access follow-up clinics and to seek medical help if problems arise. However in studies of adults attending childhood cancer late-effects clinics many patients know very little about their previous diagnosis or the treatments they received (Blackley *et al*. 1998, Byrne *et al*. 1989, Eiser *et al*. 1996). The majority of patients in such clinics feel they do not know enough and wish to receive more information in order to obtain appropriate healthcare advice and follow-up treatment.

Factors Influencing Parental Choice to Give Information to Children

There are a number of studies that have examined the factors influencing choices parents make to give or withhold information from their children.

While most health professionals advocate an open approach in giving children information about their cancer, the actual job of talking to children is often left to parents, either because parents request this, or because staff believe that parents 'know their child best' and are therefore the most appropriate people to talk about such matters. This can leave parents feeling overwhelmed and unsupported, and that they are in some way failing their child by giving bad news and not being able to prevent or protect them from what is happening. Staff have been found to seriously overestimate how often parents have actually discussed serious matters with their children, which suggests that staff themselves sometimes avoid the issue and tend to underestimate how difficult it is for parents to talk about such matters (Goldman and Christie 1993).

Parents of children with cancer are more likely to talk to their child about the cancer if the child is older (Chesler, Paris and Barbarin 1986, Last and van Veldhuizen 1996, Claflin and Barbarin 1990), and if there are older siblings in the house (Chesler, Paris and Barbarin 1986). Type of cancer, prognosis, relapse status and serious complications do not appear to influence parents' decisions to talk to their child. A number of reasons for withholding information from children have been given by parents of children with cancer and by mothers who themselves have cancer (Last and van Veldhuizen 1996, Barnes et al. 2000). Parents may believe that their child is too young to burden with frightening serious facts, that their child is too young to understand, may wish to avoid questions about cancer and death, may wish to prevent child distress, and may wish to avoid disrupting special family events. On the other hand, parents who have chosen to talk about the cancer believe that by doing so they will preserve their child's trust, and promote the child's acceptance of the illness and treatment. Such parents also share a belief that communicating about such matters will decrease their child's distress, and that their child has a right to be informed.

Parents have identified things that would help them to talk about serious matters to their children, including assistance from health professionals with information about child development, and discussion of age-appropriate strategies for telling children about cancer (Barnes et al. 2000).

Developmental Changes in Children's Understanding of Illness and of Death

Research into this area has attempted to link children's understanding of illness and death to Piaget's theory of cognitive development, and to examine the influences of other factors such as culture, illness experience, and health education on level of understanding. The majority of studies have found that children's concepts of health, illness and death are broadly linked to the child's cognitive and developmental stage, and that these schemas develop and evolve over time in a predictable fashion (Bibace and Walsh 1979, Perrin and Gerrity

1981, Koocher 1974, Hansdottir and Malcarne 1998, Thompson and Gustafson 1996). There is less agreement about the impact of personal illness on understanding, and no consistent evidence that having a chronic illness or being hospitalised increases the child's level of understanding of either experience-specific illness or general illness causality (Thompson and Gustafson 1996, Burbach and Peterson 1986, Crisp, Goodnow and Ungerer 1996, Sherman *et al.* 1985). A previous experience of the death of someone close does not necessarily result in a more accurate understanding of death by children (Thompson and Gustafson 1996, Cotton and Range 1990). These findings are perhaps to be expected, given the lack of information provided to many children who have serious illnesses, and in particular to younger children. There is, however, evidence that when children are provided with an explanation and education about illness that is targeted to their developmental stage, they demonstrate significant increases in understanding (Potter and Roberts 1984, Schonfeld *et al.* 1995).

Children's understanding of illness

A knowledge of the conceptual stages of illness understanding is important for those attempting to talk with children about illness-related issues. However, it is equally important to remember that a wide variability in the level and stage of understanding may be found in the individual child at any given age, hence the need to check first with the child what he/she understands about a particular situation or condition.

In the sensorimotor period (age 0–2 years) the young infant is unable to distinguish between self and the external physical world, and is dependent on caregivers and the developing attachment relationship for security and soothing. Preverbal infants learn to associate certain events with environmental cues and can develop conditioned responses and learn coping strategies for stressful events, but are still dependent on the caregiver for integration and interpretation of here-and-now experiences. The development of cognitive schema to explain illness requires the development of explicit or verbal memory, i.e. the conscious recollection of previous experiences, and the development of semantic or declarative knowledge. These developmental processes are linked to evolving language skills and cognitive development, and occur in the third and fourth years of life (Fundudis 1997).

The pre-operational period (age 2–7 years) is generally associated with thinking that is concrete and egocentric, and children may have difficulty distinguishing between reality and representation. Interpretation of words is often literal. They may utilise magical thinking and will often focus on one part of an event or experience, without being able to register the wider context. Illness concepts and beliefs at this stage include phenomenism – illness is caused by events or sensory stimuli that are closely temporally associated, and contagion – illness is caused by objects or environments close to the child's body at the onset of the illness.

Example

A 4-year-old girl said that she 'got leukaemia' when she came to hospital, because coming to hospital was the event that was associated with being declared 'sick' and with being subjected to unpleasant treatments and procedures.

The concrete operational period (age 7–11 years) is characterised by an increasing capacity to think logically and to understand wider contexts for events or experiences. Children can keep track of time, number, and sequence of events, and can differentiate between self and the outside world. They are able to appreciate that other people may hold differing points of view. Children at this stage believe that illness is caused by contamination – contact with germs or dirt – or by exposure to cold weather without appropriate clothing, but do not appreciate the complex interrelationship of multiple variables that might lead to illness. They believe that illness can be cured by simple measures such as taking the right medicines and staying in bed, and that medication taken by mouth has an effect on internal organs and processes (internalisation).

Example

A 7-year-old boy whose younger brother had died of disseminated abdominal neuroblastoma believed that he had caused his brother's illness because he had patted a dirty dog and then touched his brother. He was now presenting with recurrent abdominal pain and was worried that he had 'caught' cancer from his brother.

The formal operational period (age 11+ years) is associated with the capacity for abstract reasoning, deductive logic, and the ability to explore hypothetical situations. Young people at this stage can 'understand that there might be many interrelated causes of illness, that the body might respond variably to any or a combination of agents, and that illness might be caused and cured as a result of a complex interaction between host and agent factors' (Perrin and Gerrity 1981). They can conceptualise on both a physiological and psychophysiological level (Bibace and Walsh 1979).

It is not uncommon for cognitively competent people of all ages to make magical attributions regarding the causes of childhood cancer. This may be in part because the causes of childhood cancer are so poorly understood.

Example

A 12-year-old boy who had relapsed leukaemia said to a doctor: 'I was playing rugby and someone kneed me in the chest and then someone kicked me in the head and then I wasn't feeling well. And that's why I got cancer. Mum thinks so too.'

A Chinese family had become Christians a year before their daughter developed cancer. They believed at the time of diagnosis that the cancer had occurred because, as part of their move to Christianity, they had destroyed their traditional Chinese statues of gods, including the one that protects children.

Children's understanding of death

Studies examining children's beliefs about death show that these centre around evolving concepts of irreversibility, non-functionality, universality, and causality (Koocher 1974, Cotton and Range 1990). For infants up to the age of 3 years the primary focus is on attachment relationships and separation from close adults, so that death cannot be distinguished from separation or abandonment. By the age of 3 years children know that death occurs, but see death as temporary and reversible. They may show magical thinking about causes of death, and understand death as a separation from loved ones and as 'going to another place'.

Example

After a 2-year-old boy died at home, the family were choosing which of his toys to put in his coffin. His sister aged 5, who had been kept involved throughout his illness and death, was insistent that a hammer be included as he would need it to 'hammer the coffin lid off when he got to heaven'.

From 6 years onwards children develop the understanding that everyone dies at some stage including themselves, that death is irreversible, and an understanding of possible causes of death. While the concept of non-functionality also develops, children of this age can struggle still with worrying for example that someone who has died might be feeling cold after being buried.

From 12 years onwards in the stage of formal operational thinking, adolescents have an adult understanding of death. However, the sense of invulnerability that can accompany evolving adolescent individuation and autonomy may make it difficult for some adolescents to acknowledge that they themselves might die from cancer.

Example

A 16-year-old girl developed widespread metastases from a relapsed abdominal rhabdomyosarcoma and was admitted to a hospice for palliative care and pain management. She had been kept well informed about her diagnosis and her prognosis, and had actively participated in the decision to stop chemotherapy. Several weeks after admission to the hospice she told her therapist that she had 'only just realised' that she was going to die.

How do Children and Families Want Information to be Given?

There is little empirical research evaluating strategies for talking with children about their illness, or indeed for talking to adult patients. Awareness of the importance of this area has led to practical guidelines for healthcare professionals on how to break bad news to adults (Buckman 1992, Shields 1998), and how to talk to children about death (Grollman 1976, Spinetta, Swarner and Sheposh 1981, Faulkner 1993). There are also uncontrolled studies describing positive outcomes of various information-giving practices, such as the use of an analogy of weeds in a flower garden as a way of telling young children about their diagnosis of leukemia (Jankovic *et al.* 1994), and the use of a 'final stage conference' to discuss therapeutic choices with children who have end-stage cancer (Nitschke *et al.* 1982). The guidelines for adult patients developed by Buckman stress the importance of good listening and communication skills on the part of the healthcare professional, and recommend a stepwise progression that starts with ensuring that the physical setting is appropriate and that the right people are present. This is followed by finding out how much the patient knows, finding out how much the patient wants to know, sharing information, responding to the patient's feelings, and planning follow-up.

Parents whose children have cancer have been shown to have a high level of agreement with their paediatricians regarding the content of what needs to be discussed when a child is first diagnosed with cancer (Greenberg *et al.* 1984). Parents see advice on what to tell the child as ranking closely in importance to discussion about diagnosis, prognosis, and therapy.

In a study investigating what source of information was preferred by adolescent cancer patients aged 11–20 years, it was found that the majority (59%) preferred a private discussion with a healthcare professional, most often a physician (Levenson *et al.* 1982). Of these the majority (68%) wanted parents to be included in the discussion, and some of the younger patients preferred information to be given to them by their parents. Less than half of the adolescents saw pamphlets as providing an important information source.

PRACTICAL STRATEGIES IN SPEAKING WITH CHILDREN

Good communication with the child who has cancer is needed every step along the way, from diagnosis to follow-up in a late-effects clinic for those who survive, or up to the child's death for those children who do not survive.

The following guidelines are based on the authors' personal experiences working with children and adolescents with cancer, and in the light of the body of literature reviewed above. In this section we cover general guidelines in speaking with children and adolescents about their illness and treatment, specific clinical situations, other issues that may need addressing, and speaking with children and adolescents about death. We, acknowledge that there are many different ways of approaching such matters, and it is important that clinicians develop an approach that they personally feel comfortable with.

There are two important prerequisites to speaking with children. The first is learning to listen to what children say and how they say it. Only then can we understand their concerns and needs, and start to provide appropriate information and support. Good listening is essential both in formal settings where we sit down with children and speak with them about their illness, and in the unexpected moments when children indicate their thoughts and their anxieties through direct questions, conversational talk, play and drawings, or through their silence.

The second prerequisite is the provision of support to staff. Working with seriously ill children, children who die, places unavoidable emotional demands on staff. To listen to and talk with children about the difficult issues that arise when they have cancer requires a willingness to enter the child's world, to see their reality as they see it, and to hear their fears and their losses as they feel them. This is not easy, for children often cut through the defences, rationalising, and pretence that many adults use when faced by life-threatening illness in children. Children expect honest answers to honest questions. Staff may work with young patients who overwhelmingly remind them of their own children at home. Staff may also struggle to acknowledge or express their own grief and anger when children with whom they have had daily contact relapse, experience devastating disease or treatment outcomes, or die.

For staff to be able to continue to hear children and speak with children we need systems of support for staff to ensure that they can do this work without becoming too overwhelmed by, or distanced from their patients' worlds. We need a paediatric oncology team culture that acknowledges the emotional impacts of such work on staff, and the routine provision of staff supervision and support that focuses on these issues. It is only when these structures are in place that staff can safely listen to children and speak with them about serious matters.

General Guidelines

(1) Before talking with children talk to the parents to give them the information and to plan with them how best to talk with their child.
When a child has cancer, parents or primary caregivers are facing two challenging tasks simultaneously. They are having to learn about and integrate new and often overwhelming information about their child's diagnosis, prognosis and treatments, and cope with their own emotional response to the situation. At the same time they are having to support and parent as best they can, a child whose life is under threat and who is dependent on them for physical and emotional support and containment. Talking to parents first gives them an opportunity to process the information and ask questions, and space to openly express their emotions or distress, before having to focus on their child's needs. Parents are the best source of information about their child – they know what

terms or words their child uses, what sorts of experiences with illness or hospital systems the child has had previously, and how their child has coped in the past with stressful situations. They also provide important information on family spiritual and cultural beliefs that are relevant to what is said to the child and how it is framed. It is then possible to plan with the parents what is to be communicated to the child, and for what purpose.

(2) Ways that meeting with a child might then proceed:

- Meeting the child together with the parents/primary caregivers.
- Meeting with the child without parents; this is sometimes the preference of older adolescents, who might prefer another support person such as a friend or partner to be present.
- Meeting with the child and parents after the parents have talked to their child.

It may be important to give children the opportunity to talk to the doctor/nurse by themselves. Some children attempt to protect their parents from knowing how much information they have acquired, and the extent to which they understand their illness and prognosis. The child may wish to ask questions or discuss subjects that they feel unable to raise in front of their parents. This is the first step towards allowing the family to discuss openly matters that have been avoided, and to move beyond the 'mutual pretence' identified by Bluebond-Langner (1978) in children with cancer and their families.

Example

An 8-year-old boy and his parents met with the doctor to hear the diagnosis of osteogenic sarcoma and to discuss the treatment plan for chemotherapy and surgery.

After his parents left the room, the boy turned to his nurse and asked if 'children died from what he had'. The nurse told him that most children got better with the medicines and surgery, but that some children did die. She went on to tell him that everyone hoped that the treatments would make his cancer go away, but that no matter what happened, his parents and his doctors and nurses would look after him.

(3) Ensure that the setting is appropriate, i.e. private, child-friendly and safe. Arrange to have everyone seated, and if the child is confined to bed ensure that adults are not standing over the child.
Children will not feel safe if the procedures room, where invasive or unpleasant tests and treatments take place, is used for discussions.

(4) Ask the child what they know of their illness and/or treatments to date.
This helps you to know what the child understands and what terms to use. It also allows you to correct any misunderstandings that the child may have. Children invariably know from the reactions of those around them that something serious has happened, even if they are unsure of what exactly it is.

Example

A young man of 17 wrote about coming to the hospital when he was diagnosed with leukaemia 7 years earlier: 'I remember my first time. It was in the old hospital. My mum was with me. It was hot. It was summer and the fans were going and the air was stuffy and burned my nostrils when I breathed. We were waiting for a long time. My mum sat there not doing anything. My dad came along. He looked haggard.'

(5) Check with the child how much they want to know. Some children may not want to know details about their cancer or treatments, or may not want to know about more than the immediate plans.
Younger children may not be able to comprehend the time scale of extended and sequential treatment regimes. Children with marked anticipatory anxiety may need information presented in manageable sections prior to each stage, with enough time to prepare adequately for new treatments but not so far in advance that they become overwhelmed with anxiety.

Example

A boy aged 8 had several relapses of his leukaemia and required intensive treatment regimes. His mother subsequently recalled how her son coped best when he was given information openly and honestly. However, she and his treating team found that he needed to be told the immediate treatment plan only, because if they discussed all of the future options in his presence he became confused and agitated and stopped listening.

(6) Explain in terms that are appropriate to the child's level of understanding.
Use simple language, avoiding complex medical terms and abbreviations. Be aware that words which have more than one meaning may be interpreted very literally by children according to their past experiences. Children also overhear information given to their parents or to other patients, and may misinterpret what they hear or place it out of context.

Example

Mark aged 4 came back from the operating theatre with a surgical drain in place. He asked the play specialist for a specific book called 'The Little Yellow Digger' (Gilderdale 1993) which he was familiar with from preschool. The book told the story of a mechanical digger, digging a drain in the ground and had appropriate illustrations. After the story was read he said, 'I've got a drain. That's what I have got. Why have I got a drain – what's my one?' He was told that the drains that the digger put in the ground were pipes to take away water. His drain was a little pipe or tube that the doctor had put there to take away water from his chest and help him to get better.

In the following examples, children needed to have technical terms explained to them in simple language so that they could understand what was happening:

Vela aged 4 with newly diagnosed leukaemia asked the mother of another patient why they couldn't play together, and was told that the other child was 'neutropenic'. Indignantly she demanded 'Why's she got new peanuts and I haven't?'

A 7-year-old-boy whose intravenous line pump gave the alarm signal asked, 'What's that beeping? Is my confusion complete?'

When English is the child's second language it is important to use an interpreter, and to ensure that the interpreter has an understanding of developmentally appropriate concepts and language for the child. Simple pictures or diagrams may also be useful.

Example

A 2-year-old Indian girl came to a new country for medical treatment of her brain tumour, and required radiotherapy before returning home. She saw a thick cable of black electrical cords crossing the back wall of the room and attached to the radiation machine. She cried repeatedly, 'snake, snake' in Hindi. There was no common language between the child and her family and the radiation therapist, and she and her family had not had an opportunity to view the room and become familiar with the equipment before the treatment began.

Many younger children may only be able to understand complex procedures through the use of play. Using dolls to show where central lines, cannulae, or post-operative drains will be placed, or to rehearse the steps of a procedure helps the child to understand what is about to happen. Child Life Specialists or Play Specialists are trained to assist children in this manner, and the inclusion of such professionals in paediatric oncology teams is now standard practice (United Kingdom Children's Cancer Study Group 1997).

Example

A boy aged 5, while playing with the hospital Playmobile medical play figures, described his double lumen central line to the play specialist. 'My person's got a Hickman – Hickman means two. I'll show you mine, see the two (holding up his line and displaying it), they go into this one. I've got cancer medicine and other medicine.' The boy clearly understood what his central line was for, and that different medicines went down each of the two parts of the line.

Parents are the source of daily information for the child regarding what is happening and why. If parents are not well informed, they may misinterpret what they have been told. Abbreviations are used freely in a medical setting and parents hear these and may repeat them in the context of their own understanding.

Example

The mother of a child with aplastic anaemia told everyone that her child had A.L.L. – the recognised abbreviation for acute lymphoblastic leukaemia. She knew in fact that her daughter did not have leukaemia, but had heard people talk of A.L.L. and assumed that this was the abbreviation for aplastic anaemia.

Earlier findings about adolescents' disregard of pamphlets notwithstanding, providing written information in the form of handouts, pamphlets, and books for children and their parents is one way of reducing the confusion of disease names and abbreviations.

(7) Check back with the child about their understanding of the previous discussion and ask if they have any questions.

Example

A 5-year-old girl who had been given an explanation about leukaemia asked: 'Why are they called white cells when your blood is red?'

(8) Check with the child how they are feeling, and if they have any specific worries.
Children may feel unable to spontaneously volunteer concerns they have, especially if they think that their concerns or feelings will upset others. They need to be asked directly about how they are feeling.

Example

A young boy displayed a range of somatic and anxious responses after being told about plans for him to be the bone marrow donor for his sibling's transplant. When asked directly what was wrong, he replied, 'I don't want to do that bone marrow'. It was then possible to explore with him his concerns, and the reasons for his reluctance.

(9) Outline what is going to happen next, and indicate your availability for further discussions.
This should include making sure that the child can identify someone that they would feel able to talk to if they felt upset or had any questions.

Specific Situations

Limb amputation

Amputation of a limb represents a sudden and irrevocable alteration in body appearance and integrity, and parents and adolescents in particular may feel intense distress and repugnance at the thought of what will happen in surgery. Younger children may not be so concerned about changes in body appearance, or may not realise that the loss is irreversible.

Example

A 4-year-old boy whose toe had been amputated asked his father if his toe would grow back again. He was told that his toe would not grow back, and that he would always have four toes on that foot. He needed reassuring that no other parts of his body were going to be removed. He was also told that he would still be able to walk and run like before.

Children need permission to grieve for the loss of such a tangible part of themselves by way of acknowledgement and acceptance from the adults around them of their anger or sadness.

Some of the potential losses may be a more immediate concern to the parent than to the child.

Example

A father, when the surgeon explained about limb-salvage surgery to his son's upper arm, was extremely concerned as to whether his 8-year-old son would be able to fulfil his potential as a cricketer. He needed support to be able to acknowledge the loss of some of the hopes and dreams that he, as a father, had for his son, and to separate those from the more immediate issues that his son was worried about.

When mutilating surgery such as amputation is required, special care is needed in preparing the child/adolescent for the post-operative appearance of the limb. For younger children, play preparation may be invaluable in conveying to them some understanding of what will happen. Children who are not told or adequately prepared for amputation are likely to feel angry and betrayed by the adults involved.

Example

The parents of a 9-year-old boy with an osteosarcoma of the radius were unable to bring themselves to tell their son that he was to have his lower arm amputated. The boy was devastated to wake up from surgery to find his arm gone, and subsequently as an adolescent became estranged from his family, blaming his father and the surgeon for the loss of his arm.

Limb salvage procedures pose particular challenges when discussing what will happen with children and their families. Surgery such as a rotation plasty involves both loss of part of the limb, and a marked alteration in orientation or appearance of other parts of the limb in a manner that is visually and conceptually difficult to adjust to. However, when children are adequately prepared for surgery, they adapt more easily.

Example

An 8-year-old girl with an osteosarcoma of the femur was to have a van Ness rotation plasty to allow her ankle to take the place of her knee. There was much anxiety about how to present the information about the forthcoming surgery to her. However after viewing a videotape showing other children who had undergone the same procedure, she commented, 'I won't have to reach so far to smell my foot'. Her parents had stressed to her that her survival was the main priority and that was why she needed the surgery. After the surgery she would get a prosthetic (artificial) leg fitted and she would once again have two legs to stand on.

Children may want to know what happens to the amputated limb and may wish to choose what is done with the limb.

Examples

An 11-year-old girl with an osteogenic sarcoma of the humerus underwent an amputation of her arm following thorough discussion of treatment options with her and her parents. Shortly after the amputation she asked what had happened to her amputated arm and expressed a wish to see it. Her doctor undertook to investigate where the arm was, and to view the arm first prior to the girl seeing it. The girl was informed by her doctor that her arm was still in the pathology department, whereupon she then decided that she no longer wished to see it and consented to it being disposed of. When the cancer returned several years later, she asked to visit the pathology department to see the original pathological slides of the tumour. Being able to do this helped her to acknowledge and reconcile what had happened previously with what was happening now.

An adolescent boy chose to have his amputated leg cremated, and the ashes returned to him, giving him some sense of control and ownership of his leg.

Adolescents may use humour as a way of coping with loss or with challenging situations. While this can be a useful defence and coping strategy, it is important that such humour be initiated by the adolescent rather than by others. It is also important not to ignore the underlying feelings of loss.

Example

A 15-year-old boy used 'black' humour to overcome awkward situations following amputation of his leg. Soon after discharge from hospital while he was still on crutches and awaiting a prosthesis, he visited the supermarket with his mother. When people stared at him he responded: 'I seem to have lost my leg, have you seen it – perhaps I should try the meat department'.

Bone marrow transplantation

When bone marrow transplantation is planned, good explanation and communication is essential, and this is particularly so when the marrow donor is a sibling. There are many misunderstandings that can arise if this is not done carefully: siblings may not have received much information from parents or staff about cancer, and often will not have the knowledge that is obtained by children with cancer from the peer group on the ward and at special camps (Bluebond-Langner 1978).

The actual procedure may be seen by the sibling donor as involving removal of one of their bones or of all of their bone marrow to give to the recipient, and they may worry about how they will manage without it. Siblings may also have difficulty understanding the concept of human leukocyte antigen (HLA) matching.

Examples

A 4-year-old girl was a perfect HLA match to her 6-year-old sister with relapsed leukaemia. Prior to the transplant she began to worry about exactly when she would get sick, need medicines and lose her hair, because she had been told that she had the 'same blood' as her sister. She was reassured that her blood was strong and healthy, and that she was not going to get sick like her sister because she didn't have the sick leukaemia blood. She was also told that she couldn't 'catch' leukaemia from her sister. She was then told that the medicines were making her sister's sick leukaemia blood go away, and that her healthy blood would help her sister to grow strong healthy blood like hers.

A 7-year-old boy was to be the marrow donor for his older sister who had leukaemia. He had heard numbers being discussed and knew that this was important, but did not understand what the numbers referred to. While playing with the hospital Playmobile medical dolls he said: 'That's me doing the bone marrow thing for my big sister. I'm 100 out of 100 – that's why I'm doing the bone marrow. My little sister is 20 out of 10 and Mum is 60 . . . What do I do when I do the bone marrow?'

As in the previous example, he needed a careful explanation of what was to happen.

Where there are several siblings who have compatible marrow there may be sibling rivalry as to who is the preferred donor, and when a sibling is found to not be a match he/she may feel that they have failed to help. Children may also feel coerced and resentful at the prospect of being a donor, especially if there is not an opportunity to talk openly about their fear of the procedure, or their feelings towards their sibling.

Example

A teenage boy who had been in conflict with his parents over many matters, was found to be a compatible marrow donor for his younger brother. The older boy angrily told his parents that 'they only wanted him for his marrow'. An urgent family meeting was held with him and his parents at which his current distress was acknowledged, and his parents were able to tell him that they loved him.

Additional extended family supports were put in place for the boy over the transplant period when the parents would not be very available, and he and his parents were encouraged to look at other ways of resolving conflict.

There are obvious implications to the donor if the transplant fails because of non-engraftment, infection, graft versus host disease (GvHD) or relapse of the cancer. The sibling may feel personally responsible for the outcome, and fear that his or her marrow was not 'good enough'.

Fertility

The impact of certain cancer treatments on fertility is an area that should be routinely discussed in some detail with adolescents shortly after diagnosis, and with pre-adolescent children at some stage during their cancer treatment. All patients attending late-effects clinics require information about fertility and the offer of further investigation and treatment. Adolescents also need to be reassured that infertility is not synonymous with impotence.

In some adolescent boys the issue of sperm collection and storage needs to be discussed prior to commencement of chemotherapy. This can be an extremely difficult area for the young adolescent with emerging sexuality and sexual identity to discuss, especially if they have just learned that they have cancer, and needs to be approached with great sensitivity. While some parents of adolescents will have previously established open and honest communication about sexuality with their adolescent, other parents will have no communication pathways established, and thus have little idea of how best to approach this topic. As with any other discussion of serious matters, this needs to take place in a private setting, and with acknowledgement that this may be an issue that the adolescent finds difficult to discuss. It is helpful to find out how much the adolescent already understands about sexual reproduction and physiology, and the words they use to describe this. After careful explanation of the impact on fertility of treatment, the adolescent needs to be told about the possibility of storing sperm so that when he is older he can have children should he wish, and be offered the opportunity to discuss ways that sperm collection can be undertaken.

If parents are reluctant to even consider such issues with respect to their son on the basis of cultural and religious beliefs, there may still be an ethical and legal obligation to inform the adolescent of the options and consequences.

While infertility is relatively common in the general population and affects one in six couples, most people with infertility do not have to acknowledge or address these issues until they are older adults in a stable relationship. An understandable reluctance to face definite confirmation of infertility and the inherent loss for the future may result in fertility testing being declined by adolescents attending late-effects clinics.

Examples

A 19-year-old leukaemia survivor said that he was prepared to provide a semen sample, but not yet; he was still not ready for working through the issues that would arise should the sample show that he was in fact sterile.

A 15-year-old boy who had completed cancer treatment stated that he thought he might be the father of his pregnant friend's unborn child. The oncology staff knew that he was highly unlikely to be the biological father. However, he did not wish to pursue blood testing to prove paternity, and chose to maintain the hope that the child could be his.

Adolescents who have impaired fertility may feel angry that their parents gave consent to treatment that was known to impair fertility when the adolescent was younger. They may need to have the original treatment dilemmas and decisions explained to them, and have acknowledged the loss involved for them.

Specific Issues

Informed consent/assent

The type of information given to a child or adolescent may be influenced by the need for informed consent vs. assent. While it is important where possible to have a child's assent to treatment and procedures, there are many situations where treatments will proceed even without this, as long as parents are giving consent. However, in the case of older, cognitively competent adolescents, most services expect both the adolescent and their parents to give informed consent before proceeding with treatment. This requires active discussion of the advantages and disadvantages of the possible courses of action and outcomes, including the likely outcome of not treating. Such information would not be routinely given to younger children unless they were requesting it, as they can become overwhelmed and confused by the multiple possibilities and complex decision making. It is important that the adults presenting information to children or adolescents are clear before they start whether they are seeking the young person's assent or their consent, and that they make this explicit to the young person also (Leikin 1993).

Example

The parents of a 13-year-old girl who developed leukaemia decided to treat her as an adult, allowing her a large say in the treatment decisions on the basis that it was better to have her as an active participant. This led to many disagreements in which the girl became anxious and angry, and culminated in the girl informing her parents that she would not have cranial irradiation and would not complete the consolidation phase of treatment. The family then moved to another city where the new medical team, mindful of what had already occurred, was able to work with the parents to set the ground rules for the girl's ongoing management. These were based on the notion that while her assent would be sought for treatment, she was not able to give or withhold consent because she was too young to be able to make the major treatment decisions. The girl completed treatment satisfactorily and was less anxious and distressed.

Situations where adolescents and parents disagree on treatment consent are rare and can usually be resolved by careful exploration of the issues and concerns with the adolescent and with the parents. It is helpful to see the parties both alone and together, take time for discussion, and make sure that good supports are in place for the adolescent and for the parents. It may be necessary to formally assess the adolescent's level of decision-making competence, and to request legal advice. Situations where consensus is not reached are distressing for everyone, particularly if this results in a widening rift between the adolescent and parents.

Example

A young man who had been 5 years old at diagnosis with leukaemia, died at age 15 after multiple relapses. Prior to his death when conventional therapies had been exhausted, his parents were engaged in a bitter discussion about alternative therapies for their son. One parent was in favour and the other vehemently opposed. In an attempt to resolve the conflict an extended family meeting was called with appropriate cultural supports present. In the meeting he told his parents and extended family, 'no way am I taking any more pills – end of story'. This served as the catalyst to bring his parents together so that they could support him in the time he had left, and no further treatment was sought.

Siblings

Inadequate knowledge and poor parent–sibling communication about the illness have been identified as risk factors for poor emotional adjustment in the siblings of children who have cancer (Murray 2001). It is easy for healthy siblings to become almost invisible to the healthcare team, and for parents to attempt to shield them from distressing information. If the healthy sibling does not have much contact with the hospital, they also do not develop a context into which information they are given or which they overhear can be put. This highlights the need for siblings to receive ongoing information about their brother or sister's illness, and to have their anxieties and concerns listened to and addressed.

Example

An 11-year-old sister of a child who was dying with a rhabdomyosarcoma told the nurse 'my sister has cancer in some muscle thing – I don't know where, Mum doesn't tell me'. Her mother was subsequently encouraged to sit down with her daughter and a staff member and tell her more about her sister's cancer and treatments.

Community peers

The friends and classmates of children who have cancer are part of the network of support for the sick child, and can at times carry a heavy emotional load if a sick child or adolescent chooses to confide hopes, fears, and stark realities to close friends. Other adolescents choose not to tell friends about their illness, preferring to maintain what 'normality' they can for as long as possible. This also is hard for friends, who must maintain the pretence that all is well despite obvious signs that the ill friend is deteriorating. Such situations raise issues of confidentiality and respect for the ill adolescent's autonomy versus the information needs of peers to enable them to cope with their distress and grief. For many children and adolescents, this may be the first experience they have had of serious illness or death in someone close to them.

Example

A young man aged 15 was reluctant to tell friends when his treatment-resistant cancer recurred, wanted to continue 'living' as normal a life as possible – attending school, playing rugby, and being with his friends. His friends, who could see how unwell he was becoming, shielded him on the rugby field while he could still play, and spent time with him. Eventually the friends' mothers decided to tell their sons about the cancer, thus enabling their sons to continue to provide unconditional support to their dying friend. He chose not to talk about his illness or his death with friends or family. Shortly before his death, the school sought advice on how to prepare the school community for his impending death, and his funeral was subsequently held at the school. The friends 'included' him in subsequent school events, organising an annual fundraising fashion parade for CanTeen (Teenage Cancer Patient's Society) and talking about their sadness and their positive memories of him at their final school dinner two years later.

Ward peers

Treatment for a child with cancer is not something that requires one visit, one operation or a single course of chemotherapy. A treatment regimen may last many months or years, some delivered solely as an inpatient, others as a combination of inpatient and outpatient visits. Ward and clinic friendships develop, not just between the parents but the children as well, especially when the children are the same age, have the same diagnosis, or have similar treatment schedules. Families tend to link in with those families whose children were diagnosed around the same time, and families from minority ethnic groups congregate together to communicate in their own language. When treatment is not going well with a child there are ramifications beyond the family unit, and the relapse or death of a child is felt keenly by other children and families. In the ward setting children are acutely aware of what is happening with other patients, but often do not have permission to discuss this with the adults. In some instances it may be necessary to meet with the other inpatient children to talk about their anxieties and answer their questions directly. This requires delicate balancing between open acknowledgement of that which is common unspoken knowledge, and protection of the privacy and confidentiality of the index child and family.

Speaking with Children about Death

Speaking with children about death should be part of normal living, because children rapidly learn that everyone will die at some stage. Healthy children not infrequently ask parents if the parents will die, or ask if they themselves could die as a consequence of certain events. Children need honest replies to such questions to the effect that everyone, including parents, will die some day, usually when they are old and have lived a full life. Children also need the reassurance that if anything did happen to their parent, that they would be cared for.

When a child who has cancer asks, 'Am I going to die?', they need to have acknowledged that death is a possibility with any child with cancer, and that they could die. They also need to be told about the treatments that are planned, and the hope and expectation that those treatments will make the cancer go away. However, the most important thing to reassure the child of is that no matter what happens, they will be looked after, loved, and kept comfortable.

Children seem to ask this question at times when parents and hospital staff least expect it, such as in the middle of the night, or in the car in busy motorway traffic. Adults need to be prepared to answer, no matter when the question is asked. They also need to be prepared to say, 'I don't know', and acknowledge that they may not have answers for every question, but will endeavour to find answers for their child.

Sometimes in talking with children about death, it takes time to sort out exactly what the child is asking about, especially with young children who are concrete in their thinking.

Example

A boy aged 4 had never known his grandfather, but stated that he would like to see his grandfather's body. His parents were concerned that their son had a 'morbid obsession with death'. They subsequently realised that what their son wanted was to see a full-length photo of his grandfather, as all the photographs on display showed only head and shoulders – he wanted to see that his grandfather had a torso, arms, and legs.

When a Child Has Relapsed or Has Incurable Disease

(1) When a child is expected to die, how they are informed about this must take into account their age, level of understanding, previous experiences of death in the family, and cultural and religious beliefs.

(2) Reinforce how hard the child and parents and medical team have worked to 'overcome' the illness/cancer. Explain that the illness hasn't gone away and that the treatments are not able to cure the cancer. Everyone's 'job' is now to keep the child feeling comfortable and able to spend time with their family and friends.

Example

A boy aged 5 with relapsed leukaemia was playing with medical play equipment while he talked to the play specialist. He said to her: 'Mummy says this doesn't work any more. We're going home to see what love can do. Mummy says no more treatment, lots of love.'

(3) Check for questions and ask how the child is feeling now.
Children often realise that they may die, and already know the implications of their medical condition. This allows them to voice their concerns, and ask directly.

Example

A girl aged 11 years had been sick since infancy with a slow-growing tumour and had a poor prognosis. Her younger siblings, who had been given little information about her illness, met with the doctor at their parent's request, to talk about her cancer and likely outcome. After the doctor had told the siblings that sometimes cancers could not be cured and would not get better, the brother aged 8 said: 'Is that what is happening with my sister? Do children die from that, is my sister going to die?' The doctor explained to the boy and his brother that their sister was very sick and that her cancer was not going to get better, and that this was not anyone's fault. They were told that their sister was going to die sometime soon from the cancer. Both children were then able to talk with their mother and the doctor about their sadness and their parents' sadness, and to check with their parents that they would not get cancer from their sister.

(4) Explain that when someone gets very sick with this illness they die, and that this is what the doctors think will happen. Incorporate the family's spiritual and cultural beliefs about death if appropriate. Avoid using euphemisms to describe death as younger children may interpret these in a literal and concrete manner.

Example

A boy who had died of cancer was laid out on his bed at home. A young neighbourhood friend came with his parents to say goodbye. He was keen to see the dead boy's back, as he had been told that 'when someone dies they become an angel' and he wanted to see if the wings were growing yet.

(5) Reassure the child that, no matter what, they will be cared for, loved, and not abandoned, and that they will always be part of their family.

While this may seem self-evident, many children may fear that they will be left alone or abandoned, and need concrete reassurance to the contrary.

(6) Allow for hope for a different outcome if this is important to the child or family.

Example

The nursing staff caring for a 16-year-old boy who was dying with a Ewing's sarcoma became concerned that he was 'denying his impending death' and needed reassurance. The young man had acknowledged that he was dying, but sometimes talked about attending university in the future. The nursing staff were encouraged to acknowledge his hopes without challenging them, while at the same time not actively planning with him a future that was unrealistic. This enabled them to support him as he held both his loss and his hope.

(7) Explain that children and parents are often sad or angry at times like this and that this is a normal reaction.

Example

A girl developed leukaemia at 7 years, and died aged 12 after a relapse. When the doctor that told her that she had relapsed, she responded with outrage and shouted abuse at the doctor (a person she knew well and trusted). She had to have someone to blame. She was then able to move on from her anger and plan her own funeral, choosing the dress her mother was to wear, the music and words for the funeral, and writing her will leaving her prized personal possessions to family and friends.

(8) Outline ongoing supports for the child and family.

Children and adolescents often worry about how their parents will cope after their death. This may make it difficult for children to openly voice their feelings, or allow themselves to relinquish the struggle to stay alive.

Example

An adolescent girl who was dying became very agitated; it was only at the point when she was told that the hospital staff would support her distressed parents that she visibly relaxed and died peacefully.

David's Story

The following extract was written by the mother of a 5-year-old boy who died of leukaemia, and illustrates some of the issues discussed above.

'How do you explain to a 5-year-old child that he is not going to get better? How do you tell him that he is going to die? Do you in fact tell a child so young that he

is going to die? This was the agonising choice I was faced with just before my son David died.

When it became clear that David would not survive, I talked to our nurse who had been assigned to help us at home, providing us with the necessary medical advice and support that we needed. She reassured me that, despite his age, David needed to know. Nevertheless I was apprehensive about telling him.

However, we were sitting on the floor one afternoon playing – probably with his Lego, one of his favourite toys, and I felt I could broach the subject. I began by asking what he thought would happen if he didn't get better. His reply was, 'I'll be in a wheelchair for the rest of my life'. I replied that that wouldn't be the case and then explained gently that he would die and go to Heaven. He thought carefully about this for a moment or two and then said, 'Oh! Then I'll be able to say hello to the astronauts' (several days before this conversation the American Space Shuttle 'Challenger' had exploded seconds after lift-off, killing its crew of seven astronauts. David had watched photographs of the 'Challenger' enveloped in a red orange and white fireball on the television news and discussed with his parents what happened after death).

His next response was, 'Am I going to die today?'

When I reassured him that he wasn't he said, 'That's okay then'.

David left the house once in the last 6 weeks of his life. He did not want to go anywhere else. He was happy sleeping, playing with his train set and Lego when he felt able to do so, being read to, watching the occasional comedy on TV with his Dad and laughing heartily, celebrating his sixth birthday lying in bed smiling at a helium balloon floating up to the ceiling of his bedroom and trying to cope physically with his failing body.

It was a bittersweet time for all of us – his Dad, Nain (Welsh grandmother), sister and me – but those last few weeks of David's life were very special.

He died very peacefully and quickly late in the afternoon.

He had time to ask me to hold him and intimated that I was to get his Dad, who then held him in his arms as he died and both of us knew at the moment of his death that something very special had happened to him. I knew in that instance that David was well at last and it was the most profound and comforting feeling.

I cannot advise other people about what they should or should not say if they know their child is dying, but I wanted to share my experience in the hope that it may help others.

When Parents are Reluctant to Have a Child Told about the Diagnosis or Prognosis

Some parents do not want their child to be told anything about the diagnosis of cancer or the prognosis. This wish may derive from the parents' fears that honest information will damage their child emotionally and make them 'give up fighting the cancer', or may arise from strongly held cultural and spiritual beliefs and practices. Many parents, given the opportunity to talk about their fears or beliefs with the medical team will then be able to join with the staff in planning how best to proceed. It is helpful for parents to be given information about both the benefits of being open with their child, and the risks to the child's emotional wellbeing if secrecy is maintained.

Example

After an 8-year-old girl was diagnosed with metastatic cancer, a trial of chemotherapy showed the tumour to be unresponsive and aggressive. Staff were concerned that her parents had not informed her about her diagnosis and its prognosis. The family were recent immigrants, and informed the staff that it was culturally inappropriate for Chinese children to be told about a diagnosis of cancer, and that dying was never mentioned as they believed that talk of dying leads to 'a loss of interest' which hastens the death. The parents were, however, persuaded by staff that it would be helpful for their daughter to know that the treatment for her cancer was not working. They requested that her nurse, who spoke their dialect of Chinese and had established a rapport with their daughter, do the talking, and that they (the parents and older siblings) would be available but not present in the room. The girl told her nurse that she already knew exactly what her diagnosis was, and that her cancer was unresponsive and progressive. She knew that she was dying, despite no direct discussions having taken place about such matters.

What she then wanted conveyed to her parents was the fact that 'she knew what they knew'. Although further open discussions did not occur, the family was then able to provide love and support until she died. She made her will, requested that her tenth birthday be celebrated early and her friends come to visit, and the family visit the snow (a new experience).

Ten years on, her parents believe it was worth telling their daughter her diagnosis. They are grateful to the health professionals for persuading them to do so. They believe that their daughter had the right to know that she was dying, but acknowledge that they had not wanted to be the ones to tell her. Knowing openly what was happening and removing the 'mutual pretence' (Bluebond-Langner 1978) allowed her to plan her remaining life.

In the situation where parents continue to refuse permission to give the child or adolescent any information, the rights of the child to information need to be balanced against the rights of the family to choose how they manage their child during a life-threatening illness. Debate on this topic has not resolved the question of how to proceed (Higgs 1985, Hilden, Watterson and Chrastek 2000); some paediatric oncology teams have a policy of talking openly with the child from the initial point of diagnosis, others will accommodate parental views and wishes with the proviso that, if the child asks staff members a direct question about their disease or prognosis, the child will be given an honest answer.

When Adolescents Choose not to Talk about Dying

Some children and adolescents choose to not discuss their advancing disease or death, despite open information and opportunity to talk. In such instances, the young person's choice must be respected. Expressions of fear and loss, if they do occur, may be indirect or non-verbal.

Example

A young man who was 14 when he was diagnosed with a brain tumour, died 4 years later aged 18. Throughout his illness, communication with his medical caregivers was difficult as he never established eye contact and would sit with his cap pulled down around his eyes during clinic visits. Despite having a close family and an excellent relationship with his parents, he did not wish to discuss dying.

Days before he died, when his vision had failed, he dictated a letter to a friend, expressing his thanks to the friend for being there and for visiting, and hoped he would remember him after his death. He described in the letter how scared he felt, and spoke of his fear of dying. His mother was writing down the words for him; it was the first time that she had really heard how her son felt.

Importance of Cultural and Spiritual Issues

For many families their spiritual beliefs and cultural practice are the foundations on which their lives are based. Communication with the child and with the family regarding illness and death needs to be done in a manner that is congruent with and respectful of the family beliefs. Staff should if necessary seek advice and guidance from cultural workers and spiritual leaders in order to be able to work appropriately with the child and family. They do not, however, have to share the same faith themselves to be able to communicate well and provide good care.

Example

Mary was 14 years old when diagnosed with an osteosarcoma. Treatment involved surgery (amputation) and chemotherapy. Five years later a local recurrence with metastatic spread was diagnosed. Surgery was not an option and she declined palliative chemotherapy, but accepted, after extensive family meetings, radiotherapy. Even though at 19 she was legally an adult, she needed approval from her father as head of the family before agreeing to the radiotherapy. This provided temporary shrinkage of the rapidly expanding tumour recurrence.

Her devout Christian faith and close community of family and friends provided her with strength and support during her terminal illness.

After her death her social worker wrote:

Mary and her family had a profound and sincere faith and they never really gave up hope that Jesus would save Mary. Initially Mary said that she didn't want treatment because she did not want to lose her hair. In our travelling to and from appointments in the car she talked about her very strong belief that Jesus would make the right decisions for her and that her parents wanted her to put the utmost faith in him. Mary and her parents (particularly her father) prayed for hours every day. Mary had a goal – to go to her parents' homeland to see their religious leader. Initially it was for her and her father, then for her and her mother and then towards the end just for her mother. Acknowledging that she would not be going was the final acceptance that her death was now inevitable.

Mary talked about her beliefs so openly because she had trust in her medical team, borne out of long association. Throughout those last months of her life, although the tumour moved rapidly at its own pace, Mary always talked at her pace – sometimes about her faith, often about her hopes of visiting her parents' homeland and of attending university. Her valedictory at school was that she had made it to university, the first to do so in her extended family. Sometimes she talked about her illness and her tiredness. I also recall visiting a few days before she died and just sitting on the floor next to her when she was on the sofa – she just rested her hand on my head and said that she was all right. Her parents and I talked about allsorts; Mary never took her hand away, just drifted in and out of the conversation until it was time for me to go. When she said, 'Goodbye and thank you', I knew that I would not talk to her again.

The things that were important for Mary and her family were their trust, the preservation of her and her parents' dignity, caring for her family and community, acceptance of her faith, and moving at her pace. These all came together to enable a 'conversation' with a terminally ill young woman that often didn't need words.

Talking about funerals

Some children and adolescents, faced by the knowledge that they are dying, choose to plan their own funeral. They may want to discuss in great detail the issues of service format, cremation vs. burial, and giving away their possessions. Such discussion can be difficult for the adults involved, who might hold different views about what should happen after death, and who may have difficulty facing the child's stark view of reality. However, for young people this process can give them a sense of control over one part of their existence, while still having to deal with advancing disease over which they have no control.

Attendance of children at funerals varies according to cultural, religious, and family tradition and practice. Included in these traditions are beliefs about whether children should be encouraged to visit and spend time with the body of the dead person prior to the funeral, whether children will attend open-casket funerals, and inclusion or exclusion of children from religious ceremony and rituals.

When a child with cancer dies, fellow patients and their families often choose to attend the funeral but may not have much knowledge of the funeral customs that they will witness or be expected to participate in. Older children and adolescents often make a conscious decision to attend or not attend a particular funeral, whereas younger children may attend because their parents wish to show support to the family, but may have even less understanding of what is going to happen. Children need an explanation of what will happen at the funeral, what they will see and hear, and how other people might react emotionally. It will also help if they understand a little about the religious beliefs and rituals practised by the dead child's family.

Example

At the graveside of a classmate, a group of 5-year-olds were peering into the grave as the coffin was lowered into the ground. The officiating priest told them not to look into the ground but up at the sky, because their friend had become an angel. The children, fascinated, looked upwards but were extremely bewildered and disappointed when they saw nothing – no angel flying.

CONCLUSION

In this chapter we have tried to suggest ways in which the serious issues for children and adolescents with cancer can be talked about. It is by listening to children and speaking with them truthfully about their illness, their treatment, and for some their death, that we give them the solid ground from which they and their families can find a way through whatever lies ahead.

> *Speak, speak. When the time comes*
> *do not be silent but know the time.*   (Helen Shaw)

ACKNOWLEDGEMENTS

Our thanks to the children and their families encountered while working in paediatric oncology for the lessons we have learned from them.

We would also like to thank our colleagues in the multidisciplinary paediatric oncology and consultation liaison teams at Starship Children's Hospital for their constructive comments on this chapter and for their support, and in particular to thank Barbara Mackay for allowing us to use some case illustrations drawn from her paper (Mackay 1999) and her clinical work.

The names of children in the case examples have been changed to protect their privacy.

310   PSYCHOSOCIAL ASPECTS OF PEDIATRIC ONCOLOGY

REFERENCES

Barnes, J., Kroll, L., Burke, O., et al. (2000) Qualitative interview study of communication between parents and children about maternal breast cancer. *BMJ* **321**, 479–482.
Bibace, R, Walsh, M.E. (1979) Developmental stages in children's conceptions of illness. In Stone, Cohen & Adler (Eds) *Health Psychology*. San Francisco: Jossey-Bass, pp. 285–301.
Blackley, A., Eiser, C., Ellis, A., et al. (1998) Development and evaluation of an information booklet for adult survivors of cancer in childhood. *Archives of Disease in Childhood* **78**, 340–344.
Bluebond-Langner, M. (1978) *The Private Worlds of Dying Children*. Princeton, NJ: Princeton University Press.
Bluebond-Langner M., Perkel D., Goertzel T., et al. (1990) Children's knowledge of cancer and its treatment: Impact of an oncology camp experience. *Journal of Pediatrics* **116**(2), 207–213.
Buckman, R. (1992) *How to Break Bad News. A Guide for Healthcare Professionals*. John Hopkins University Press, Baltimore.
Burbach, D.J., Petersor, L. (1986) Children's concepts of illness: A review and critique of the cognitive-developmental literature. *Health Psychology* **5**, 307–325.
Byrne, J., Lewis, M.E.S., Halamek, L., et al. (1989) Childhood cancer survivors' knowledge of their diagnosis and treatment. *Annals of Internal Medicine* **110**(5), 400–403.
Chesler, M.A., Paris, J., Barbarin, O.A. (1986) 'Telling' the child with cancer: Parental choices to share information with ill children. *Journal of Pediatric Psychology* **11**(4), 497–516.
Claflin, C.J., Barbarin, O.A. (1990) Does 'telling' less protect more? Relationships among age, information disclosure, and what children with cancer see and feel. *Journal of Pediatric Psychology* **16**(2), 169–191.
Cotton, C.R., Range, L.M. (1990) Children's death concepts: Relationship to cognitive functioning, age, experience with death, fear of death, and helplessness. *Journal of Clinical Child Psychology* **19**, 123–127.
Crisp, J., Goodnow, J. J., Ungerer, J. A. (1996) The impact of experience on children's understanding of illness. *Journal of Pediatric Psychology* **21**(1), 57–72.
Eiser, C., Levitt, G., Leiper, A., et al. (1996) Clinic audit for long term survivors of childhood cancer. *Archives of Disease in Childhood* **75**, 405–409.
Faulkner, K.W. (1993) Children's understanding of death. In Armstrong-Dailey, Goltzer (Eds), *Hospice Care for Children*. New York: Oxford University Press, pp. 9–21.
Fundudis, T. (1997) Young children's memory: How good is it? How much do we know about it? *Child Psychology & Psychiatry Review* Vol 2(4), 150–158.
Gilderdale, Betty and Alan (1993) *The Little Yellow Digger*. Ashton Scholastic Ltd.
Goldman, A., Christie, D. (1993) Children with cancer talking about their own death, with their families. *Pediatric Hematology and Oncology* **10**, 223–231.
Greenberg, L.W., Jewett, L.S., Gluck, R.S., et al. (1984) Giving information for a life-threatening diagnosis. *AJDC* **138**, 649–653.
Grollman, E.A. (1976) *Talking About Death: A dialogue between parent and child* (revised edn). Boston, MA: Beacon.
Hansdottir, I., Malcarne, V.L. (1998) Concepts of illness in Icelandic children. *Journal of Pediatric Psychology* **23**(3), 187–195.
Higgs, R. (1985) A father says 'Don't tell my son the truth'. *Journal of Medical Ethics* **11**, 153–158.

Hilden, J.M., Watterson, J., Chrastek, J. (2000) Tell the children. *Journal of Clinical Oncology* **18**(17), 3193–3195.

Jankovic, M., Loiacono, N.B., Spinetta, J.J., *et al.* (1994) Telling young children with leukemia their diagnosis: The flower garden as analogy. *Pediatric Hematology and Oncology* **11**, 75–81.

Koocher, G.P. (1974) Talking with children about death. *American Journal of Orthopsychiatry* **44**(3), 404–410.

Kroll, L., Barnes, J., Jones, A.L., *et al.* (1998) Cancer in parents: Telling children. *BMJ* **316**, 880.

Last, B.F., van Veldhuizen, A.M. (1996) Information about diagnosis and prognosis related to anxiety and depression in children with cancer aged 8–16 years. *European Journal of Cancer* **32A**(2), 290–294.

Leikin, S.L. (1993) The role of adolescents in decisions concerning their cancer therapy. *CANCER Supplement* **71**(10), 3342–3346.

Levenson, P.M., Pfefferbaum, B.J., Copeland, D.R., *et al.* (1982) Information preferences of cancer patients ages 11–20. *Journal of Adolescent Health Care* **3**, 9–13.

Mackay, B. (1999) When your brother or sister has cancer: Supporting siblings' rights to know. Paper presented at the Children's Issues Centre's 3rd Child and Family Policy Conference, July, Dunedin, New Zealand.

Murray, J.S. (2001) Social support for school-aged siblings of children with cancer: A comparison between parent and sibling perceptions. *Journal of Pediatric Oncology Nursing* **18**(3), 90–104.

Nitschke, R., Humphrey, G.B., Sexauer, C.L., *et al.* (1982) Therapeutic choices made by patients with end-stage cancer. *Journal of Pediatrics* **101**(3), 471–476.

Perrin, E.C., Gerrity, P.S. (1981) There's a demon in your belly: Children's understanding of illness. *Pediatrics* **67**(6), 841–849.

Potter, P.C., Roberts, M.C. (1984) Children's perceptions of chronic illness: The roles of disease symptoms, cognitive development, and information. *Journal of Pediatric Psychology* **9**, 13–27.

Rosenheim, E., Reicher, R. (1985) Informing children about a parent's terminal illness. *Journal of Child Psychology and Psychiatry* **26**, 995–998.

Schonfeld, D.J., O'Hare, L.L., Perrin, E.C., Quackenbush, M., Showalter, D.R., Cicchetti, D.V. (1995) A randomised, controlled trial of a school-based, multifaceted AIDS education program in the elementary grades: the impact on comprehension, knowledge and fears. *Pediatrics* **95**(4), 480–486.

Shaw, H. (1995) *I listen – reflections and meditations.* Edited by Deborah Grossman Knowles. Auckland: Puriri Press.

Sherman, M., Koch, D., Giardina, P., *et al.* (1985) Thalassemic children's understanding of illness: A study of cognitive and emotional factors. *Annals of the New York Academy of Sciences* **445**, 327–336.

Shields, C.E. (1998) Giving patients bad news. *Primary Care* **25**(2), 381–390.

Slavin, L., O'Malley, J., Koocher, G., *et al.* (1982) Communication of the cancer diagnosis to pediatric patients: Impacts on long term adjustments. *American Journal of Psychiatry* **139**, 179–183.

Spinetta, J.J., Swarner, J.A., Sheposh, J.P. (1981) Effective parental coping following the death of a child from cancer. *Journal of Pediatric Psychology* **6**, 251–263.

Tebbi, C.K. (1993) Treatment compliance in childhood and adolescence. *CANCER Supplement* **71**(10), 3441–3449.

Tebbi, C.K., Cummings, K.M., Zevon, M.A., *et al.* (1986) Compliance of pediatric and adolescent cancer patients. *Cancer* **58**, 1179–1184.

Thompson, R.J., Gustafson, K.E. (1996) Developmental changes in conceptualizations of health, illness, pain, and death. In *Adaption to Chronic Illness in Children.* Washington, DC: American Psychological Association, pp. 181–195.

United Kingdom Children's Cancer Study Group (UKCCSG) (1997) Requirements of a Children's Cancer Treatment Centre Wishing to Participate within the UKCCSG, May.

13

Psychosocial Interventions: the Cognitive–Behavioral Approach

BOB F. LAST AND MARTHA A. GROOTENHUIS

Emma Kinderziekenhuis, Academic Medical Center, Psychosocial Department, University of Amsterdam, The Netherlands

INTRODUCTION

Childhood cancer in the family is an obviously stressful situation. Much research has been conducted in which the emotional reactions and coping strategies of children with cancer and their parents were investigated. For both children with cancer and their parents different findings are reported.

Several studies that investigated the psychological and social adaptation of children with cancer found that they did not differ significantly from healthy controls (Kaplan *et al.* 1987). Some studies have even reported lower levels of depression in children with cancer compared to healthy controls (Canning, Canning and Boyce 1992, Worchel *et al.* 1988). In a review about young childhood cancer survivors it is also shown that overall emotional adjustment of the survivors as a group was within normal limits (Stam, Grootenhuis and Last 2001). However, one-third of the adolescent survivors met criteria for lifetime PTSD, which is a greater percentage than in the general population (Spirito *et al.* 1990).

Many studies have been conducted among parents of children with cancer and different reactions have been reported for different periods of treatment (Grootenhuis and Last, 1997c). Researchers who focused on parents of newly diagnosed children with cancer, or children who are in treatment, report increased emotional distress such as anxiety or depression of parents against

Psychosocial Aspects of Pediatric Oncology. Edited by S. Kreitler and M. Weyl Ben Arush
© 2004 John Wiley & Sons Ltd: ISBN 0 471 49939 0

normative data (Dahlquist *et al.* 1993, Manne *et al.* 1995). In longitudinal studies also increased negative emotions such as anxiety, depression, insomnia or somatic and social dysfunctioning shortly after diagnosis are found (Fife, Norton and Groom 1987, Sawyer *et al.* 1993). Brown *et al.* (1993) found that 34% of the mothers of children with cancer in various phases of their child's disease were diagnosed with a psychiatric disorder. Little depression of parents of children with cancer in treatment has been found as well (Dahlquist *et al.* 1993, Mulhern *et al.* 1992).

Contradictory findings among children and parents can partly be attributed to the inappropriateness of instruments to measure the impact of childhood cancer (Van Dongen-Melman *et al.* 1995). Studies focusing on illness-related psychosocial consequences instead of depression and anxiety, found that problems for parents concerned uncertainty and loneliness (Van Dongen-Melman *et al.* 1995, Grootenhuis and Last 1997a), or regarded concerns about the child's future, health and relapse (Leventhal-Belfer, Bakker and Russo 1993).

Other explanations for the scarcity of serious adjustment problems are children's and parents' capacities to develop strengths and abilities to 'bounce back', which is called resilience (Patterson 1995). Another possible explanation could be 'response shift', which means that the experience with cancer has changed children's conceptualization of problems. As a result of this response shift, problems are being underreported. Response shift has also been described in adults with cancer (Sprangers and Schwartz 1999). In other words, the reliance on different coping strategies such as avoidance, social support, and open communication play an important role in the emotional adjustment of children with cancer (Phipps, Fairclough and Mulhern 1995, Worchel *et al.* 1992) and their parents (Shapiro and Shumaker 1987, Speechley and Noh 1992). Several intervention studies showed possibilities of improving coping strategies and reducing feelings of distress in children with cancer (Jay *et al.* 1987, Katz *et al.* 1988). Empirical evaluations of intervention programs for parents are, however, rare and report no significant effects on adjustment (Kupst *et al.* 1982, Hoekstra-Weebers *et al.* 1998).

The purpose of this chapter is to put in order the understanding of the emotions and coping strategies, and behavioral reactions of children with cancer and their parents. First, the cognitive approach will be outlined with the theoretical background of cognitions and emotions. This will include a description of the emotions in the light of different situational meaning structures which determine the appraisal of the situation for children with cancer and their parents. Situational meaning structures which are important for children and parents are, for example, uncertainty about the outcome of the disease, responsibility for the cause and the course of the illness, and the uncontrollability of the situation. Thereafter, the process of coping is discussed and a conceptual framework is presented as a tool to comprehend children's and parental reactions to childhood cancer. Because the coping process of children with cancer and their parents is greatly influenced by the uncontrollability of the situation, we chose the model developed by Rothbaum, Weisz and Snyder (1982) in addition to the traditional approach. Their model describes control strategies which can be used to understand the coping behaviors of children with cancer and their parents. The traditional approach of learned stimulus–response relationships is outlined with examples of behavioral therapeutic techniques. Based on the concepts of the cognitive and behavioral approach of emotions we suggest an integrated model for psychosocial intervention. Three cases will be presented to show how the psychosocial intervention model can be applied in pediatric oncology.

COGNITION AND EMOTIONS

Appraisal

Through cognitive appraisal processes, people evaluate the significance of events for their wellbeing. Lazarus and Folkman (1984) distinguish three kinds of cognitive appraisal: primary, secondary, and reappraisal. Primary appraisal is the first assessment of the situation. If the situation is considered stressful it can have three forms: harm/loss, threat, and challenge. At this moment, the person decides whether the situation is an emotional one or not (Frijda 1986). This results in a number of emotions, or psychological reactions to events, depending on the relevance for the concerns of a person (Frijda 1986). Positive emotions are evoked by events which correspond to what a person desires (e.g., safety, absence of pain). Negative emotions are evoked by events, which do not correspond to the needs or desires of a person (uncertainty, fear of loss, pain). In recent emotion theory, cognition is a determinant of emotional response through processes of 'appraisal' or 'meaning-analysis' (Frijda 1986). Each specific emotion corresponds to a different appraisal, a different situational meaning structure. Every situation consists of different components. The component which is dominant for a person determines which emotion will arise. Shifts in dominance within the situational meaning structure leads to shifts in emotional experience. Negative outcome of medical examinations will raise uncertainty in a cancer patient and by those feelings of fear, whether focusing on the progress in cancer treatment evokes subsequently feelings of hope.

   In the cognitive approach of emotions the appraisal process not only refers to actual stimulus conditions but also to the associations of a person with the actual situation (Davey 1989). These associations are the cognitive representations referring to the component that dominates in the situational meaning structure. For instance, a cancer patient who experienced the death of a fellow-patient after he or she was removed to a certain room may easily be seized with fear memorizing this event when replaced to this room some time later. This associative process can be understood in terms of classic conditioning. Associative learning is conceived as a basic principle in contemporary classical conditioning. For instance, empirical study on the acquisition of phobic fears revealed that cognitive representation of a conditioned stimulus (CS) with an unconditioned stimulus (UCS) evokes a conditioned response (CR) – not only in a sequential (an event predicts the occurrence of an other event) but also as a referential (an event activates the memory to an earlier event) relationship (Davey 1989, 1992). Therefore analysis of the cognitive representations present in the appraisal of the situational meaning structure of a person is of importance in psychodiagnostics, prior to psychosocial and/or psychotherapeutical interventions (Davey 1992, Korrelboom and Kernkamp 1993).

Appraisal by Children with Cancer and their Parents

The components, which are important in the appraisal of the situation for children with cancer and their parents, are uncertainty, uncontrollability of the situation, responsibility, the restriction of freedom, and the long duration of the situation (Van Veldhuizen and Last 1991). In the case of children, the appraisal of the situation is highly dependent on the rapidly shifting developmental level (Peterson 1989).

Uncertainty about the course and the outcome of the disease is a condition related to hope and fear. Indications pointing to a remission of the disease contribute to a feeling of hope and trust, while indications of a relapse or recurrence of the disease evoke feelings of fear that all efforts will be unsuccessful. Feelings of uncertainty about the future and fear of a relapse are often reported by parents of children with cancer (Leventhal-Belfer, Bakker and Russo 1993). In the first major study about surviving childhood cancer (Koocher and O'Malley 1981), it was shown that uncertainty of parents was one of the major concerns. Parents of childhood cancer survivors were mainly uncertain about the long-term effects of the treatment and the possibilities for a relapse.

Being confronted with cancer means being confronted with *uncontrollability*, which easily evokes feelings of helplessness. Children and parents cannot influence the disease or the treatment process very much. This is in the hands of doctors and nurses. The child has to undergo many painful medical procedures while parents stand by helplessly. In reaction children can easily develop avoidant and/or resistant behavior in order to 'flight' from the noxious stimuli (Humphrey *et al.* 1992). Moreover, young children in particular are subject to cognitive distortions that can influence the appraisal (Manne and Andersen 1991). In the case of medical procedures, children can have immature conceptualizations about bodily processes, such as a fear that one's blood will leak out during a venepuncture (Peterson 1989). Another example of a cognitive distortion is the idea of children that the disease is contagious. Distress in children of all ages undergoing medical procedures has been documented repeatedly (Manne and Andersen 1991). Determination of the controllability of the situation determines whether individuals feel insecure or confident. Parents of children with cancer with lower survival perspectives, that is, children with cancer who have had a relapse, reported more feelings of helplessness (Grootenhuis and Last 1997a).

The child is frequently not able to attend school, to participate in sports, and/or to play with friends. Parents have to make arrangements for work, housekeeping, holidays, support for the siblings, and so on. These *limitations of freedom of action* evoke feelings of frustration and anger. Families with a child with cancer also often have financial problems due to additional costs such as travel and extra meals (Aitken and Hathaway 1993). These additional problems further restrict families.

The answer to the question who or what is *responsible* for the situation is related to feelings of guilt if the person feels he/she is to blame, or anger if someone else is to blame. Eiser, Havermans and Eiser (1995) investigated feelings of responsibility of parents of children with cancer. Both mothers and fathers frequently blamed the general practitioner. Pride may play a role if the child or parent feels they are able to hold on in spite of all difficulties. This is an example of a positive emotional consequence. Positive psychosocial conse-quences should not be overlooked because the ability of children and parents to have an improved outlook on life or enhanced relationships are also part of the illness experience. Greenberg and Meadows (1991) reported that children and parents often express gratitude for the child's survival.

Long duration of the threatening situation is associated with feelings of exhaustion and depression if the child or parent does not perceive an end to the suffering. High levels of depression have been reported for mothers of children in relapse (Grootenhuis and Last 1997a).

Besides actual conditions, associative cognitive representations are also central in the appraisal process of children with cancer and their parents. For instance, for a child with cancer, the stimulus 'take your medicine' can easily be associated with traumatic memories of a 'struggle' with an impatient nurse in the hospital and may evoke anxiety originally emanating from uncontroll-ability. For parents, seeing their seriously ill child with symptoms comparable to a fellow patient can be associated with images about a fellow patient dying and evoke thoughts about the possible death of their own child.

Coping

Emotions are not only evoked by appraisal of what a situation may do to a person, but also by the appraisal of what a person can do to change that situation. Cognitive appraisal and reappraisal is the first stage in coping. How a person deals with a stressful situation is called coping. One's perceptions, or cognitive appraisals, are an important element in regulating distress (emotion-focused coping) or managing the problem causing the distress (problem-focused coping). Problem-focused coping involves direct efforts to ameliorate the problem causing the distress, whereas emotion-focused coping is directed towards regulating affects surrounding a stressful experience (Lazarus and Folkman 1984). Coping should not be equated with mastery over the environment: many sources of stress cannot be mastered, and effective coping under these conditions is that which allows the person to tolerate, minimize, accept, or ignore what cannot be mastered. It should also be recognized that coping is, to some extent, a temporally and situation-specific process. Consequently, coping is defined by Lazarus and Folkman (1984, p. 141) as 'constantly changing cognitive and behavioral efforts to manage specific external and/or internal demands that are appraised as taxing or exceeding the resources of a person'. The definition is process-oriented: the efforts and strategies are constantly changing. Considering the situation-specific process, it may also be presumed that coping is susceptible to changes and sensible to interventions. Frijda (1986) stresses the importance of regulation. People do not only have emotions, they also handle them. Regulations refer to all processes that have the function of modifying other processes induced by a given stimulus situation. Parents of children with cancer have few possibilities to regulate events, but they have the ability to regulate appraisal. The appraisal of a situation can be regulated by selective attention and self-serving cognitive activities. These appraisal regulations are comparable to emotion-focused coping strategies. Appraisal regulations are part of the emotion process.

One of the best-known appraisal regulations is the use of denial. Individuals facing a life-threatening illness often go through a phase of denial; they try to protect themselves from painful or frightening information related to external reality (Breznitz 1983). Whether denial is a negative force or can be considered as adaptive is a point of controversy. Denial can be useful, but in the long run, denial can also lead a patient to conceal serious physical complaints. This is the difference between denial of facts and denial of implications (Lazarus 1983). Patients who are able to function effectively and are able to maintain a high degree of optimism, behavior which may be viewed as denial, can also be viewed, from a cognitive viewpoint, as 'selective information processing' or can be considered as healthy denial (Druss and Douglas 1988). The term 'resilience' has been introduced to bridge the gap between the differing viewpoints. It describes the strengths and abilities of patients and families who can 'bounce back' from the stress and challenges they face and eliminate, or minimize, negative outcomes (Patterson 1995, Druss and Douglas 1988). It is the experience of many healthcare providers to see that patients or families show the ability to adapt to stress and to be able to cope with a threatening situation.

This capacity to keep on going is what is meant with 'being resilient'. In relation to this Folkman and Moskowitz (2000) stress the importance of positive affect which co-occurs with distress. Especially positive appraisal (cognitive strategies for reframing a situation to see it in a positive light) appears to be an important kind of coping which determines positive affect.

Another area which has received considerable attention in the research on coping with cancer is the importance of turning to others or social support. Social support affects coping in several ways. Social resources can reinterpret the meaning of the situation so it seems less threatening, or it may influence the use of other coping strategies, e.g., provide distraction. Social support is therefore considered as a coping resource by several researchers (Rowland 1989).

Control Strategies

Rothbaum, Weisz and Snyder (1982) emphasize the concept of uncontrollability in their two-process model of perceived control, separating primary and secondary control strategies. Primary control strategies are classified as attempts to gain control by bringing the environment into line with their wishes (e.g., seeking treatment, changing one's own and other people's behavior). Secondary control strategies are attempts to gain control by bringing themselves into line with environmental forces (e.g., seeking explanations and changing expectations or attitudes). This is similar to the classification of problem- and emotion-focused coping strategies (Lazarus and Folkman 1984). Rothbaum, Weisz and Snyder (1982), however, made a further classification into four strategies: (1) predictive, (2) vicarious, (3) illusory, and (4) interpretative control, all possibly used in primary or secondary form (Figure 13.1). These four control strategies lend themselves to the purpose to describe frequently occurring reactions of children with cancer and their parents.

Predictive control

Strategies of primary predictive control are gaining knowledge about the expected course of the disease, of the treatment schedule, and the side effects of treatment. The gaining of knowledge in the case of primary predictive control focuses on everything that can contribute to prediction and can satisfy the need to know what to expect. In predicting events, a feeling of control over the situation is created. Secondary predictive control is used in attempts by child or parents to predict events to avoid disappointments. Most striking in this way of coping with the threatening situation are parents who react with 'anticipatory mourning' while the treatment of their child is still curative. By predicting and grieving about a 'certain' loss, they prevent themselves from feeling the shock

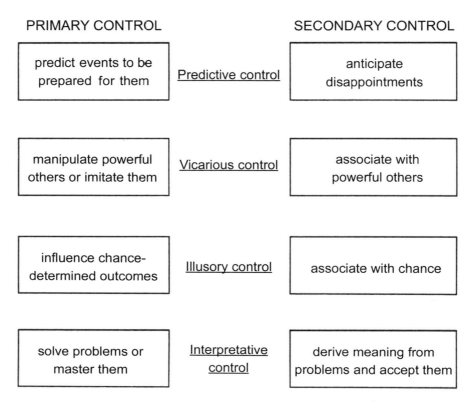

Figure 13.1 Primary and secondary control strategies

and pain related to the unexpected death of their child. This type of parental coping is regularly met in clinical encounters, but was not representative for the group of parents of children with cancer participating in our own study (Grootenhuis *et al.* 1996), in which the parents protected themselves more by being optimistic than by preparing themselves for disappointment. Secondary predictive control can apparently manifest itself in two ways. On the one hand, parents can protect themselves against disappointments by expecting the worst, but, on the other hand, they can also protect themselves by having positive expectations. By living day to day and by being optimistic, children and parents may try to control their emotions. Such manifestations of secondary predictive control can also be considered as forms of healthy denial or attempts to reframe the situation in a positive light (Folkman and Moskowitz 2000). In our own study (Grootenhuis and Last 1997b), we found that persistence in being hopeful, that is having positive expectations, proved to be the major predictor of positive emotional outcome for parents of children with cancer.

The same findings were shown for children with cancer (Grootenhuis and Last 2001b). We found no differences between children with different prognosis (in remission or with a relapse) either on measures of anxiety and depression, or on measures of cognitive control strategies. Emotional adjustment of the children was predicted by defensiveness and by positive expectations about the course of the illness. These findings demonstrate again that having positive expectations about the course of the illness are of major importance for the emotional adjustment of children with cancer.

Vicarious Control

Vicarious control can be exercised by trying to imitate or manipulate powerful others (primary form) or by attempts to associate with them (secondary form). Children with cancer and their parents are highly dependent on doctors. Their attempts to influence the doctor's choices can especially be seen when treatment is not successful and the survival perspective is reduced. Trying to evade a dreadful fate, parents may try to convince the doctor not to terminate treatment, and even to use experimental therapies. The secondary manifestation of vicarious control is demonstrated by attributing special power to the doctor, on whom all hope is focused. In this case, a sense of control is derived from the perception that others, such as the medical caregivers, can exert control. We know from clinical experiences and written diaries how important medical caregivers are for parents and children. An example of this is present in a diary of a girl treated for leukaemia (Floortje Peneder 1994) who writes after having heard the diagnosis: 'I am in the best hospital now, with the best professor in the Netherlands' (p. 15).

Illusory Control

Illusory control is used to attempt to influence chance-determined outcomes or as a secondary process, to associate with chance. Attempts to influence the chance-determined outcome of the illness can be sought in changes in lifestyle, eating habits, or alternative healthcare. These actions offer children and parents the possibility to do something themselves, and thus promote a sense of control. Our finding of increased use of alternative treatment by families of children with cancer in relapse can be considered as indicative of the use of this type of control (Grootenhuis et al. 1998b). Secondary illusory control is present in children and parents when they take the side of fate, admitting that fate is more powerful, but create the illusion that fate will be kind to them. Hoping for a miracle, wishful thinking, or attributing special characteristics to the child as a proof that the child is one of the survivors are illustrations of illusory control in its secondary form. An example of this is a mother who says: 'I am sure my son will survive his illness. I know this because his astrological sign is the lion'. Bull and Drotar (1991) found that children with cancer who are off-treatment frequently used intrapsychic coping strategies. They often used praying, wishful thinking, or self-encouraging statements to deal with cancer-related stress, which can be considered as secondary illusory control.

In a recent study we administered a questionnaire measuring all four cognitive control strategy scales to several children with chronic diseases and their parents participating in research on our department. Based on these findings we know that parents of children with cancer rely more on illusory control than parents of children with other chronic illnesses (Grootenhuis and Last 2001). Reliance on wishful thinking appears to be very important to them.

By attributing positive characteristics to their child, parents create an image of the child as being vital, hence fostering the illusion that fate will be kind to them. The parents need to believe that the child is strong, because if the child can handle the situation, it increases their confidence that the child will survive. We found support for parents' attribution of positive characteristics to their children with cancer. We discovered that parents of children with cancer attributed more cheerful behavior to their children than parents of children with asthma and healthy children do (Grootenhuis et al. 1998a).

Interpretative Control

Primary interpretative control is focused on understanding problems so as to able to solve them or otherwise master them. Gaining information about the disease and the different treatment modalities is often seen in children and parents and is very obvious around the time of the diagnosis. Empirical research confirms that a majority of older children (>8 years) prefer to be informed about their disease and treatment (Orr, Hoffmans and Bennets 1984, Last and Van Veldhuizen 1996). Secondary interpretative control refers to the search for meaning and understanding. Finding an answer to questions like 'What caused cancer in my child?' and 'Why did this happen to me?' serves the process of acceptance and helps children and parents to find meaning in the cancer experience. Attempts of parents to search information on the internet is also an example of interpretative control.

In our study on the use of the four secondary control strategies by parents of children with cancer, we found that all the parents (Grootenhuis et al. 1996) used secondary interpretative control most frequently. The use of interpretative control appears to be important, regardless of educational level and survival perspective. Although the mothers of children with cancer relied more on interpretative control than the fathers did, interpretative control seemed to be meaningful for all the parents.

THE BEHAVIORAL APPROACH

The cognitive approach of emotional reactions is additional to the traditional behavioral approach. In the behavioral approach all behavior is conceived as learned stimulus–response relationships. The process of learning is governed by principles of classic conditioning (Pavlov 1927), operant conditioning (Skinner 1969) and imitation (Bandura 1969). In classical conditioning a reflexive response to a stimulus is brought under control of another stimulus by *contiguity* of both stimuli. An example in pediatric oncology of this principle is present in the child already vomiting at home at the moment he has to go to the hospital to get a chemotherapeutic cure with nausea-evoking drugs. In operant conditioning a specific stimulus is brought under control by consistent reinforcement of a response that follows the specific stimulus. In operant conditioning, behavior is determined by its consequence, using the principle of *contingency*. This principle is working in the child having learned that he will hear his favorite story after taking his medicine. Observation of behavioral sequences in others can also establish behavior. The observer learns to associate certain responses with the observed conditions, providing a basis for *imitation* when the observer is in a similar position as the model. Children with cancer learn a lot from their fellow-patients. Observing another child at the ward during chemotherapy can serve as a role model in a positive but also in a negative way.

Application of Behavioral Therapeutic Techniques

The use of the learning principles underlying the behavioral approach, has shown to be beneficial to the child with cancer in particular in handling anxiety- and pain-provoking treatment procedures (e.g. venapuncture, bone marrow aspiration, lumbar-puncture, infusion of chemotherapeutic drugs and/or operations). Besides improvements in using anesthetics and nausea-reducing drugs, the application of behavior therapeutic techniques remains important in many cases. The possibilities of the behavioral approach have been extensively described (e.g. van Broeck 1992, Jay *et al.* 1987, LeBaron 1992, Eiser 1990). The main techniques used are summarized in Figure 13.2.

Pre-exposure prevents the child from aversive conditioning through exposure to possible anxiety-provoking stimuli at a moment the child is quiet and relaxed. This technique is useful as a method of preparation and only applicable in situations with a high probability of occurrence and low stress intensity, as for instance in children who will get radiotherapy or general anesthesia. Showing a book of photographs of a medical procedure and/or showing the room and apparatus of examination or treatment are supportive in using this type of intervention.

With positive reinforcement parents and medical caregivers can encourage cooperative behavior. Social reinforcement through approval can be completed

Pre-exposure

Positive Reinforcement

Relaxation and Breathing Exercises

Modeling

Systematic Desensitization

Guided Imagery

Figure 13.2 Anxiety- and pain-reducing techniques

with material reinforcers after undergoing medical examination or treatment. Relaxation and breathing exercises are useful in decreasing the activity of the sympathetic and motor nervous system in more tense situations. In learning and encouraging the child to use these techniques during medical procedures the level of experienced anxiety and pain can be reduced. Modeling films are used to inform the child about a stressful medical procedure and also to teach the child techniques (like relaxation or self-distraction) to remain in control during the event. In looking with the child to the film the child is encouraged to imitate the behavior of the model-child shown in the picture.

Systematic desensitization (SD) is used in case of a child reacting with extreme avoidant behavior. SD involves the composition of a hierarchy of increasingly anxiety-provoking stimuli. Step-by-step exposure to these stimuli together with an antagonistic response like relaxation reduces the level of anxiety and the tendency to react with avoidance. With guided imagery the child's attention is being distracted from the aversive medical procedure towards a fantasy story unrelated to the painful event. This technique has proven to be successful in children and adolescents who are sensitive to suggestions. It is preferable to agree with the child on a story he or she likes. If a child is attracted to Superman, invite him to identify with Superman solving all kinds of bizarre problems.

In practice, the mentioned techniques are often used in combination (Rudolph, Dennig and Weisz 1995). For instance pre-exposure to the radiotherapy room is often followed by instructions on how to relax. In doing so it can be agreed with the child to tell a distracting story during therapy and positively reinforce the child after treatment.

THE PSYCHOSOCIAL INTERVENTION MODEL

Framework

The main characteristics of the situation, the different emotions, the types of primary and secondary control and the history of learned behavior are brought together in a model for psychosocial intervention (see Figure 13.3). This model

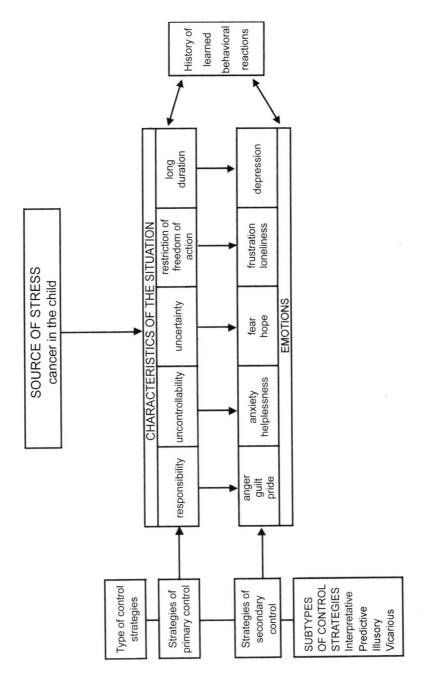

Figure 13.3 The psychosocial intervention model

offers a framework for psychosocial intervention. It shows us the main features of the situation, the related emotions, the role of primary and secondary control and also the history of learned behavior. In coping with a stressful situation, children and parents use the various control strategies in their specific way. Psychosocial intervention is indicated if control fails and subsequently, child and/or parents need support in rebuilding their defenses or to reduce or eliminate unpleasant behavioral reactions.

Using this scheme, we can analyze and understand the emotional reactions of the child and his/her parents and use it as a guide to psychosocial interventions. In working with this model, we ask the following questions: (1) What situational components and emotions are dominant for the child and the parents? (2) Which control strategies are especially used by the child and by the parents? (3) What is the history of learned behavioral reactions related to the disease and the treatment? (4) To what extent do the child and the parents use their control strategies effectively? If, for instance, child and/or parents are very anxious about the course of the disease and mainly attempt to use interpretative control in reducing uncertainty, we have to look critically at the information they got about the disease and the treatment. If child and/or parents fear a negative outcome of the disease and show little confidence in the medical doctor, it may be necessary to enhance their vicarious control. And also, if the child remains very anxious about a treatment procedure, it makes sense to look at his history of learned behavioral reactions and use specific behavioral therapeutic techniques to overcome this fear (as is shown in the case of Jim).

Case Illustrations

Maria

Maria is a 7-year-old girl and has been treated for osteosarcoma. She has had an operation and has had post-surgical chemotherapy. She lost her hair due to the chemotherapy. The tumor was removed and she is in remission. She only comes to the hospital for check-ups and whether the disease will remain in remission is uncertain. Maria is bald, but very vital. She goes to school with pleasure. Her parents came to the Pediatric Psycho-Social Department with the complaint that Maria has trouble sleeping. She calls for her parents from her bed, and ends up sleeping with her parents. Her parents are not able to sleep well, and especially her father is exhausted.

In Maria's case we wondered why she was afraid to be alone in her bed. We also asked ourselves the aforementioned questions. Are there associations which make it difficult for her? Furthermore, we wondered what associations the parents have with Maria going to bed and what associations they have when Maria calls them in the night.

Situational components

Because Maria is young, her feelings of certainty are very dependent on her parents. After inquiry, it turns out that Maria woke up from her operation earlier than expected and that her parents found her very upset. Consequently, when she is alone in her bed, she feels uncertain. The appraisal of the situation as uncertain concurs with Maria's association of being alone in her bed and the uncertainty about whether her parents are available. Maria's father appraises the situation as very uncertain. Will Maria survive her illness? Because her illness started with pain in her belly, before going to bed, father urges Maria to call him if she feels something in her belly. Maria's mother has confidence in Maria's treatment and her uncertainties mainly relate to her husband's worries and Maria's sleeping problems.

Control strategies and effectiveness

Maria does not know whether her parents are available, and she is not sure about her illness. It seems that she has little possibility of relying on interpretative control. Maria's mother is confident (secondary predictive control: positive expectations) that Maria will survive her illness. She says that Maria is an optimistic and strong girl who will be able to survive her illness (secondary illusory control: attribution of positive characteristics). Maria's father worries about her illness and he is anticipating a negative outcome. He thinks Maria will not survive (secondary predictive control: negative expectations). After inquiry, it turns out that his father (Maria's grandfather) died of cancer 6 months earlier and that Maria's father has not come to terms with this. There also appears to be an important association influencing the appraisal for the father: 'When I see Maria sleeping, it is like seeing my father on his death-bed'. For the father, Maria's going to sleep appears to be a conditioned stimulus triggering anxiety arising originally from uncertainty about the outcome of the disease. Maria's father appears to have in interest in Maria coming out of her bed; it reassures him temporarily.

Intervention

Having analyzed the situation, we now know more about the cognitive representations and emotional reactions of Maria and her parents. In the first place, Maria should be helped to increase her feeling of safety, and it should be explained that she is in remission and not ill right now (increasing her interpretative control). She should know more about her illness. The main psychosocial support should be directed at the father. His mourning for his father should be discussed and supported to break the association between his dying father and his sick daughter. Maria's symptoms should no longer be negatively predicted by the father.

Michael

Michael is a 12-year-old boy suffering from a non-Hodgkin lymphoma. He is tall for his age and looks older. His cancer is being treated with intensive chemotherapy over a long period of 53 weeks. At the moment of referral to the Psychosocial Department he was in the 22nd week. Michael is rebellious in the hospital and is non-compliant with protective rules of his therapy (e.g., brushing his teeth and rinsing his mouth). He is also abusive to his mother and the nurses in the ward. His parents feel helpless and are tired of all the quarrels.

Situational components and emotions

Michael is a popular teenager who feels very frustrated by the restrictions imposed on his freedom by his illness. He is directing his frustration and anger especially at his mother. His mother has the feeling she cannot control the situation and feels helpless. She also feels responsible towards the nurses for Michael's behavior, which makes her feel guilty, together with being angry at Michael. Michael's fathers admits that he is very uncertain about Michael's survival chances and the father admits he only cries when he is alone.

Control strategies and effectiveness

Because Michael seems older than he is, it is easy to assume he understands his illness and treatment. Michael does not really know the consequences of his disease (little interpretative control) and he relies little on vicarious control, resulting in rebellious behavior against the hospital staff. Because Michael is non-compliant with his treatment schedule, his treatment protocol cannot be followed as well as it should be. Little primary predictive control is therefore possible for his mother. Mother has a great deal of confidence in the hospital (secondary vicarious control). That Michael's father is the most pessimistic of the family shows that he is anticipating disappointment (secondary predictive control).

Intervention

The family needs a better understanding of the treatment, survival chances, and consequences of non-compliance. Therefore, a meeting with the physician was organized. This enhances the interpretative control and vicarious control of all family members. In this round-table discussion, the effects of the medication Michael is taking were also discussed. The use of dexametason is known to cause mood disturbances. Because Michael has difficulties with the restriction of his freedom he was supported in finding an alternative for playing football. He is being supported in doing something together with his father.

Jim

Jim is a 6-year-old boy highly anxious and angry about undergoing his chemotherapy. 'I don't want it', he cried. The doctors gave Jim sedative medicines before the infusion was installed. Nevertheless he remained very upset and frequently tried to eliminate the infusion. Psychological intervention was requested.

In discussion with Jim and his parents it became clear that Jim had experienced a traumatic sequence with his first chemotherapy. His mother was late at the ward because of a traffic jam, the doctors had already started Jim's first infusion. A nurse and a play therapist prepared Jim as well as possible, but Jim was angry and felt alone. When his mother arrived he was very upset and shouted at her.

Situational components

It seemed that as a consequence of his first traumatic experience in the hospital Jim appraises every hospitalization as highly uncertain and uncontrollable. He experienced associated memories to the event of staying alone and undergoing a sudden painful procedure. A high level of arousal motivated by separation anxiety blocked any information needed for building up a certain sense of control in the situation.

Response and consequences

Jim reacted with crying and shouting and attempts to escape from the situation. This behavior resulted in a struggle and the anger of the nurses and his parents to get the job done in the end. Sometimes the procedure was postponed, which reinforced his rebellious behavior.

Intervention

An intervention was designed aimed at enhancing Jim's feeling of self-control and reduction of stress in the short period of time, before the next chemotherapy. The first session was focused on a ventilation of feelings about the traumatic event using talking and painting. Moreover, a hierarchy of low, middle and highly anxiety provoking stimuli was composed. His mother took part in the sessions. As an antagonistic response Jim learned breathing exercises by blowing at a little kite and learned muscle relaxation by getting weak as a pudding. Jim enjoyed the training and played with hospital materials. Together we looked at a model film in which a 7-year-old boy used the exercise in getting a venepuncture. In this film the boy also uses distraction by counting little stars in the eyes of his mother while the doctor inserts a needle in a blood vessel. Jim was encouraged to do the same. In the final session Jim practiced the instruction in a simulated infusion procedure. He was encouraged for his efforts and improvements. Mother rewarded him with an ice cream in the main hall of the hospital. On the day of the next cure Jim arrived more relaxed. Also his mother showed more confidence knowing how she could support her son. Jim cried for a short while but was cooperative.

IN CONCLUSION

The model for psychosocial intervention presented in this chapter is meant to be a helpful instrument in arranging and analyzing the findings from previous diagnostic efforts. The model presented emphasizes the importance of the characteristics of the situation, the main primary and secondary control strategies, and the history of learned behavioral reactions. These aspects are involved in analyzing the emotional and behavioral reactions of children with cancer and their parents. It is important that healthcare providers understand emotional and behavioral reactions, and coping strategies, because with this knowledge they can respond more appropriately. If healthcare providers respond adequately, this will be beneficial for children's and parents' emotional adjustment. The focus on the described control strategies is not meant as an exclusive point of view. Children and parents also rely on other coping strategies (e.g. classical defence mechanisms) or other coping resources (social and financial support).

To understand emotional and behavioral reactions, careful diagnostics are necessary. In many cases the child's and/or the parents' emotional problems or problems of adjustment cannot easily be converted to cause and consequence. We also have to keep in mind that parents and children may rely on more than one control strategy at the same time and that the same person or situation may generate different feelings of control. This is also important to realize when arranging interventions. The model serves as a guideline to put one's thoughts into hypotheses about the occurrence and origin of psychosocial adjustment problems of the child with cancer and his parents. Based on these hypotheses focused interventions can be initiated.

REFERENCES

Aitken, T.J., Hathaway, G. (1993) Long distance related stressors and coping behaviors in parents of children with cancer. *Journal of Pediatric Oncology Nursing* **10**, 3–12.
Bandura, A. (1969) *Principles of behavior therapy*. New York: Holt, Rinehart & Winston.

Breznitz, S. (1983) The seven kinds of denial. In Breznitz, S. (Ed.) *The Denial of Stress*. New York: International University Press, pp. 257–280.

Brown, R.T., Kaslow, N.J., Madan-Swain, A., Doepke, K.J., Sexson, S.B., Hill, L.J. (1993) Parental psychopathology and children's adjustment to leukemia. *Journal of the American Academy of Child and Adolescent Psychiatry* **32**, 554–561.

Bull, B.A., Drotar, D. (1991) Coping with cancer in remission: stressors and strategies reported by children and adolescents. *Journal of Pediatric Psychology* **16**, 767–782.

Canning, E.H., Canning R.D., Boyce, W.T. (1992) Depressive symptoms and adaptive style in children with cancer. *Journal of the American Academy of Child Psychiatry* **31**, 1120–1124.

Dahlquist, L.M., Czyzewski, D.I., Copeland, K.G., Jones, C.L., Taub, E., Vaughan, J.K. (1993) Parents of children newly diagnosed with cancer: anxiety, coping, and marital distress. *Journal of Pediatric Psychology* **18**, 365–376.

Davey, G.C.L. (1989) UCS Revaluation and conditioning models of acquired fears. *Behavioural Research Therapy* **27**, 521–528.

Davey, G.C.L. (1992) Classical conditioning and the acquisition of human fears and phobias: a review and synthesis of the literature. *Advising Behavioural Research Therapy* **14**, 29–66.

Druss, R.G., Douglas, C.J. (1988) Adaptive responses to illness and disability. Healthy denial. *General Hospital Psychiatry* **10**, 163–168.

Eiser, C. (1990) *Chronic Childhood Disease*. Cambridge: Cambridge University Press.

Eiser, C., Havermans, T., Eiser, J.R. (1995) Parents' attributions about childhood cancer: implications for relationships with medical staff. *Child: Care, Health and Development* **21**, 31–42.

Fife, B., Norton, J., Groom, G. (1987) The family's adaptation to childhood leukemia. *Social Science and Medicine* **24**, 159–168.

Floortje Peneder (1994) *Het dagboek van Floortje Peneder*. Amsterdam: Nijgh and Van Ditmar.

Folkman, S., Moskowitz, J.T. (2000) Positive affect and the other side of coping. *American Psychologist* **55**, 647–654.

Frijda, N.H. (1986) *The Emotions*. Cambridge: Cambridge University Press.

Greenberg, H.S., Meadows, A.T. (1991) Psychosocial impact of cancer survival on school-age children and their parents. *Journal of Psychosocial Oncology* **9**, 43–56.

Grootenhuis, M.A., Last, B.F. (1997a) Parents' emotional reactions related to different prospects for the survival of their children with cancer. *Journal of Psychosocial Oncology* **15**, 43–62.

Grootenhuis, M.A., Last, B.F. (1997b) Predictors of parental adjustment to childhood cancer. *Psycho-Oncology* **6**, 115–128.

Grootenhuis M.A., Last, B.F. (1997c) Adjustment and coping by parents of children with cancer: A review of the literature. *Supportive Care in Cancer* **5**, 466–484.

Grootenhuis, M.A., Last, B.F. (2001a) The cognitive control strategy scale for children with a chronic disease and their parents. *Psycho-Oncology* **10**, S35.

Grootenhuis, M.A., Last, B.F. (2001b) Children with cancer with different survival perspectives: defensiveness, control strategies, and psychological adjustment. *Psycho-Oncology*, **10**, 305–314.

Grootenhuis, M.A., Last, B.F., De Graaf-Nijkerk, J.H., Van Der Wel, M. (1996) Secondary control strategies used by parents of children with cancer. *Psycho-Oncology* **5**, 91–102.

Grootenhuis, M.A., Last, B.F., Van Der Wel, M., De Graaf-Nijkerk, J.H. (1998a) Parents' attributions of positive characteristics to their children with cancer. *Psychology and Health* **13**, 67–81.

Grootenhuis, M.A., Last, B.F., De Graaf-Nijkerk, J.H., Van der Wel, M. (1998b) Use of alternative treatment in pediatric oncology. *Cancer Nursing* **21**, 282–288.

Hoekstra-Weebers, J.E., Heuvel, F., Jaspers, J.P., Kamps, W.A., Klip, E.C. (1998) Brief report: an intervention program for parents of pediatric cancer patients: a randomized controlled trial. *Journal of Pediatric Psychology* **23**, 207–214.

Humphrey, G.B., Van De Iel, H.B., Boon, C.M., Van den Heuvel, C.F. (1992) Stress reduction interventions in pediatric oncology. Could coping strategies play a role? In Last, B.F. & Van Veldhuizen, A.M. (Eds) *Developments in Pediatric Psychosocial Oncology*. Lisse: Swets & Zeitlinger, pp. 113–116.

Jay, S.M., Elliot, C.H., Katz, E.R., Siegel, S. (1987) Cognitive-behavioral and pharmacologic interventions for children undergoing painful medical procedures. *Journal of Consulting and Clinical Psychology* **55**, 860–865.

Katz, E.R., Rubenstein, C.L., Hubert, N.C., Blew, A. (1988) School and social reintegration of children with cancer. *Journal of Psychosocial Oncology* **6**, 123–140.

Kaplan, S., Busner, J., Weinhold, C., Lenon, P. (1987) Depressive symptoms in children and adolescents with cancer: a longitudinal study. *Journal of the American Academy of Child Psychiatry* **26**, 782–787.

Korrelboom, C.W.K., Kernkamp, J.H.B. (1993) *Gedragstherapie*. Muiderberg: Dick Coutinho.

Kupst, M., Schulman, J.L., Honig, G., Maurer, H., Morgan, E., Fochtmann, D. (1982) Family coping with childhood leukemia: one year after diagnosis. *Journal of Pediatric Psychology* **7**, 157–174.

Koocher, G.P., O'Malley, J.E. (1981) *The Damocles Syndrome. Psychosocial consequences of surviving childhood cancer*. New York: McGraw-Hill.

Last, B.F., Van Veldhuizen, A.M.H. (1996) Information about diagnosis and prognosis related to anxiety and depression in children with cancer aged 8–16 years. *European Journal of Cancer* **32A**, 290–294.

Lazarus, R.S. (1983) The costs and benefits of denial. In Breznitz, S. (Eds) *The Denial of Stress*. New York: International University Press, pp. 1–30.

Lazarus, R.S., Folkman, S. (1984) *Stress, Appraisal, and Coping*. New York: Springer.

LeBaron, S. (1992) The use of images and suggestion in the treatment of pain in children. In Last, B.F., Van Veldhuizen, A.M. (Eds) *Developments in Pediatric Psychosocial Oncology*. Lisse: Swets & Zeitlinger, pp. 137–146.

Leventhal-Belfer, L., Bakker, A.M., Russo, C.L. (1993) Parents of childhood cancer survivors: a descriptive look at their concerns and needs. *Journal of Psychosocial Oncology* **11**, 19–41.

Manne, S.L., Andersen, B.L. (1991) Pain and pain-related distress in children with cancer. In Bush, J.P., Olson, A.L., Boyle, W.E., Evans, M.W., Zug, L.A. (Eds) Overall function in rural childhood cancer survivors. *Clinical Pediatrics* **32**, 334–342.

Manne, S.L., Lesanics, D., Meyers, P., Wollner, N., Steinherz, P., Redd, W. (1995) Predictors of depressive symptomatology among parents of newly diagnosed children with cancer. *Journal of Pediatric Psychology* **20**, 491–510.

Mulhern, R.K., Fairclough, D.L., Smith, B., Douglas, S.M. (1992) Maternal depression, assessment methods, and physical symptoms affect estimates of depressive symptomatology among children with cancer. *Journal of Pediatric Psychology* **17**, 313–326.

Orr, D., Hoffmans, M., Bennets, G. (1984) Adolescents with cancer report their psychological needs. *Journal of Psychosocial Oncology* **2**, 47–59.

Patterson, J.M. (1995) Promoting resilience in families experiencing stress. *Pediatric Clinics of North America* **42**, 47–63.

Pavlov, I.P. (1927) *Conditioned Reflexes*. New York: Oxford University Press.

Peterson, L. (1989) Coping by children undergoing stressful medical procedures: some conceptual, methodological, and therapeutic issues. *Journal of Consulting and Clinical Psychology* **57**, 380–387.

Phipps, S., Fairclough, D., Mulhern, R.K. (1995) Avoidant coping in children with cancer. *Journal of Pediatric Psychology* **20**, 217–232.

Rothbaum, F., Weisz, J.R., Snyder, S.S. (1982) Changing the world and changing the self: a two-process model of perceived control. *Journal of Personality and Social Psychology* **42**, 5–37.

Rowland, J.H. (1989) Interpersonal resources: social support. In Holland, J.C., Rowland, J.H. (Eds) *Handbook of Psychooncology. Psychological care of the patient with cancer*. New York: Oxford University Press, pp. 58–71.

Rudolph, K.D., Dennig, M.D., Weisz, J.R. (1995) Determinants and consequences of children's coping in the medical setting: Conceptualization, review, and critique. *Psychological-Bulletin* **118**(3), 328–357.

Sawyer, M.G., Antoniou, G., Toogood, I., Rice, M., Baghurst, P.A. (1993) A prospective study of the psychological adjustment of parents and families of children with cancer. *Journal of Paediatric Child Health* **29**, 352–356.

Shapiro, J., Shumaker, S. (1987) Differences in emotional well-being and communication styles between mothers and fathers of pediatric cancer patients. *Journal of Psychosocial Oncology* **5**, 121–131.

Siefert, K., Wittmann, D., Farquar, S., Talsma, F. (1992) Similarities and differences between children with asthma and children with cancer: Implications for preventive intervention. *Journal of Primary Prevention* **13**, 149–159.

Skinner, B.F. (1969) *Contingencies of Reinforcement*. New York: Appleton-Century-Crofts.

Speechley, K.N., Noh, S. (1992) Surviving childhood cancer, social support, and parents' psychological adjustment. *Journal of Pediatric Psychology* **17**, 15–31.

Spirito, A., Stark, L.J., Cobiella, C., Drigan, R., Androkites, A., Hewett, K. (1990) Social adjustment of children successfully treated for cancer. *Journal of Pediatric Psychology* **15**, 359–371.

Sprangers, M.A.G., Schwartz, C.E. (1999) Integrating response shift into health-related quality of life research: a theoretical model. *Social Science Medicine* **48**, 1507–1515.

Stam, H., Grootenhuis, M.A., Last, B.F. (2001) Social and emotional adjustment in young survivors of childhood cancer. *Review Supportive Care Cancer* **9**, 489–513.

Van Broeck, N.G.A. (1992) Behavioral therapeutic techniques as preparation for aversive medical procedures. In Last, B.F., Van Veldhuizen, A.M. (Eds) *Developments in Pediatric Psychosocial Oncology*. Lisse: Swets & Zeitlinger, pp. 117–136.

Van Dongen-Melman, J.E.W.M., Pruyn, J.F.A., De Groot, A., Koot, H.M., Hählen, K., Verhulst, F.C. (1995) Late psychosocial consequences for parents of children who survived cancer. *Journal of Pediatric Psychology* **20**, 567–586.

Van Veldhuizen, A.M., Last, B.F. (1991) *Children with Cancer. Communication and emotions*. Amsterdam: Swets & Zeitlinger.

Worchel, F.F., Nolan, B.F., Willson, V.L., Purser, J.S., Copeland, D.R., Pfefferbaum, B. (1988) Assessment of depression in children with cancer. *Journal of Pediatric Psychology* **13**, 101–112.

Worchel, F.F., Rae, W.A., Olson, T.K., Crowley, S.L. (1992) Selective responsiveness of chronically ill children to assessments of depression. *Journal of Personality Assessment* **59**, 605–615.

14

Complementary and Alternative Medicine Use in Children with Cancer

CYNTHIA D. MYERS, JONATHAN BERGMAN AND LONNIE K. ZELTZER
David Geffen School of Medicine at University of California at Los Angeles, CA, USA

INTRODUCTION

Population studies in the United States and abroad have shown that the use of complementary and alternative medicine (CAM) is common among adults and children for the intended purposes of cancer prevention, slowing cancer progression, and palliation of symptoms and side effects of cancer treatment. The purpose of the current chapter is to inform healthcare professionals about the topic of CAM in general and specifically for pediatric cancer by (1) describing recent developments at the National Institutes of Health with regard to CAM in the United States and at the World Health Organization with regard to traditional medicine and CAM use internationally; (2) reviewing the literature on the prevalence of the use of CAM generally and for pediatric cancer; (3) compiling reports of clinical trials of CAM modalities in the context of pediatric cancer; and (4) describing the clinical use of hypnosis, as one example of clinical application of a CAM modality in pediatric oncology.

CAM AT THE NATIONAL INSTITUTES OF HEALTH

CAM is described by the National Center for Complementary and Alternative Medicine (NCCAM) at the US Department of Health National Institutes of

Psychosocial Aspects of Pediatric Oncology. Edited by S. Kreitler and M. Weyl Ben Arush
© 2004 John Wiley & Sons Ltd: ISBN 0 471 49939 0

Health as 'a group of diverse medical and health care systems, practices, and products that are not presently considered to be part of conventional medicine' (National Center for Complementary and Alternative Medicine 2003a). 'Conventional medicine' in this context is defined as 'medicine as practiced by holders of MD (medical doctor) or DO (doctor of osteopathy) degrees and by their allied health professionals, such as physical therapists, psychologists, and registered nurses'. What is considered to be CAM is debated (Friedman *et al.* 1997), and changes as therapies that are proven to be safe and effective become integrated into conventional health care.

NCCAM groups CAM therapies into five categories, or domains. One domain is 'Alternative Medical Systems', which are built upon complete systems of theory and practice. Examples include homeopathic medicine, naturopathic medicine, Ayurveda, and traditional Chinese medicine, among others. Homeopaths aim to stimulate the body's defense mechanisms and healing processes by administering minute doses of plant extracts and minerals. Naturopaths work to restore health through nutrition, homeopathic remedies, herbal medicine, hydrotherapy, physical therapies, counseling, and pharmacology. Acupuncture, a component of traditional Chinese medicine, illustrates the way in which the field of CAM changes over time. Whereas acupuncture was once considered unorthodox in Western medicine, scientific evidence has accumulated to support its safety and effectiveness, and it has been assimilated broadly into Western medical practice for specific indications such as managing chronic pain and nausea associated with chemotherapy.

A second CAM domain, according to NCCAM, is the 'Biologically Based Therapies', which use substances found in nature, such as herbal remedies that employ plant preparations for therapeutic effects, vitamins and other dietary supplements, and foods and special dietary modifications. A third domain comprises the 'Manipulative and Body-Based Methods', including, for example, chiropractic, osteopathic manipulations, and massage.

Included in NCCAM's fourth CAM domain are the 'Energy Therapies', of which there are two types. The first type of energy therapy is exemplified by Reiki and other therapies that intend to manipulate energy biofields within and around the human body. These biofields have not yet been scientifically proven to exist. The second type of energy therapy is the bioelectromagnetic-based therapies involving the unconventional use of electromagnetic fields, such as pulsed fields, alternating current or direct current fields.

Finally, the 'Mind–Body Interventions' comprise a fifth domain of CAM therapies. Included here are a variety of techniques designed to enhance the mind's capacity to affect bodily function and symptoms. Examples of mind–body interventions, according to NCCAM, include meditation, prayer, guided imagery and hypnosis. Like acupuncture, hypnosis is an example of a CAM modality for which there is substantial scientific evidence of effect as well as integration into conventional medicine.

For most CAM therapies, there are key questions regarding safety and efficacy that are yet to be answered through scientific studies. In 1992, the Office of Alternative Medicine (OAM) was established within the National Institutes of Health (NIH) Office of the Director with the mission of providing the American public with reliable information about the safety and effectiveness of CAM practices. A 1998 congressional mandate expanded the OAM into the National Center for Complementary and Alternative Medicine (NCCAM). The OAM's 1993 budget of $2 million grew to NCCAM's 2001 budget of $89.1 million. NCCAM's developing programs include extramural and intramural research funding, development of scientific databases, providing a public information clearinghouse, and facilitating national and international cooperative efforts in CAM research and education. Additional information about NCCAM may be found online at http://nccam.nih.gov/ (National Center for Complementary and Alternative Medicine 2003b). Also in 1998, the National Cancer Institute (NCI) established the Office of Cancer Complementary and Alternative Medicine (OCCAM) to coordinate and enhance the activities of the NCI in the arena of CAM. Additional information about OCCAM may be found at http://www3.cancer.gov/occam/about.html (Office of Cancer Complementary and Alternative Medicine 2003). Facilitating the evaluation of the safety and efficacy of CAM is a key objective of both NCCAM and OCCAM.

CAM AT THE WORLD HEALTH ORGANIZATION

Several therapies often referred to as CAM have their origins in traditional medical practices that predate modern medicine. The World Health Organization (WHO), recognizes that the use of traditional medicine varies greatly from country to country and region to region, and that many Member States consider traditional medicine a priority for healthcare in their regions. Accordingly, the WHO released a global plan in 2002 to address several issues on the usage of traditional medicine and CAM. These issues include safety, questions of policy, regulation, evidence, biodiversity, and preservation and protection of traditional knowledge. The strategy provides a framework for policy to assist countries to regulate traditional medicine or CAM to make their use safer, more accessible to their populations, and sustainable. Additional information about the WHO policy statement on traditional medicine and CAM can be located on the internet at www.who.int/medicines/ organization/trm/orgtrmmain.shtml (World Health Organization 2003).

PREVALENCE OF CAM USE

Landmark national surveys conducted by Eisenberg and colleagues have been credited with first informing the medical community about the extent of the use of CAM therapies in the United States. Eisenberg *et al.* conducted parallel nationally representative telephone surveys in 1990 (Eisenberg *et al.* 1993) and 1997 (Eisenberg *et al.* 1998) concerning healthcare practices including CAM use, broadly defined. Participants in the 1990 survey numbered 1539, and in 1997 numbered 2055. These studies estimated that a third of the US adult population used at least one of 16 CAM therapies, broadly defined, in 1990, increasing to 42.1% in 1997. Use of 10 out of 16 alternative therapies had increased significantly from 1990 to 1997, with the largest increases in the use of herbal medicine, therapeutic massage, megavitamins, self-help groups, folk remedies, energy healing, and homeopathy. Visits to chiropractors and massage therapists accounted for nearly half of all visits to practitioners of CAM therapies administered by a professional, as opposed to self-administered practices or products. CAM therapies were used most frequently for chronic conditions, and more among women and those between 35 and 49 years old with some college education and with annual incomes above $50,000.

In both surveys, the majority of respondents using CAM (96%) also saw a medical doctor during the prior twelve months; however, only a minority of the CAM treatments (39.8% in 1990, 38.5% in 1997) were disclosed to physicians. Five hundred and seven respondents reported their reasons for non-disclosure of use of CAM therapies. Common reasons for non-disclosure were 'It wasn't important for the doctor to know' (61%), 'The doctor never asked' (60%), 'It was none of the doctor's business' (31%), and 'The doctor would not understand' (20%). Fourteen percent of respondents thought their doctor would disapprove of or discourage CAM use, and 2% thought their doctor might not continue as their provider if they revealed their use of CAM. The investigators concluded that these national survey data did not support a commonly held perception that patients turn to CAM out of dissatisfaction with conventional care. Rather, the data indicated that most respondents perceive the combination of CAM and conventional care to be superior to the use of either approach alone (Eisenberg *et al.* 2001).

In another major survey, Paramore (1997) reported responses obtained from a national probability sample of 3450 persons to the National Access to Care Survey, which included questions about chiropractic, relaxation techniques, therapeutic massage, and acupuncture. With a response rate of 75%, results indicated that in 1994, nearly 10% of the US population (almost 25 million persons) saw a professional for at least one of the listed CAM therapies. Unlike Eisenberg *et al.*'s (1993, 1998) studies, neither sex nor race/ethnicity predicted CAM use. Astin (1998) reported results from a random sample national mail survey completed by 1035 people. CAM use was predicted by anxiety, back problems, chronic pain, and urinary tract problems. Dissatisfaction with conventional medicine did not predict CAM use, nor did sex, age, income, or race/ethnicity.

CAM USE FOR CANCER AND SIDE EFFECTS OF CANCER TREATMENT BY ADULTS

CAM use by adult cancer patients has now been surveyed in several studies. A summary of 26 such surveys concluded that the prevalence of CAM use ranged from 7% to 64%, with an overall prevalence of 31.4% (Ernst and Cassileth 1998). A recent survey of 453 adults attending outpatient clinics at MD Anderson Cancer Center, with a 51.4% response rate, found that 83.3% had used at least one CAM approach, including spiritual practices (80.5%), vitamins and herbs (62.6%), and others (Richardson *et al.* 2000). Patients' motivations for using CAM included improving quality of life (76.7%), boosting immunity (71.1%), prolonging life (62.5%), and relieving symptoms (44%). Of note, fully a third of patients were motivated by hope for curing their disease (37.5%). Patients most often continue to be treated with conventional medicine in addition to CAM, and most patients do not disclose CAM use to their treating physician. These findings highlight the great need for evidence-based guidelines with which informed healthcare providers can sensitively query patients about CAM use and advise accurately with regard to potential risks and benefits of CAM use and the integration of CAM with conventional treatments for cancer.

CAM USE FOR CANCER AND SIDE EFFECTS OF PEDIATRIC CANCER TREATMENT

The utilization of CAM in pediatric oncology patients has been studied in the United States as well as internationally. In most cases, CAM was used to complement rather than replace traditional treatment, usually to treat symptoms or side effects, although there are controversial exceptions wherein parents discontinue their child's conventional treatment in favor of unproven alternative therapies (Burgio and Locatelli 2000). Telephone interviews conducted in Washington State with parents of 75 children with a primary neoplasm about the child's use of CAM indicated that 73% utilized one or more CAM therapies (Neuhouser *et al.* 2001). Thirty-five percent used herbal preparations, 28% used high-dose dietary supplements such as vitamins C or E, and 21% saw a specialized CAM practitioner such as an acupuncturist or naturopathic doctor. Most parents (75%) were very satisfied with their child's physicians; however, CAM utilization was highest in children whose parents were not fully satisfied. Parents generally attributed substantial improvements in their child's health and well-being to CAM, although there were exceptions including two parents who attributed significant adverse side effects to use of herbal preparations.

Kemper and Wornham (2001) prospectively studied 70 pediatric patients (43 of them oncology patients) who were referred for CAM consultation as part of their treatment at an urban tertiary care teaching hospital in Boston, Massachusetts. The most frequent goals for CAM therapy were treatment of pain, nausea, insomnia, or agitation, and the most common CAM modalities employed included herbs, dietary supplements, diet and nutrition, biofeedback and massage. Several families also engaged in prayer or Reiki and other energy healing techniques or were interested in learning more about these.

In a parent interview study of 75 pediatric cancer patients receiving conventional care at an urban academic hospital, 84% of respondents reported the child had used one or more CAM therapies, most commonly changes in diet or nutrition, herbal preparations, and mind–body approaches, in conjunction with conventional treatment (Kelly *et al.* 2000). Utilization of CAM was not predicted by cancer diagnosis, race, ethnicity, socioeconomic status, or educational attainment. Fifty percent of the therapies used were not reported to the treating physician. Among patients using CAM, 85% were concurrently enrolled in clinical trials of experimental medical therapies for cancer, highlighting the unmeasured effect of CAM modalities on symptoms, quality of life, and other outcomes that may be targeted in clinical trials and thus comprise a potential confound in cancer research.

Friedman, T. *et al.* (1997) assessed the prevalence of CAM utilization in 81 pediatric cancer patients and 80 children attending a continuity care clinic for well-child check-ups or non-cancer acute care. Sixty-five percent of the cancer patients and 51% of the non-cancer patients utilized CAM. Parents who discussed CAM with their child's primary physician or oncologist were most often parents of cancer patients (53%), of higher income (59%), and white (47%).

CAM treatment for pediatric oncology patients is also popular outside the United States. In the Netherlands, Grootenhuis *et al.* (1998) interviewed and administered questionnaires to 84 pediatric cancer patients and their parents. Forty-three of the children were in first continuous remission, and 41 had relapsed or had a second malignancy. Overall, 31% utilized one or more CAM modality, with patients in relapse utilizing CAM more often (46%) than patients who were in remission (16%). Approaches that were described by the authors as 'autonomous medical concepts', including homeopathy and the macrobiotic system of diet and philosophy, were the most popular of the CAM modalities, used in 58% of the families. Next in popularity was a group described as 'physical and bioelectric', including massage, applied kinesiology, and light therapy, used by nine families. Use of imagery healing, psychic healing, and faith healing were the third most popular, used by six families.

Australian parents of 48 pediatric oncology patients age 4 to 16 years old diagnosed with cancer excluding brain tumors reported that 46% of the children had utilized at least one CAM modality as part of their treatment regimen (Sawyer *et al.* 1994). The most common CAM modalities employed were imagery, hypnotherapy, relaxation, diets, and multivitamins. Spiritualism, faith healing, meditation, megavitamins, and other approaches were also used, although less commonly. Use of CAM was discussed with the treating physician only 44% of the time.

Fernandez *et al.* (1998) conducted a retrospective questionnaire population-based survey of 583 parents of children diagnosed with cancer in British Columbia from 1989 to 1995. Parents of 366 patients responded, reporting that 42% of the children had used CAM for cancer. Most often employed were relaxation/imagery strategies, massage, therapeutic touch, herbal teas, plant extracts, and therapeutic vitamins. Predictors of increased use included prior CAM utilization, a positive attitude towards CAM, information from family or friends, information from alternative caregivers, high risk of death at diagnosis, and advanced education of at least one parent. Reasons for non-utilization included lack of knowledge about CAM and fear of interference with the primary therapy. Consistent with other studies on adult and pediatric samples, CAM therapies were most often used in conjunction with (as opposed to in replacement of) conventional treatment. More than half (54.3%) of parents believed that CAM had ameliorated effects of cancer or its treatment, and another reported benefit to parents was feeling that they were doing everything possible for their child.

Yeh *et al.* (2000) interviewed parents of 63 pediatric oncology patients in Taiwan to study the use of traditional Chinese medicine as well as popular folk remedies in conjunction with Western conventional oncology medicine. Seventy-three percent of children had utilized at least one traditional Chinese medicine therapy or folk remedy in conjunction with Western care. Most common was the use of formulated functional food, consisting of generally expensive packaged liquid or powder remedies purported to be high in nutritional value and able to limit side effects, increase immune function, and improve prognosis. Herbal remedies were also used. The potential toxicity of such products when used concurrently with conventional treatment was not known. Spiritual practices including temple worship or consulting a shaman were also used to complement Western treatment. Nineteen percent of children had been treated by practitioners of Western medicine and practitioners of traditional Chinese medicine. Use of traditional and popular approaches was not predicted by education or the family's social status. Only 10 parents disclosed the concurrent use of traditional or popular therapies to the Western oncologist. Parents were concerned that to do so might be interpreted as implying distrust or dissatisfaction with standard treatments. Parents also perceived negative attitudes of oncologists toward alternative therapies, and were concerned about jeopardizing important relationships with these individuals. Very little communication was reported between the primary oncologist and practitioners of traditional or popular therapies.

CLINICAL TRIALS OF CAM

Reports of clinical trials of CAM therapies in relation to pediatric oncology were sought in the PUBMED and the CINAHL electronic databases. CAM search terms were gleaned from prevalence studies and paired with child, pediatric, and cancer. Results will be presented using the organizing framework provided by the five domains of CAM delineated by NCCAM. Reports were sparse or nonexistent for most categories; therefore, literature summarizing the evidence for safety and efficacy in studies of adults will also be referenced. In particular, the reader will be referred to a recent, highly informative review paper by Weiger *et al.* (2002) summarizing current evidence for effects on cancer progression and palliation, in adult samples, of selected CAM therapies including dietary modifications and supplementation, herbal products and other biological agents, acupuncture, massage, exercise, and psychological and mind–body therapies. Wieger *et al.* conducted an exhaustive search collecting references from multiple databases and other sources, and used stringent criteria to evaluate the quality of the evidence and the associated risks for these therapies, upon which they made recommendations to treating physicians on how to advise adult patients who seek CAM therapies for cancer. They also tabulated information on ongoing federally and non-federally funded clinical trials of CAM therapies in samples of adults with cancer.

ALTERNATIVE MEDICAL SYSTEMS

The search terms acupuncture, Ayurvedic, homeopath, and naturopath did not produce any records of clinical trials using Alternative Medical Systems in pediatric oncology samples. In their review paper regarding CAM therapies for adult cancer patients, Weiger and colleagues concluded that randomized, controlled trials of acupuncture to date, although limited in size, suggest that it is reasonable to accept the use of acupuncture in conjunction with standard anti-emetics to control chemotherapy-related nausea and vomiting. Further, although fewer data are available on the use of acupuncture in palliation of chronic cancer-related pain in adults, the data suggest it is reasonable to accept this approach if patients elect to try it. Adverse events have been documented in conjunction with therapy, but these are judged to be unlikely when accepted techniques are used by competent practitioners (Weiger *et al.* 2002).

BIOLOGICALLY BASED THERAPIES

The search terms cartilage, diet, herbal, Laetrile, megavitamin, melatonin, mistletoe, phytotreatment, plant, and vitamin did not lead to records of clinical trials of biologically based therapies in pediatric oncology samples. One comprehensive tutorial paper on herbs and supplements used to treat childhood cancers was located (Kemper 1999). This article contains a great deal of information useful in educating consumers and clinicians about potential risks and benefits of remedies many patients are using, while underscoring the need to test these therapies systematically in children. Weiger *et al.* critically reviewed several studies of dietary, herbal, and biological CAM therapies used with adult samples, and provided extensive information about interactive effects and risks associated with use of these substances in conjunction with conventional cancer therapies (Weiger *et al.* 2002).

MANIPULATIVE AND BODY-BASED METHODS

Searching the terms chiropractic, osteopath, manipulation, and massage led to one clinical trial of massage therapy conducted at the Touch Research Institute at the University of Miami. Twenty children, mean age 6.9 years, with acute lymphoblastic leukemia were randomly assigned to receive daily massages for one month from one of their parents in addition to medical care, or to be on a waiting list while continuing with medical care. Negative affect was assessed in parents and children before and after the first massage and on the last day of the clinical trial. The child's complete blood count was also assessed on the first and last days of the study. Results of this preliminary study suggest that massage was associated with short-term reduction in negative affect for children and parents, reduced negative affect over the one-month trial in parents, and increased white blood cell count in children (Field *et al.* 2001).

Weiger and colleagues' (2002) review of studies with adult patients concluded that two small randomized, controlled studies found massage to be associated with reduced anxiety. Of three randomized, controlled trials of standardized massage protocols with adults, only one found relief of cancer-related pain. Weiger *et al.* noted that massage directing treatment to the painful areas, as might be expected in actual clinical practice, has not been tested. One small randomized, controlled trial found that massage was associated with reduced nausea in patients undergoing autologous bone marrow transplantation. Two small trials (one randomized and one quasi-randomized) found manual lymph drainage effective as an adjunct to compression bandaging in patients with arm lymphedema after surgery for breast cancer.

With regard to risks, no studies indicated that massage promoted tumor metastasis; however, Weiger *et al.* recommended that massage be avoided directly over known tumors or even predictable metastasis sites without known disease. They also urged caution regarding massage in the following situations: (1) patients with bony metastases who may be prone to fracture, (2) tissues damaged by surgical or radiation therapy, (3) thrombocytopenic patients or those on anticoagulants where hematomas may develop from pressures that would otherwise be well tolerated, (4) hypercoagulability and thrombus formation, and (5) avoiding stents or other prosthetic devices because of potential displacement. With these precautions observed, Weiger *et al.* concluded that the available evidence with adults suggests that it is reasonable to accept and consider recommending massage for relief of anxiety and as an adjunct for lymphedema. They further concluded that although evidence on massage effects on cancer-related pain is mixed, it seems reasonable to accept this approach if patients elect to try it (Weiger *et al.* 2002).

ENERGY THERAPIES

Searching the terms energy, healing, magnetic, and Reiki led to no clinical trials of energy therapies in pediatric oncology samples. (This category of CAM therapies was not reviewed in the Weiger *et al.* (2002) paper on CAM therapies for adult cancer patients.)

MIND–BODY INTERVENTIONS

Several clinical trials for symptom control in pediatric samples were located with the search terms imagery and hypnosis. No clinical trials were located with the search terms faith, meditation, prayer, religion, or spirituality. (Weiger *et al.* (2002) did not review studies on spiritual and religious approaches to cancer treatment or palliation.)

Wall and Womack (1989) compared the effects of hypnotic and cognitive distraction strategies on pain and anxiety associated with bone marrow aspiration or lumbar puncture (BMA/LP). Twenty pediatric oncology outpatients ages 5 to 18 years were assessed for anticipatory and procedural pain and anxiety in relation to their scheduled BMA/LP procedures. Patients were then taught one or the other strategy during two practice sessions. At their next scheduled BMA/LP, participants employed their strategies and assessments were again made pre- and post-procedure. Results indicated that both strategies were associated with pain reduction, and neither was associated with anxiety reduction. The degree of hypnotizability did not correlate with pain reduction.

By contrast, a study using a multiple baseline design with subjects as their own control found that hypnosis was associated with both reduced anxiety and reduced discomfort in 16 adolescent oncology patients (mean age 14, SD ± 1.6) undergoing bone marrow aspirations, lumbar punctures, and chemotherapeutic injections (Kellerman *et al.* 1983). In another study, hypnosis was compared to non-hypnotic techniques, including deep breathing and distraction, for reduction of pain and anxiety in 33 pediatric oncology patients ages 6 to 17 years (mean age 10.06, SD $\pm$ 3.17). Pain and anxiety were assessed by independent observers as well as by patients during bone marrow aspirations and lumbar punctures. Pain during bone marrow aspiration was reduced by hypnosis and non-hypnotic techniques, with a greater degree of reduction in the hypnotic group; anxiety was reduced by hypnosis alone. Pain during lumbar puncture was reduced only by hypnosis, while anxiety was reduced by both hypnosis and non-hypnotic techniques, with a greater reduction in the hypnosis group (Zeltzer and LeBaron 1982). Katz, Kellerman and Ellenberg (1987) studied hypnosis in the reduction of pain and distress in pediatric cancer patients. Thirty-six children ages 6 to 11 years with acute lymphoblastic leukemia, all of whom had undergone at least three bone marrow aspirations (BMA) prior to enrollment and were scheduled for repeated BMAs, were randomized to a hypnosis or play comparison group. Hypnotic intervention included training in hypnosis and self-hypnosis. Hypnosis and play were both associated with reduced self-report of pain and distress associated with BMA, but not with reduced observational measures, highlighting the importance of multi-modal assessment.

Hypnosis proved useful in controlling nausea, vomiting, and distress in pediatric oncology patients undergoing medical procedures. In a randomized, controlled trial, the effects of hypnosis and non-hypnotic relaxation/distraction techniques were compared to an attention-placebo in 54 pediatric cancer patients ages 5 through 17 years reporting significant chemotherapy-related nausea and/or vomiting during baseline assessment. Anticipatory and post-chemotherapy distress, nausea, vomiting, and functional disruption were assessed by observation and interview. Children receiving placebo intervention had generally increased symptoms over time, those receiving cognitive distraction/relaxation maintained symptoms at a steady level, and those receiving hypnosis showed general reduction in symptoms over time (Zeltzer et al. 1991).

In another study, 19 patients ages 6 to 17 years with mixed diagnoses receiving matched chemotherapy doses were randomized to supportive counseling or hypnosis for the reduction of symptoms of nausea and vomiting related to treatment. Both hypnosis and supportive counseling were associated with reduced nausea, vomiting, and the extent of distress due to these symptoms, and symptomatic improvement was maintained after the procedure. Although baseline differences between the two groups were noted, the efficacy of both procedures was approximately equal (Zeltzer, LeBaron and Zeltzer 1984).

CLINICAL APPLICATION: HYPNOTHERAPY AS AN EXAMPLE

Hypnotherapy is often used as a mind–body therapy embedded within a psychological framework. The goals of any psychological intervention for children with pain are fourfold: (1) instill a new paradigm regarding reasons for the pain; (2) reduce focus on self; (3) enhance perceptions of controllability of the pain; and (4) facilitate increased functionality. Before beginning to use hypnotherapy, it is helpful to reframe the pain in terms of pain mechanisms. A simple age-appropriate overview of pain transmission and inhibition, including the impact of emotions and beliefs on this neural system, can be readily accomplished, sometimes with the aid of a schematic diagram (e.g., the affected body part, connections to spinal cord, and brain). This neural definition can then be applied to the child's particular pain problem. The goal of hypnotherapy then, as explained to the child, is to use certain parts of his/her brain to increase the effectiveness of his/her own natural pain control system. In this way, both the child and parents can understand the potential impact of hypnotherapeutic intervention on circuitry in the brain that relates to pain perception.

Hypnotherapy is a psychological intervention that helps the child to have a narrowed and channeled focus of attention, so that the child can be open to possibilities of altered sensations, emotions, and beliefs. Muscle relaxation is often an accompaniment of a hypnotic state but is not necessary for hypnotherapy to occur. The primary focused goals of hypnotherapy are to: (1) capture attention, (2) reduce distress, (3) reframe the pain experience, and (4) help the child to dissociate from the pain. This process typically involves three stages: (1) 'induction' (help the child to dissociate from the environment), (2) 'deepening' (enhance the dissociation), and (3) suggesting that the child find a 'favorite place' (that is safe, fun, interesting, and in which the child feels in control). Images can be suggested to enhance imaginative involvement and the child can be asked to notice the sights, smells, texture of clothes, sounds, etc., around him/her. Helping the child to use his/her sensory system often helps to enhance involvement of the child in his/her favorite place.

For acute pain experiences such as medical procedures, exciting and challenging events can happen within this imaginative involvement. For example, a child might see himself or herself playing basketball and making the winning basket for the team and 'saving the team', or the child might be playing soccer and noticing the goal ahead and the ball in front of his/her feet, while the rest of the team is right behind him/her. Sometimes the use of focal hypnoanesthesia can be helpful to reduce pain during a medical procedure. For example, a 'magic glove' can be 'placed' on a hand that is to have an intravenous line placed. Recall of past anesthetic experiences (e.g., a foot or hand numbed when placed in snow) can also be used.

For children with chronic pain, a 'central sensory control station' can be suggested as being located in the part of the brain that 'thinks with pictures'. This can be described as the center for control of sensory signals coming from the body. Various suggestions for what this might 'look like' can be provided (e.g., colored lights, knobs, and switches, such as what a pilot might see at the front of a plane). The child can be asked to signal with a finger when he/she 'finds' the central control station, and to signal again when he/she finds the 'switch or lever' that controls the feelings coming from the affected body part (e.g., foot, stomach). At that point, it can be suggested that the switch is like a rheostat (dimmer switch) rather than an on/off switch and that the child can slowly turn the switch until he/she has 'just as much feeling (in that body part) as he/she wants to have'. It might be suggested that if he/she turned the switch 'all the way off', that body part might become numb, and so he/she should turn it 'just enough'. It can also be suggested that, as these changes begin to take place, as evidence of a change in the whole system, the child might notice new sensations, such as tingling, in his/her hands or feet (children typically will notice this before they notice decreased sensation in the part that hurts). It can be suggested that the brain is now beginning to learn what 'it' needs to do to help quiet the pain signals to help that part of the body feel better. Analogies can be given, such as learning to ride a bicycle. 'In the beginning, it took work and concentration. But, after a while, the brain learned what it needed to do and the you could ride without thinking about it.' Post-hypnotic suggestions could then be provided for the beginning of change and ease of entering this special state of mind whenever the child needed to, or perhaps at bedtime.

As a relationship is developed with the child and the hypnotherapy becomes part of the longer-term therapeutic process, additional types of imagery may be suggested to the child. For example, the child might begin to find his/her 'wise person' or guide within. This might look like an animal or whatever the child might 'see'. The child can then learn to begin to trust this guide within and begin to listen to this inner wisdom. Many children use their imagery experiences in symbolic fashion to work through other issues to develop an enhanced sense of competence. For example, an adolescent with acute myelogenous leukemia who was in palliative care following relapse was angry and withdrawn, but sometimes would yell at the nurses when they tried to get him to respond to them. Dr. Zeltzer began to get to know him when she was called in for a pain consult to review his palliative care plans. She learned from him that he had wanted to be a 'famous architect' and even had a house in mind that he had planned to build some day. He was angry and felt 'cheated' out of being able to ever build his house. As Dr. Zeltzer asked for more details about the house, she and the patient gradually embarked on the building of his house in imagery sessions. At the start of each session, after the sessions spent in drawing the plans (in imagery), the patient would imagine getting the tools and materials that he would need for the work that day. He became very involved in the development and building of this house and would describe in great detail what he was working on and how it looked. As he became more absorbed in the house building, he needed less analgesia to feel comfortable. He began to sleep better at night and his mood became less depressed and angry than previously. After about two weeks of this, he announced that his 'house was built' and he appeared proud. He then began to describe the house to his family and anyone who showed interest. He died two days later.

Ultimately, hypnotherapy can be an effective tool for changing the mind/ body dualism to a new paradigm in which all systems are connected. This treatment can facilitate feelings of control and the belief that physical changes are possible. This paradigm shift heralds the beginning of reduction of pain and enhancement of functioning. Hypnotherapy can play a major role metaphorically in increasing feelings of control, competence, and hope.

CONCLUSIONS

Popular interest in and use of complementary and alternative therapies clearly has outpaced scientific evaluation of these modalities. At present, significant gaps in the available scientific knowledge base limit the ability of health professionals to guide parents and pediatric patients with regard to complementary and alternative approaches to treatment of cancer or the side effects of cancer treatment. Most CAM approaches, especially in pediatric samples, remain relatively or completely unstudied from the standpoint of controlled clinical trials research. Increased resources are currently being allotted to their evaluation in adult samples at the local, national, and international levels, and several clinical trials are currently underway. The popularity of CAM interventions for children with cancer renders the scientific evaluation of their safety, efficacy, and effectiveness for children key research objectives.

ACKNOWLEDGEMENT

Supported in part by the Sue Stiles Program in Integrative Oncology at UCLA.

REFERENCES

Astin, J.A. (1998) Why patients use alternative medicine. *JAMA* **279**, 1548–1553.
Burgio, G.R., Locatelli, F. (2000) Alternative therapies and the Di Bella affair in pediatrics. A questionnaire submitted to Italian pediatric oncologists and hematologists. *Haematologica* **85**(2), 189–194.
Eisenberg, D.M., Davis, R.B., Ettner, S.L., Appel, S., Wilkey, S., Van Rompay, M., Kessler, R.C. (1998) Trends in alternative medicine use in the United States, 1990–1997. *JAMA* **280**, 1569–1575.
Eisenberg, D.M., Kessler, R.C., Foster, C., Norlock, F.E., Calkins, D.R., Delbanco, T.L. (1993) Unconventional medicine in the United States: prevalence, costs, and patterns of use. *N. Eng. J. Med.* **328**, 246–252.

Eisenberg, D.M., Kessler, R.C., Van Rompay, M.I., Kaptchuk, T.J., Wilkey, S.A., Appel, S., Davis, R.B. (2001) Perceptions about complementary therapies relative to conventional therapies among adults who use both: results from a national survey. *Ann. Intern. Med.* **135**(5), 344–351.

Ernst, E., Cassileth, B.R. (1998) The prevalence of complementary/alternative medicine in cancer: A systematic review. *Cancer* **83**, 777–782.

Fernandez, C.V., Stutzer, C.A., MacWilliam, L., Fryer, C. (1998) Alternative and complementary therapy use in pediatric oncology patients in British Columbia: prevalence and reasons for use and nonuse. *J. Clin. Oncol.* **16**(4), 1279–1286.

Field, T., Cullen, C., Diego, M., Hernandez-Rief, •., Sprinz, P., Kissell, B., Beebe, K., Bango-Sanchez, V. (2001) Leukemia immune changes following massage therapy. *Journal of Bodywork and Movement Therapy* **5**, 271–274.

Friedman, R., Sedler, M., Myers, P., Benson, H. (1997) Behavioral medicine, complementary medicine and integrated care. Economic implications. *Prim. Care* **24**(4), 949–962

Friedman, T., Slayton, W.B., Allen, L.S., Pollock, B.H., Dumont-Driscoll, M., Mehta, P., Graham-Pole, J. (1997) Use of alternative therapies for children with cancer. *Pediatrics* **100**(6), E1.

Grootenhuis, M.A., Last, B.F., de Graaf-Nijkerk, J.H., van der Wel, M. (1998) Use of alternative treatment in pediatric oncology. *Cancer Nurs.* **21**(4), 282–288.

Katz, E.R., Kellerman, J., Ellenberg, L. (1987) Hypnosis in the reduction of acute pain and distress in children with cancer. *Journal of Pediatric Psychology* **12**(3), 379–395.

Kellerman, J., Zeltzer, L., Ellenberg, L., Dash, J. (1983) Adolescents with cancer. Hypnosis for the reduction of the acute pain and anxiety associated with medical procedures. *J. Adolesc. Health Care* **4**(2), 85–90.

Kelly, K.M., Jacobson, J.S., Kennedy, D.D., Braudt, S.M., Mallick, M., Weiner, M.A. (2000) Use of unconventional therapies by children with cancer at an urban medical center. *J. Pediatr. Hematol. Oncol.* **22**(5), 412–416.

Kemper, K.J. (1999) Shark cartilage, cat's claw, and other complementary cancer therapies. *Contemporary Pediatrics* **16**, 101.

Kemper, K.J., Wornham, W.L. (2001) Consultations for holistic pediatric services for inpatients and outpatient oncology patients at a children's hospital. *Arch. Pediatr. Adolesc. Med.* **155**(4), 449–454.

National Center for Complementary and Alternative Medicine (2003a) What is CAM? http://nccam.nih.gov/health/whatiscam/Accessed Feb. 5.

National Center for Complementary and Alternative Medicine (2003b) About NCCAM, General Information. Available at http://nccam.nih.gov/ Accessed Feb. 5.

Neuhouser, M.L, Patterson, R.E., Schwartz, S.M., Hedderson, M.M., Bowen, D.J., Standish, L.J. (2001) Use of alternative medicine by children with cancer in Washington State. *Prev. Med.* **33**(5), 347–354.

Office of Cancer Complementary and Alternative Medicine (2003) http://www3.cancer.gov/occam/about.html Accessed Feb. 6.

Paramore, L.C. (1997) Use of alternative therapies: estimates from the Robert Wood Johnson Foundation National Access to Care survey. *J. Pain. Symptom Management* **13**, 83–89.

Richardson, M.A., Sanders, T., Palmer, J.L., Greisinger, A., Singletary, S.E. (2000) Complementary/alternative medicine use in a comprehensive cancer center and the implications for oncology. *J. Clin. Oncol.* **18**, 2505–2514.

Sawyer, M.G., Gannoni, A.F., Toogood, I.R., Antoniou, G., Rice, M. (1994) The use of alternative therapies by children with cancer. *Med. J. Aust.* **160**, 320–322.

Wall, V.J., Womack, W. (1989) Hypnotic versus active cognitive strategies for alleviation of procedural distress in pediatric oncology patients. *Am. J. Clin. Hypn.* **31**(3), 181–191.

Weiger, W.A., Smith, M., Boon, H., Richardson, M.A., Kaptchuk, T.J., Eisenberg, D.M. (2002) Advising patients who seek complementary and alternative medical therapies for cancer. *Ann. Intern. Med.* **137**(11), 889–903.

World Health Organization, policy statement on traditional medicine and complementary/alternative medicine (2003) www.who.int/medicines/organization/trm/orgtrmmain.shtml Accessed Feb. 12.

Yeh, C.H., Tsai, J.L., Li, W., Chen, H.M., Lee, S.C., Lin, C.F., Yang, C.P. (2000) Use of alternative therapy among pediatric oncology patients in Taiwan. *Pediatr. Hematol. Oncol.* **17**(1), 55–65.

Zeltzer, L.K., Dolgin, M.J., LeBaron, S., LeBaron, C. (1991) A randomized, controlled study of behavioral intervention for chemotherapy distress in children with cancer. *Pediatrics* **88**(1), 34–42.

Zeltzer, L., LeBaron, S. (1982) Hypnosis and nonhypnotic techniques for reduction of pain and anxiety during painful procedures in children and adolescents with cancer. *J. Pediatr.* **101**(6), 1032–1035.

Zeltzer, L., LeBaron, S., Zeltzer, P.M. (1984) The effectiveness of behavioral intervention for reduction of nausea and vomiting in children and adolescents receiving chemotherapy. *J. Clin. Oncol.* **2**(6), 683–690.

15

Fantasy, Art Therapies, Humor and Pets as Psychosocial Means of Intervention

SHULAMITH KREITLER

*Psychooncology Unit, Tel-Aviv Medical Center
and Department of Psychology, Tel-Aviv University, Israel*

DANIEL OPPENHEIM

Department of Pediatric Oncology and Unit of Psycho-oncology, Institut Gustave Roussy, Villejuif, France

ELSA SEGEV-SHOHAM

Pediatric Oncology Unit, Haemek Medical Center, Afula, Israel

INTRODUCTION

It is now acknowledged that medical and nursing tasks are important but not the only care children and adolescents with cancer require. Many wards are now attentive to the quality of the therapeutic environment they can offer. Their objective is to assuage the difficulties of this traumatic ordeal and mitigate the risk of psychological problems in the course of the treatments and following them, to help the patients to live through their childhood and their adolescence, preserving their capabilities and their rights to play, to learn, to think, to laugh, and to be active.

The present chapter describes various forms and modalities of art therapy, practiced in different wards around the world, each presented by expert practitioners. Each type of therapy is characterized by a particular

Psychosocial Aspects of Pediatric Oncology. Edited by S. Kreitler and M. Weyl Ben Arush
© 2004 John Wiley & Sons Ltd: ISBN 0 471 49939 0

methodology and is targeted to attain specific goals. Yet, in practice each type of therapy is often used for attaining different goals, similar to those targeted by other types of therapy. Moreover, often several therapy types are applied together, either at the discretion of the therapist, tailored to the needs and possibilities of a particular patient, or in prestructured multimodal comprehensive packages (Hilgard and LeBaron 1984; Jay *et al.* 1991).

In general, there are in this broad domain many detailed case reports (e.g., Rudloff 1985, Cotton 1985), descriptions of particular projects and elaborate presentations of technique and relatively few well-designed studies with a sufficient number of participants focused on any one of the described therapy modalities or on comparing the effects of two or more therapies. One reason for this is the tendency to apply various techniques together; another reason may be the need for great flexibility in view of the necessity to adapt the therapies to a great variety of children, in difficult medical situations (Prager 1995). This state of affairs renders it difficult to provide evidence-based support in the strict sense of the term for the particular effects of any of the therapies.

The most frequently cited objectives of the different therapies are the following: distraction of attention, blocking or inhibiting of distress reactions, mitigating side effects of medical procedures or treatments (e.g., pain, nausea, fatigue), reducing fear of the unknown, reducing negative emotions (e.g., distress, fear, etc.), inducing positive emotions (e.g., joy, security, love, confidence and pride), increasing self-esteem, strengthening sense of control, and promoting cooperation with the medical procedures (Luzzatto and Gabriel 1998).

A. FANTASY INVOLVEMENT

The sedative and possibly healing power of imagery has been recognized in many cultures since ancient times (Kunzendorf 1991). In recent years there has been growing use of images as a therapeutic modality in medical contexts, with children no less than with adults. Fantasy could be considered as a component that plays a role in all the expressive and affective interventions. It is often coupled with hypnosis which provides the relaxation or concentration part and uses imagery for presenting suggestions in the course of hypnosis and post-hypnotically. Also without hypnosis it is usually applied in the context of art therapy and only rarely as a single modality (Hockenberry 1989). When used alone, it represents a therapy that focuses on engaging the child in some imaginary activity. The child is asked to imagine some kind of experience, object, event or situation. All the child's senses may be involved, namely, not only visual sensations which are most common, but also sounds, tastes, smells, or a combination of these. When the focus is on visual imagery, the child may be asked to imagine being in a favorite room or place, in a flower garden, watching some kind of sport activity, or animals, TV or movies; when the focus is on auditory imagery, the fantasy may involve hearing conversations with significant others, favorite songs, playing a musical instrument, environmental sounds (waves etc.), or listening to music; when the focus is on movement imagery, the child is requested to imagine flying, swimming, skating, amusement ride, or any other pleasurable activity (Hockenberry-Eaton *et al.* 1999). When applied in regard to pain, the focus is either on providing distraction, in which case any pleasant absorbing fantasy will do, or on combating pain by changing the perception of the pain, for example, imagine that you blow the pain away, or that it fades out (French, Painter and Coury 1994). The process of imagining may range from completely free unstructured suggestions to imagine anything one desires, to providing step-by-step instructions about how to proceed. Precise instructions would include steps, such as the following: "we are going to make a journey to a nice place which you will greatly enjoy; please sit comfortably and close your eyes; breathe slowly; now choose a place in which you want to be; now that you have reached it, observe carefully who is there in that place; then focus on the objects in that place; try to see the colors and the forms; try to hear the sounds; are there any smells, etc.; you may now come back from that place". Not only the process of imagining but also the image itself may be subjected to different degrees of guidance or shaping by the therapist. For example, in order to initiate the procedure of imagining, the therapist may show the child a cartoon on TV and introduce the child to a particular character or location. Also the theme of the image may be suggested to the child, for example, a road, a wheel, a circus. In other contexts, the therapist would wait for the child to come up with an image and would shape it by suggestions so that it exerts its optimal therapeutic impact or at least does not develop into an anxiety-laden negative image, as may sometimes be the case. The goals of guided imagery are mostly reduction of anxiety and stress, promoting positive feelings and sometimes 'fighting cancer' (i.e., promoting healing). Studies showed that guided imagery has significant effects in reducing distress in children undergoing diagnostic procedures (Zeltzer and LeBaron 1982) or chemotherapy (Cotanch, Hockenberry and Herman 1985, Genuis 1995). One session of imaginative involvement with children 3–10 years old reduced more distress than standard care in bone marrow aspirations (Kuttner, Bowman and Teasdale 1988). Another study with 25 pediatric oncology patients, found that 21 agreed to use the exercises of guided imagery and 19 showed substantial reductions in pain and nausea associated with their practice, especially if they begin the exercises at the time of their initial diagnosis (Olness 1981). There is evidence that children project their disease concerns and anxieties onto the images they produce (Achtenberg and Lawlis 1984). Studies demonstrating the effect of guided imagery on immune function in adults (Schneider, Smith and Witcher 1983) have yet to be replicated in children. Also, there is a need for research focused on the processes accounting for the beneficial effects of imagery.

B. GUIDED IMAGERY COMBINED WITH COMPUTERIZED ART THERAPY

A special variety of guided imagery was developed by using computerized animation (Magen and Ben Arush 1999). The goal was to help pediatric oncology and hematology patients to meet the challenges of serious illness regardless of distance from the hospital, language, time and religion, by providing them a safe environment in which to express their feelings in a nonverbal way. This was attained by constructing a graphic program, adapted for use of children from the age of 4 years onward, which allows the child creative exploration and discovery. It was created by using a digital camera, video-phone and scanner, with hand-painted drawings and graphics, computerized video animation, computer CD games and audio-cassettes with music, sounds from nature and voice. The program, called 'The Bridge', is based on nonverbal communication, which aids in projecting unconscious imagery. It stimulates the five senses and awakens the child's imagination. The computerized program is introduced to the child in the hospital under the supervision of an art therapist. Each child receives an art therapy menu, adapted to his/her emotional, psychological and medical condition. The program allows freedom of choice of colors, forms and even medium, and encourages the child to produce images by using the different expressive options. The scanned images are transferred to the home computers. Patients are requested to print and/or transfer the images into diskettes. Siblings and parents are invited to participate if necessary, so that family interactions and communication are promoted. The program may be activated by the child at home so that it assists the medical staff with home medical management.

C. VISUAL ARTS

Introduction

Art therapy based on the visual arts is probably the most widely applied modality of art therapy. It uses painting, drawing, sculpture, photography, ceramics, and the fabric arts in order to enable the children to express their conscious and unconscious concerns about the disease and to externalize their fears and anxieties, as well as to promote self-awareness and self-confidence and to try out new solutions to their problems in a safe environment. A variety of materials are used (e.g., different colors, clay, wood, beads, buttons, cloth, paper), in a variety of forms (e.g., finger painting, drawing, face painting, sponge painting, instructing others to produce the image, using even computer graphic programs), with a variety of produced outputs (e.g., paintings, sculpted objects, drawn images, embroidery, photographs, masks, and dolls).

The three poles of this therapeutic modality are the therapist, the patient and the image, whereby the art therapist is often called upon to act in the triple role of artist, teacher and therapist. The emphasis is on creativity and expressiveness, often coupled with spontaneity and improvising. This therapeutic modality is characterized by three major dimensions: (a) the expressive–creative dimension, based on the relation between the patient and the image, wherein the therapist fulfills the role of facilitator in the image production process; (b) the cognitive–symbolic dimension, based on the relationship between the therapist and the patient through and about the produced image, wherein the therapist helps the patient to understand the image; and (c) the interactive–analytic dimension, which is based on the direct communication between the therapist and the patient, wherein the therapist uses the image and its meanings in order to help the patient understand himself or herself (Luzzatto and Gabriel 1998).

Art therapy is being practiced in different forms. It may take place in the hospital, in the child's home or in the therapist's clinic; it may consist of individual sessions or group sessions; it may or may not be accompanied or followed by analysis of the art work and discussion in the group setting or between the therapist and the child. During each session the therapist may offer techniques, subject-matter, media and/or free choices in line with the changing needs of the patient and the therapeutic goals. The child may decide consciously what to convey through the art work, or simply start in a random fashion to produce something.

Varieties

Special kinds of art therapy have been developed. For example, structured art therapy consists in asking the children to draw specific themes, once or even more than once in consecutive sessions. Standard themes would be the 'mandala' (color–feeling wheel), the 'change-in-family' drawing and the 'scariest' drawing. The structured aspect of these drawings allows the therapist to ask highly focused questions and interpret the drawings within the context of the individual's reality (Sourkes 1991).

Another interesting kind of art therapy focuses on mask making. Jones (1997) described its application with five pediatric oncology patients, in the course of treatment, in a public hospital. The masks were produced from papier maché. All children completed their masks over a period of 5 to 8 weeks. The project included a video recording of each patient's mask making process, photographs of each mask, and a closing semi-structured interview. Analysis of the masks and the video recordings showed that the project promoted creativity, individual expression, symbolization, objectification of feeling, expression of disease-related concerns, while supporting adaptive denial, self-representation, expression of wishes, fantasy development and production of a transitional object. It also enabled the children to gain control of some aspect of their time in the hospital. According to the observation of the oncologists, the mask making decreased the children's anticipatory anxiety, possibly by providing distraction, but did not increase the children's social interaction.

Recent years have witnessed the emergence of a new kind of art therapy, which can be called computer-assisted art therapy (Collie 1998a, 1998b, Malchiodi 2000). This variety of art therapy is based on using computer technology for creating and sharing images. The special features concern the production, storing and communication of the products. Concerning production, computer-assisted art therapy provides the following possibilities: to use computer drawing by applying different graphic software; to use image banks for selecting images, constructing new images out of given graphic elements or improving on self-produced images; to create animated graphics; to combine drawings and photographs; to add to the images multi-media components, e.g., sounds, music, and motion. It is of special importance to emphasize that the use of computers obviates the need to rely on the use of materials (e.g., colors, cloth) which may jeopardize pediatric oncology patients whose immune systems are compromised. Concerning storing of the products, computer-assisted art therapy enables easy storage of the products, in multiple locations, and easy access to the products stored on diskettes or CDs. Possibly the most innovative developments occur in regard to communication. Computer-assisted art therapy enables sharing the products with sick and healthy children in other countries, cultures and continents. It also presents the possibility for electronic exhibitions, open to actually any interested or accidental spectator around the globe. Most importantly, it enables on-line interactive communication between the art-producers and the art-therapist, one or more, in real time. This enables not only computer support for art therapy at a distance, but also bridges the gap between producing static images and dynamic performance. All these features seem to indicate that we may be on the verge of a revolution in art therapy whose future is difficult to outline.

A Report from the Department of Pediatric Oncology, Institut Gustave Roussy, Villejuif, France

Each year, 35% to 50% of the children (above the age of 6 years) and adolescents in the ward participate in the fine arts workshop (Géricot and

Perrignon 2000) receiving tuition and training from a specialized teacher. This is not an academic activity but an opportunity to give free rein to creativity. They make greeting cards for Christmas, wooden figures (doctors, nurses, children, volunteers) and a long streamer with their self-portraits which decorate the walls. Thus, they contribute to making the ward pleasant to look at and affirm that it is also theirs, and does not belong only to the staff. The art teacher, who is a professional, proposes the themes, provides the children with the technical means, tools, and examples of old or recent paintings, and offers advice so that they can create a beautiful work of art, in their own style and own objective. She notices how the children's work or behaviour are related to their inner world and the situation they are currently experiencing (in a setting of this kind even the slightest detail in these works of art is meaningful), but does not discuss these aspects with them (there is no confusion with psychotherapy). She does, however, talk to the psychoanalyst when she witnesses excessive distress in the child, or disarray in herself.

Themes

Children work on successive themes, illustrating them with paintings, sculptures, collages, or photographs. Here are some examples of what they have produced:

- '*Castles*': children painted fortified castles, a house of cards, luxury castles, the hospital, a jail, their own house, thus expressing their feelings of insecurity and a plea for protection, their ironic revolt against the caregivers, as well as their longing to be at home.
- *Collages*: they made figures and scenes with pieces of photographs cut out of magazines. They thus played at being mad surgeons, cutting and remodelling strange, horrific or beautiful faces and bodies.
- *Photographs of the ward*: they took photos of different kinds, such as documentary pictures (the everyday life in the ward), ironic ones (children glimpsed at through the aquarium, like fishes), cruel ones (crutches with plaster), and poetic ones (a smiling face drawn on a bald skull). Other photos expressed themes, such as anger, an effort to control fear, lassitude, or yearning for tenderness.
- *Self-portraits*: This was the theme the children appreciated most of all. All the portraits show some obvious or discrete signs of the cancer, such as a deformed face or body, baldness (sometimes hidden by luxurious hair 'invading' the face), and thinness (sometimes the body looks as if it has undergone erosion). Some of the bodies have no defined limits. However, in those cases when the bodies have limits, they are exaggerated, for example, they are drawn in the form of a protective band which is so large that it invades the inside of the body as the tumour did, though there is always a

little hole indicating that such protection is somehow missing. Some bodies look like an unstable tower, on the verge of collapsing, while others appear to be controlling this danger by excessive rigidity which is not always efficient. The clothes play a role in these contradictory attitudes: some emphasize a fragile appearance (stripes that give the impression that the body has been cut into slices, or a necklace giving the impression that the head has been cut off), some try to hide the body, some look like strong armour.

It is possible to divide into two groups all the portraits, regardless of the identity, the age or the artistic skill of the children. The first group includes portraits reflecting the efforts of the children to control their image. In portraits of this kind the signs of cancer and fragility are violently and provocatively displayed or masked (a paraplegic boy drew himself walking in a landscape), but often a detail reveals that these efforts were in vain. The eyes are often void, lifeless. The spectators of these portraits feel compelled to express pity, curiosity, fascination, or an indulgent compliment, but remain outside their world. These portraits can be contemplated several times, but they do not change. It is as if the child were saying: 'I'm only showing what I want to show, you won't see or know any more'. The second group includes portraits which authentically express the child's disarray. Portraits of this kind display violent colours, and are done with large and brusque brush strokes, and the eyes are full of life. The spectators feel caught in a dialogue with the portraits, they can penetrate deep inside of them, explore them time and again, and each time discover new things and new emotions, probably much like what the children themselves were experiencing while they did the paintings.

What do they expect from this activity?

Naturally, the children expect compliments, but not forced praise. They know they need a true appreciation of their skills, an honest look at their image and at themselves. People who only see the image and not the children's face are discredited and the same goes for those who do not accept the children's disguise and try to remove their mask.

The works of art belong to the children, but may be exposed in the ward, in the hospital, at art fairs, in schools, or in festivals all over the country. Thus the children present a proud image of sick children, and establish active links between the world of paediatric oncology and illness and the 'normal' outside world. Through the paintings they are no longer 'passive and sick children' but children who have preserved a sense of beauty and of creativity, which in the course of their illness has not been forgotten but rather has been confronted in a positive manner. They know their portraits also express their inner world of thoughts and emotions related to their illness, but without words. Furthermore, the artistic work helps them to perceive themselves in a different light:

they can avoid directly complaining and expressing their sufferings or terrifying fantasies. It also protects them from looking at themselves and at their faces and bodies directly. Last but not least, these works are objects to be remembered and precious traces left by the children of their suffering and fight. Years later the children, or the parents and the caregivers will be able to look at them and remember.

Severe illness does not transform the children into artists. It may reveal that some of them are truly gifted, but that would by no means apply to all children. Yet, because the artistic setting is exciting and safe, it thrusts all the children into expressing their inner world in a rich and intense way, regardless of how gifted or skilled in the arts they may be. Accordingly, all products can be admired as authentic works of art, requiring the same kind of appreciation and criteria, although only some of them attain the level of what could be called 'works of art'. The self-portraits talk about cancer but also about many other things and, most of all, about the children, their values, and their dignity.

D. BIBLIOTHERAPY

Bibliotherapy is a therapy that uses literary products (i.e., books) as a therapeutic means for providing relief, enhanced self-understanding, promotion of coping skills and personal growth. Bibliotherapy is an interactive process with three essential components: the client or patient, the trained facilitator or therapist and literary products of different kinds (e.g., stories, poetry, plays, folktales, legends, proverbs). In the context of pediatric oncology, different kinds of books are used for a variety of goals – for example, for distraction during medical procedures; for providing health-relevant information about the procedures, treatments and the disease; for fun (e.g., humor, adventure books); for relaxation and reduction of anxiety; and for psychotherapeutically relevant goals, such as enhancing the child's self-esteem and self-identity. The most salient and interesting is the psychotherapeutic use. The underlying philosophy is that 'the world is made up of stories, not facts' (Remen 1996). The patient is exposed to a structured selection of literary themes designed to encourage self-exploration and self-expression. The theoretical rationale for this type of psychotherapy is the assumption that life is a narrative and that psychotherapy is the production and improvement and understanding of this narrative. The characteristic processes applied in bibliotherapy are the following: transcending the patient's enclosure within the confines of his or her own narrow set of problems; coping within an imaginary protected setting; attaining a timeout period that enables release from one's own problems by identifying with the problems of the literary figures; promoting self-awareness by encouraging the child to talk freely about one's problems and feelings while discussing those of the literary figure that may resemble one's own; providing emotional relief by identifying emotionally with problems and solutions of the depicted figures; coping with taboo issues, such as death, loss, abandonment that embody the child's innermost fears by presenting the themes symbolically and sometimes by providing in fantasy wish fulfillment of taboo desires through the explicit or implicit narrative. Even a short-term application of bibliotherapy is expected to facilitate integration of the traumatic event or situation and to help identify sources of strength, thus promoting self-esteem, the experience of a continuity of life events, social functioning and increased life satisfaction (Borden 1992).

The basic technique used in bibliotherapy consists in the therapist telling the child a story in his/her own language or reading to the child a story out of some printed text. There are, however, many possible variations of the basic technique. The story may sometimes but not always be accompanied by showing relevant pictures. The reading is often followed by a discussion of the themes by the therapist and the child. Sometimes the story is told or read to a group of children and is followed by group discussion. Another variation includes the following three phases: first the therapist tells or reads a story to the child, then the child tells it back to the therapist, and finally they discuss it. Sometimes the reading of the story is amended or amplified by fantasy, for example, the child is asked to suggest additions or changes in the story, or the child and therapist exchange presents between themselves in the form of stories (Gardner 1986, Mair 1989).

The story told or read by the therapist may refer directly to cancer (there is a set of books about children with cancer in most languages, e.g., Cothern (1994) and Noonan (1992)), but may also deal with other themes, selected by the therapist as pertinent to the child's current needs.

There are specializations within bibliotherapy – poetry therapy (Leedy 1985, Lerner 1994), folktale or mythology therapy etc. according to the preferences and needs of the clients. Each type of literature contributes something unique, e.g., poetry provides special images, rhymes and rhythms; folktales provide metaphors and generally applicable 'lessons'; stories provide absorbing plots with figures with whom one may identify; etc. Books of humor and jokes constitute a special subcategory that is sometimes conceptualized as 'humor therapy' (see section K of this chapter).

There is empirical evidence that telling the child a story with one's beloved or admired hero, who helps the child cope with the situations gradually increasing in difficulty, reduces the children's distress during treatments (Jay et al. 1991; see also Chapter 13 of this book). Storytelling incorporated within a multimodal treatment package was shown to reduce distress as well as nausea, vomiting and the bother of other side effects (Hilgard and LeBaron 1984). In a study with leukemia patients, 6–19 years old, undergoing bone marrow transplantation, even after one intervention of storytelling there was already less self-reported pain and anxiety (Hilgard and LeBaron 1982). The therapeutic effect of books and stories may be exercised simply by reading the material, but the effect is usually enhanced when the material has been also discussed.

E. WRITING

Introduction

Writing is a form of therapy that consists in the patients' writing of poetry, stories, personal memoirs, testimonials, or diaries (also called journaling). Writing may be considered as representing the creative part of bibliotherapy. Patients often feel the need to write. Some patients tend to write or respond well to the suggestion to write either because they are basically verbal types or because they feel that nonverbal means of expression are too infantile for them or not common in their culture (e.g., Arab children). Some patients start writing on their own initiative, whereas others need to be encouraged. Again, some do it on their own, others dictate it to others, while still others need the help of someone else who acts as a therapist. The written products sometimes assume the form of metaphorical stories (e.g., fighting a cruel dictatorial ruler who kills away most of his citizens, because he acts under an ancient curse that he can only be evil), at other times they are outright documentations (e.g., a girl, 11 years old, diagnosed with advanced brain tumor wrote almost a day-by-day account, starting the morrow of the diagnosis and ending a week prior to her death). Often patients write poems of a classical or modern type. Some patients produce a written product only once, or only during a certain period of time; others write sporadically, and still others keep on writing all through.

Part of the beneficial effect of writing is the emotional relief it provides. Another factor may be the sense of control and freedom it provides the writer who is hemmed in in a situation in which he/she may feel overwhelmed, helpless and dominated by external factors (e.g., the disease, the treatments, hospital regulations). In a series of studies on the effects of writing in people in general it was shown that those who were asked to write about consequential events felt in the short term worse than those who were asked to write about trivial events, but in the long run they had fewer health problems and better immunological functioning. This and similar findings were explained as being due to two factors. The first was obviating the need for inhibition. Inhibition requires hard work on the part of the inhibitor and increases stress. Hence, writing has a beneficial effect because it makes inhibition unnecessary. The second factor is the use of language. Language enables distancing from the event and assimilating it while processing it and organizing the material. Hence writing has a beneficial effect because it makes use of language (Pennebaker

Kiecolt-Glaser and Glaser 1988, Booth, Petrie and Pennebaker 1997, Esterling *et al.* 1999).

A Study with Arab Patients in Israel

Arab patients may find it difficult to use the media of visual art therapy due to cultural attitudes. Hence it was considered to be of prime importance to try the use of verbal art therapy with them. Storytelling in writing functions for the children as a means for expressing themselves, both directly and through metaphors and artistic distance. This setting provides safety and legitimacy for dealing with negative emotions and taboo themes. It is assumed that the expression itself has a therapeutic impact. Furthermore, storytelling provides the therapists with information about the concerns of the children that trouble them and that they may ignore or be too shy to disclose publicly. According to the Lahad (1992) method that was applied, the child is asked to write a story on the basis of memory or fantasy, in line with six basic guiding questions. It is assumed that the six recurrent questions provide the child a steady framework which enhances the sense of protective security. The child can actually write the story or dictate it to the therapist. The method was applied with seven pediatric oncology patients, 12–18 years old. They were all from Muslim orthodox families, living in Arab villages in the Galilee. The storytelling went on for 8 months, in a continuous though sometimes irregular manner, due to treatment limitations. All children reported that the stories they told helped them to feel better and stronger.

The children produced 34 stories over the months of treatment. This material was subjected to content analysis in order to identify the major themes bothering the children. The themes identified by the judges were grouped and formed nine bipolar clusters. The following three clusters appeared in all the stories: the need for love, belongingness and acceptance versus fear of loneliness and abandonment; longing for life and health versus fear of death; and the need for control versus feeling helpless and powerless. Three further themes appeared in many of the stories: longing for strength versus feeling weak (90%), wishing for success versus experiencing failure (65%), and striving for independence versus feeling dependent (42%). Finally, there were three further clusters which appeared only in a minority of the stories: the contrast between feeling hatred and feeling love (25%), the contrast between one's internal feeling and external appearance and behavior (20%) and the contrast between trust and distrust of others (10%).

Notably, all themes express the children's distress, their conflicts, their fears and frustrations, as well as their struggle for strength, control, health and life. The unique properties of the stories were that they reflected the manner in which the children experienced these problems and the solutions that reached through the harsh experiences they were undergoing. These conclusions are illustrated by the following examples of stories produced by the children. The first story was told by A., a sick boy 12 years old. He wrote a story about the sick TV set, which became exhausted and almost collapsed and stopped functioning because it was being used continuously by the children. The sick TV set confessed its fears to its friend, the remote control, which came to its help and asked the kids to reduce the time they used the TV set. This story applies projection and expresses by means of artistic distance the need for help through a technician. The story reflects a sense of helplessness, fear of death, and distrust coupled with a desire to be helpful and useful to others. Four years later the boy still recalled the story and admitted that it was the one which best reflected his state at the time.

The second story was told by a 16-year-old boy, two months before his death. His story was about the rain which threatens to put out a candle, his candle. The metaphor of life as light is well-known. This story expressed the patient's fear of death and sense of approaching death, but mainly the futility of fighting for the light when there is so much rain that threatens to put out the weak and helpless candle.

The third example is a story produced by a 7-year-old child. He told a story about a dog one of whose spots fell away from his body without his being aware of it. Since he became different he was chased away by everyone in the village. This story expresses the experience of a child who suffers because he is different from the other children who are healthy. More specifically, it reflects the sense of rejection and abandonment due to a physical symptom which one completely ignores. Having the sickness without yet knowing about it is a frightening experience of many cancer patients that undermines their sense of security and control.

F. PLAY

Play is a means that is being used for alleviating distress, pain and various side effects of chemotherapy. One study showed that even adding to the medical procedure an expandable whistle-like toy ('party blower') makes crying less likely and enables relaxation by paced breathing (Manne *et al.* 1994). Another study examined the effects of playing video games on children (9–20 years old, with various cancer diagnoses) in the course of chemotherapy. Most (69%) of the children in the experimental group who played the games reported a sizable reduction in nausea as compared with 23% in the control group who got no video games. Further, in the second part of the study, the introduction and withdrawal of the opportunity to play video games were followed by reduction and exacerbation of nausea, respectively. Notably, playing video games was associated with an increase in systolic blood pressure, indicating an increase in arousal (Redd *et al.* 1987). Another study with three participants, 11–17 years old, suffering from acute lymphocytic leukemia, showed that playing video games in the course of chemotherapy was associated with self-reported reductions in anticipatory symptoms (e.g., insomnia, biting nails 24 hours prior to treatment) and state anxiety, observer-rated distress due to side-effects (e.g., dizziness, nausea), and self-reported as well as observer-rated post-chemotherapy side effects. The mentioned distress signs were exacerbated when the games were withdrawn; the signs were reduced again when the video games were reintroduced (Kolko and Rickard-Figueroa 1985). A study with children undergoing bone marrow transplantation for acute lymphocytic leukemia, showed that non-directed play was as effective as hypnosis (including the use of imagery, muscle relaxation, and suggestions of mastery) in reducing the children's self-rated pain and fear (Katz, Kellerman and Ellenberg 1987). Playing games forms part of several intervention packages in pediatric oncology which reported overall positive effects on the wellbeing of the treated children or adolescents (Hilgard and LeBaron 1984, LeBaron and Zeltzer 1984, McGrath and de Veber 1986, Wall and Womack 1989, Zeltzer and LeBaron 1982). It is likely that computer games will be increasingly used, complementing the common video games. The beneficial effect that playing has on children in treatment for cancer is mostly attributed to the distraction of the children's attention from the painful procedures they are undergoing (e.g., Hilgard and LeBaron 1984, Kolko *et al.* 1985). However, it seems likely that further processes may play a role, such as gaining a sense of control, and overcoming distress by fantasy. The possible involvement of fantasy indicates a likely blurring of boundaries between proper play and play therapy (see section G of this chapter).

G. PLAY THERAPY

Play therapy is a therapeutic medium which uses playing with dolls and other toys or objects in order to provide support to children in distress and help them resolve problems that impair their wellbeing (Walker 1989). Play therapy is designed to assist the child in coping with stressful situations, enhance the child's sense of mastery, help the child establish an atmosphere of normality under conditions that deviate from normality, and reduce helplessness and anxiety. Playing is an integral part of the child's normal world and can therefore be expected to have the potential for a strong therapeutic impact. The goal of play therapy is often to help the child adapt the reality to the self and the self to reality.

Play therapy may be conducted in the form of individual sessions or group sessions with several sick children, whereby mutual support and the possibility for creating social ties are provided (Cooper and Blitz 1985, Lingnell and Dunn 1999). Significant others, for example, parents, siblings or members of the medical staff, may act as observers watching the child's play. They may gain thereby a better understanding of the child's means of coping, as well as feelings and perceptions of the situation and even of the observing figures themselves.

Play therapy may be carried out in different forms. Toys and dolls can be given to the child who is left alone with them, to play as he or she wishes. This non-directive procedure can be amended by suggesting a general playing theme to the child, such as 'this is a hospital ward' or 'this is a kindergarten' or 'they are all going on a trip'. Play therapy may be enacted also in a directive–interactive manner, whereby the therapist lets the child start out with the play, offers an interpretation or suggestion for the next step, and so on, closing up with a discussion between the therapist and the child. The number of sessions also varies in line with the needs of the child and the particular play therapy technique used by the therapist.

Here are some examples of play therapy sessions in the context of the hospital ward. A 4-year-old girl, diagnosed with Hodgkin's disease, used to play for hours with a set of dolls presented to her by the therapist. The play changed from one session to the other but one element kept recurring: she used to hide one doll somewhere in her bed and would start crying because she 'lost' it. When this happened, the therapist asked what was the matter, whereby the girl would urge her to help to find the missing doll. When the doll was found, which was invariably the case, the girl would cry with joy and make a big party for the dolls. In one of the follow-up visits to the hospital she volunteered of her own accord the meaning of the game: 'even when you die, they will look for you and find you'. Apparently the play she devised helped her deal with the fear of death. The theme of coping with one's own pending death recurs in accounts of play therapy with pediatric oncology patients (e.g., Manheimer 2000, McCall 2000, Tacata 2000).

A 9-year-old girl, diagnosed with leukemia (ALL), who met with a play therapist for several sessions, focused on one theme which she evolved over three sessions until she was apparently satisfied with the ending (= solution?). The theme was the conflict of a little truck between telling and not telling the big truck that it was broken. In the first session, the little truck suppressed its moans and sighs, and hid in a dark corner, concealing from the big truck the fact that it was broken. In the next session, the little truck lay in the center of the playground with its wheels turned upward, displaying in public its state, for everyone to see. The big truck was so overwhelmed that it turned its back on the little one. In the third session, the little truck ran on purpose against the big truck and by colliding with it attached itself to the big truck so that they could move only if they kept together. At the end of each session the therapist offered a one-sentence summary of the events (e.g., 'Little truck shows everyone how sick he is but no one takes notice').

Another patient, an 8-year-old boy diagnosed with Ewing's sarcoma, used to play military games. Once he arranged the toys in the form of an attacking army; on another occasion he staged an attack on a castle which was eventually conquered; and on still another occasion he had airplanes dropping bombs on the cover of his bed which represented 'the enemy territory'. When asked by the therapist to describe what was going on he explained that there was a war, a serious war, 'a war for life and death', which necessitated investing all one's resources in order to win the war. This set of plays afforded the expression of aggression the child may have felt because of the restrictions imposed by hospitalization and the disease. But in addition, it seems that it also served the purpose of mobilizing all the child's resources in order 'to win the battle for health'.

Examples of further themes that recur in play therapy with pediatric oncology patients are misunderstanding of the child why he or she was at all in the hospital (Tacata 2000), family relations under the threat of death (McCall 2000), and loneliness due to difficulty of interpersonal relations with friends (Goodman 1999).

Notably, most examples illustrate the use of projection and symbolization by the children in their endeavors to find a solution to a bothering problem by means of therapist-guided play therapy.

H. DRAMA THERAPY AND PSYCHODRAMA

Drama therapy is a mode of therapy which uses dramatization and dramatic forms of expression as a therapeutic medium (Clayton 1993). The best known form of drama therapy is psychodrama, developed originally by Jacob L. Moreno (1994). It employs guided dramatic action, supplemented by action methods and role playing, in order to facilitate insight into the patient's problems, promote the patients' awareness and understanding of themselves and reality, and enable the learning of new skills and the enhancement of emotional wellbeing. Like some other forms of art therapy (e.g., bibliotherapy), psychodrama enables the patients to approach real-life problems and emotionally-laden themes through the safe distance of fictionalized situations and characters. In addition, the dramatic medium and the largely nonverbal form of expression combine to lower the patients' control, so that they may reveal about themselves more than they would otherwise. The special characteristic components of psychodrama are acting-out and fantasy. The patient is encouraged to engage in acting out in a protected setup, and to give free rein to his/her fantasy in a spontaneous, creative manner. The product is a creative expression of imagination which assumes through action a concrete form in reality. Thus, there is a breaking up of restricting structures coupled with the production of new structures which often spell out new solutions to both old and new problems.

Accordingly, psychodrama provides a safe, supportive environment to practice new and more effective roles and behaviors, rehearse new roles, try out solutions, and explore new options. In general, it offers the opportunity to see reality from different points of view. Finally, since it relies on action, it is often more empowering than traditional verbal therapies. The overall procedure includes the steps that lead the patient from reality to fiction to a better reality.

The basic components of psychodrama are the protagonist, the auxiliary egos (= others who play significant others or inner forces within the person), the audience, the director (= therapist), the stage (physical space). The three major structural components involved in psychodrama are warm-up, action, and sharing (= discussion) (Dunne 1992).

Drama therapy may be enacted according to a script discussed before the enactment or produced spontaneously in the course of the enactment. It can be enacted in line with a script produced by the child spontaneously, or by the therapist, or by both, sometimes even in line with a script out of a book or play. The drama may be enacted by the child or children and sometimes with puppets (dolls or marionettes). The boundary between theater and drama therapy becomes blurred sometimes, so that psychodramatic elements are embedded within the context of theater presenting therapeutically relevant themes, thus combining entertainment, catharsis, and therapy. One example is the STOP GAP drama therapy workshops of California that go around in hospitals doing theater and psychodrama.

Drama therapy can be applied in any space, small or large, closed or open, in the presence of others (adults, children) or without them. However, essentially the presence of spectators, be they an active or passive audience, is conceptualized as an integral component of drama therapy. Others may often be called upon to fulfill various roles in the unfolding drama. For example, in one session with a 12-year-old child suffering from leukemia, psychodrama was enacted in the sick room in the hospital, in the presence of two additional patients. The child assumed the role of 'the sick child', whereas the two other patients played in turn the roles of 'two doctors' discussing the case of 'the sick child' and concluding that he will recover, then the roles of 'the fear' and 'the hope' dwelling within 'the sick child', fighting it out between themselves until 'the hope' won the upper hand. This psychodramatic enactment served the goal of confronting the child's fears and strengthening his hope. In a series of psychodramatic sessions with a group of survivors of childhood cancer, the enacted themes were problems of being accepted again in the group of children, the sense of having missed out because of the long time spent in the hospital, the feeling of being different from other children, not being understood by others, and means of making others understand.

Drama therapy is often applied in order to prepare the child for medical procedures, undertaken for diagnostic or treatment purposes. This use of drama therapy, which is sometimes called behavioral rehearsal, consists in going with the child through the different steps of the procedure he or she is expected to undergo, whereby the child may assume in turn the roles of patient, nurse, and doctor. Puppets may sometimes be introduced into the drama. The dramatic enactment, which may be repeated more than once, allows the child familiarization with the situation, reduction of fear of the unknown and strengthening the sense of mastery and control (DuHamel, Johnson Vickberg and Redd 1998, p. 963). This kind of application of drama therapy has been reported to have highly beneficial effects on the mood and cooperation of the child (Ancelin-Schuetzenberger, 1991).

Dramatic Play Therapy in the Hospital Setting

Dramatic play therapy represents a special variety of drama therapy. It combines the therapeutic advantages of drama and of play to form a unique tool to address the sick child's special needs. Its enactment requires the patient, a drama therapist, one or more other individuals (adults or children), dolls or puppets and often other toys and objects too. The drama unfolds in line with a script that has been prepared in advance or is being improvised on the spot. Change of roles often takes place. Dramatic play therapy is of special importance in the context of hospitalization. Hospitalization is traumatic for children and causes radical changes in their lives. They are forced to leave their known world and forgo their freedom and privacy. Further, they have no control over the situation and have to undergo frightening and painful procedures.

There are several clear-cut advantages of dramatic play therapy in the hospital setting. It enables children (a) to re-enact familiar activities and thus reduce the strangeness and threat of the unknown environment; (b) to reorganize their life and thus gain a better understanding of what is happening to them; (c) to assume in the play an active role and thus regain the sense of control that has been impaired by the disease and the hospitalization; (d) to express aggression under controlled conditions and thus attain a modicum of relief for the sustained frustration; and (e) to express their dreams, needs and feelings, by projecting them onto the dolls and puppets.

As mentioned earlier, dramatic play therapy is often used in order to help prepare children for diagnostic or therapeutic medical procedures (even surgery) both by providing them information about what is going to take place and by reducing fear and tension through the enactment of the events. In this context, the actual use of real accessories, such as gloves or syringes, is of great help. The following example illustrates the use of dramatic play therapy in preparing a child for a medical procedure. The patient was a 6-year-old girl diagnosed with histiocytosis at the age of 2.3 years. She has undergone many medical tests pre- and post-diagnosis, mostly under general anesthetic. The recurrent painful tests made her highly anxious. Her anxiety was further exacerbated through the anxiety of her parents who felt that the girl had terminal disease. The goal of the play therapy was to prepare the girl for an MRI test without anesthetic. The play therapy was based on using two glove puppets representing mother and father, a small doll representing a baby, and a plastic tube representing the MRI machine. The major protagonists of the play were Mother, Father, and Baby. The Doctor joined in later. The patient and the drama therapist were present all through. In the first session the patient was a spectator. In the beginning the Father and Mother decided not to tell Baby that they were going for an MRI but instead to deceive her by telling her that they were going on a trip. At this point the patient interfered and the first session ended with her admitting to the drama therapist that she knew the show was about her. In the second session, the patient assumed a more active role. She chose for herself the role of the mother and for the drama therapist the role of the baby. Baby started to question Mother about where they were going. When she was told about the MRI test she wanted to know why and how it would be done. Mother showed her by simulation with the plastic tube how the MRI test would be performed. At this point Baby raised concerns about frightening sounds in the course of the medical test (made sounds) and asked to be hugged. The Doctor joined the play and explained that the patient would be put to sleep so that she does not move in the course of the test. Baby resisted this suggestion because she was afraid that she would not wake up. The Doctor suggested that when she gets to the clinic for the MRI, she could ask not to be put under anesthetic. The session ended with Mother holding Baby. Following the suggestion of the drama therapist, the patient and her mother took the dolls home for the weekend in order to play with them. The therapy was highly successful: the girl underwent MRI without anesthetic. She lay completely still for 45 minutes, with her mother holding her hand. The girl and her mother were strengthened by the success, learned to cope with different procedures and even helped other parents.

I. CINEMA AND VIDEO THERAPY

Focus on Viewing

Cinema therapy is the use of cinema in order to diagnose and help individuals in distress. Conservative cinema therapy consists in showing the patient a readymade film selected by the therapist especially for the patient with the intent of illustrating or highlighting some particular problem or issue relevant for the patient. For example, the film *Life is Beautiful* (by Robert Begnini) portrays a father who turned the stay in a concentration camp into a kind of game for the child and thus helped him survive the horror with a minimum anxiety and without paying too high a price in mental health. Other examples include *The Miracle Maker* about Helen Keller (by Arthur Penn), Charlie Chaplin's *The Kid* and the more recent *Patch Adams* demonstrating humor therapy. Films involve powerful sensory experiences, appealing to various senses and portraying situations that often resemble those in actual daily life. Hence they may be used profitably in order to transmit to patients, also children, various therapeutically important messages, such as 'you are not the only one hit by the trouble from which you are suffering', 'others struggling with difficulties similar to yours or other serious problems have survived it', 'various problem solving options are open to people in trouble', and 'every cloud has a silver lining'. The transmission of the messages is enhanced by means of the experiential impact of film, and the indirect way in which it is communicated. The film may be watched by the child alone or in the company of an adult (e.g., parent, sibling, other patients), at home or in the hospital, once or several times, and with a variety of screening devices (e.g., movie screening machine, DVD, video). Further, viewing the film may or may not be preceded by some kind of focusing by the therapist and may or may not be followed by discussion with the therapist. Conservative cinema therapy resembles bibliotherapy and may be considered as a film-based variety of bibliotherapy.

Focus on Producing

Another variety of cinema or video therapy consists in actually producing a film. The underlying assumption is that the film-making process offers various artistic and organizational activities that resemble those used by therapists and which may provide useful and challenging psychological exercises. This variety of cinema therapy requires a film-making expert, a therapist and a patient. Working together this team produces a film primarily for the benefit of one single spectator, who is the patient.

Video therapy consists in encouraging and helping a child to produce a video film. Snap shot and video cameras, tape, CD and computers are used, along with traditional art therapy tools, such as storytelling, music, and painting. The focus is on producing video animation, but further means such as sculpting, modeling and drawing may also be often used in these projects. The children are induced to invent the plot, write the script, draw and sculpt the background scenario, design and decide where, when and how the video takes place, and then film and edit the film. In this kind of video art therapy the child assumes alternately the roles of director, actor, author and producer of his or her own movie. Five major stages are involved in the process: (a) text-writing (scenery-preparation), in which the child learns how to prepare a 'story board'; (b) directing, in which the child directs others, who may be children or patients, the child's parents or siblings, and members of the medical staff; (c) filming, in which the child chooses whether to film, photograph or act in front of the camera; (d) editing, in which the child introduces into the film the changes he or she considers appropriate in order to shape a product with a specific purpose, for example, a movie that can be used as a therapeutic tool in the future; and (e) screening, in which the child assumes control of when, where and to whom the movie would be screened.

When the video film is finished, the child is encouraged to take it home as his or her own. However, it can also be used for discussion in individual sessions or group sessions, in order to improve the children's or the care-takers' insight.

Video art therapy is assumed to have unique contributions to the child's wellbeing. First, it provides distraction which helps in alleviating pain and anxiety. This is achieved by involving the child in an interesting and totally engrossing activity, satisfying insofar as it appeals to the child's narcissistic needs, and with enough variety to hold the child's attention for longer periods of time. Second, it provides catharsis by enabling the child to express his or her innermost fears, problems and anxiety by means of unconscious projection and symbolic representations in the video plot and images. Third, it contributes significantly to improving the child's mood and quality of life by providing satisfaction, fun and entertainment. Fourth, it promotes interaction between the child and his or her family by involving the whole family in the video production, which of course stays with the family as a document commem-orating happy moments to remember in the future out of this difficult period. Fifth, it contributes to strengthening the child's ego by providing activities and encouraging creativity that may help to reveal new strengths and discover new talents. Ego-strengthening is particularly important both because the circumstances increase the child's sense of helplessness, and because through the newly acquired strength the child may find new ways of coping. Sixth, it contributes to improving the child's body image by involving the child in bodily activities.

Video therapy is appropriate for use with very young as well as older children. In the Department of Pediatric Oncology/Hematology at the Rambam Medical Center it has been applied successfully in recent years with over 80 children, ranging in age from 5 to 22. All have admitted that engaging in video therapy has made a significant contribution to their overall wellbeing. Many have mentioned that video therapy has given them moments of happiness despite all the suffering they have undergone in the hospital.

J. CLOWN THERAPY

Twice a week, two clowns come to the ward (Oppenheim, Simonds and Hartmann 1997), like others do in ten paediatric departments in France (e.g., the 'Rire Médecin', and also in the United States, Canada, Brazil and Germany (e.g., 'The Big Apple Circus Clown Care Unit' at the Yale–New Haven

Children's Hospital, the so-called 'therapeutic clown' David Langdon at the Winnipeg Children's Hospital in Canada) (Darrach 1990). They work in the corridors and the waiting hall area as well as in the rooms, with children and adolescents, even with the terminally ill, individually or collectively in a group, but also with the parents and the caregivers. Each clown has his or her own style, personality, and particular skill: they play music, perform magic tricks, dance, speak too fast, stutter, or mime, etc. They come in different varieties – big or small, fat or lean, with long hair or bald heads, skilful or clumsy, but all wear red noses. Their names are Dr Giraffe, Dr Basket, Dr Cauliflower, Dr Lulu Leek, etc. They perform brief and improvised shows in the corridors by themselves or by drawing into the dance, the game or the little scene a child, or anyone else who happens to be in the vicinity. The children become spectators or actors, and eventually receive a red nose. The clowns wear a decorated white coat, carry props in their doctor's bags, some of which are made with medical or nursing devices (e.g., balloons made of gloves, whistles or telephones made of syringes or stethoscopes).

The clowns' work

The clowns offer joy and laughter, but do much more than simply amuse the children. Children know about their illness and the complex and precise treatments they need. They usually accept these constraints which are nonetheless hard to endure. This is why they enjoy the anarchy, nonsense and fantasy introduced by the clowns as a means of revenge, through their clothes, the way they walk or dance, the way they talk or shout, telling fake and horror stories, disturbing the parents and nurses. Playful and musical noises are heard, instead of silence or aggressive noises (pagers, pump alarms, sometimes cries, etc.) The clowns are fully aware of the fact that the children may sometimes feel frustration because they have to endure painful treatments and operations. Therefore they readily provide the children an outlet to engage in aggressive behavior: the children can bite and be bitten, they can tear off Giraffe's 'Velcroed' tail, they can push a clown, and so on. The clowns also transform the function of a place from its intended use: the nurse's room turns into a dance hall, a child's room becomes a ring or a circus, and the whole ward turns into a playground, in addition to its original function to provide medical care services.

The clowns help the children to regain possession of and pride in their bodies by showing that they are proud of their own strange and distorted bodies, when they demonstrate how to put a handicap to good use, when they grimace together with the child, when they transform a child's neck brace into a royal necklace. They express openly the emotions the children may feel (fear, terror, love, anger, etc.) and show how these can be understood and integrated in a play and in a story. Thus, the children know that even their most intense or violent emotions have a place in the ward and that they can also do something positive with them.

Illness plays a key role in the clowns' games. Illness is the implicit theme in the background when ropes are cut and magically restored, when a ball disappears in the nose and reappears in the mouth, when a child removes Giraffe's horn and puts it on his own nose, or on the nurse's head. Pranks of this kind may illustrate the child's etiopathological theories, e.g., 'Where does my illness come from? Somebody has put it inside me. If I could give it to someone else, or if only it could disappear magically'. The games enacted by clowns allow the children to express their illness theories, without fully believing in them or feeling bound to explain them, and to maintain them, without getting into conflict with the medical theories which they know and accept. When the clowns parody the caregivers, they allow the children to revolt under safe conditions. This may give the children not only an emotional outlet, but may also help to avoid non-compliance.

The clowns' objective

Through their appearance, pranks, games, and jokes the clowns help the children to stay active, creative, and 'authentic' children, rather than being merely children with cancer undergoing aggressive treatment. More specifically, they enable the young patients to preserve their joy, despite the toughness of their situation, as well as to think freely and maintain their capacity to use their imagination, despite sometimes burdensome worries, fear of the present, of the future, and of the unknown. The clowns also help the caregivers and the parents to widen their perception of themselves and their roles in regard to the children. This may help to delay burnout, and prevent feelings of guilt they may have when confronted with children's sadness.

Under what conditions is the clowns' work possible?

Clowns do not simply compensate for or cover-up the absence of medical and nursing competence and of psychological support. They participate in the care of the child, working in close collaboration and harmony with the medical staff, fully aware of the risk that both the children and the nurses may contrast the 'good doctors' (the clowns) to the 'bad and naughty ones' (the pediatricians and nurses). They have to determine the specific role they intend to play in midst of all the other professionals (psycho-oncologists, teachers, art therapists etc.). They must be experienced professional clowns, trained for this specific setting, functioning in line with a strict code of ethics. They have regular meetings with a psycho-oncologist who can help to shed light on some of the problems and intricacies of the situation in pediatric oncology. Being a clown in this setting is a serious and difficult task. If the clowns are not aware of and do not know how to deal with the intense emotions, and with the deep, complex and sometimes violent thoughts which can be vented under the mask of play, then the relation of the clowns with the child may be dangerous for both parties.

K. HUMOR THERAPY

The potentially beneficial effects of laughter and humor on health have long been surmised and were expressed in sayings, such as 'The arrival of a good clown exercises a more beneficial effect upon the health of a town than 20 asses laden with pills' (Sir Thomas Sydenham) or 'If it were not for laughs, we would be sicker than we are' (William Frey, both professor of medicine and researcher of humor). A growing body of research is beginning to provide empirical evidence supporting the contribution of humor and laughter to strengthening the immune system, moderating the effects of stress, and serving as an efficient coping and defense mechanism (Lefcourt 2001, Martin 2001, Vaillant 2000). The popular screenplay *Patch Adams* has put a spotlight on the healing aspects of laughter in the medical context, whereas the show 'Andre Vincent is Unwell' (in Edinburgh, 2002), which enacted the suffering of a cancer patient in the form of stand-up comedy, has contributed to breaking the notion that cancer is a taboo subject in comedy. In recent years there have been notable initiatives to bring humor therapy into the oncology wards, e.g., The Hamptons Comedy Festival (2002), the East Coast's premier comedy organization dedicated to using comedy to fight cancer, has launched in 2002 the *Comedy Fights Cancer/ Laughter Promotes Healing* initiative, and brings comics to cancer patients in hospitals in the form of large shows or bedside performances. At Loma Linda University Cancer Institute humor-based treatment complements chemotherapy so that during the treatments the patients are encouraged to watch videos or read literature from the Laughter Library, with the SMILE (Subjective Multidimensional Interactive Laughter Evaluation) software guiding their choices of material. 'Humor carts' (conceived by humor therapist Judy Goldblum-Carleton) exist in over 40 hospitals in the USA, bringing to pediatric oncology wards humor therapists who have learned how to create fun and laughter in the sick children. The largest and most ambitious project is Rx Laughter [created by Dunay Hilber and led by Margaret Stuber and Lonnie Zeltzer, and conducted by the Johnson Cancer Center, the Mattel Children's Hospital at UCLA and the UCLA Neuropsychiatric Institute and Hospital] which applies for therapeutic entertainment carefully selected cartoons and TV classic films in order to study how best to use humor for pain reduction and prevention or treatment of diseases in children and adolescents.

Research shows that children (5–10 years) with cancer do not differ in humor from healthy children and that they more often rated a cartoon as funny even without understanding the joke, which indicates they had a tendency for humor (LaRue and Zigler 1986). A study with 43 school-aged children with cancer showed that children scoring high on the Multidimensional Sense of Humor Scale had better psychological adjustment than those scoring low, regardless of the amount of cancer stressors, insofar as coping humor moderated the daily hassles of living with cancer. Moreover, the high scorers had a lower incidence of infections when the number of reported cancer stressors increased, and better immunological functioning (as assessed by salivary IgA levels and absolute neutrophil counts; Dowling 2001). Major involved mechanisms are partly physiological (e.g., muscular relaxation) and partly psychological (e.g., better coping) (Buckman, 1994). Both types of effects appear to be mediated by the cognitive changes brought about by humor (Kreitler, Drechsler and Kreitler 1988, Kreitler and Kreitler 1970). Humor consists of shifts in the meanings assigned to the situation and the major protagonists. The shifts express awareness both of the problem inherent in the situation and of its insolubility, at least for the time being. Hence, humor renders it easier to accept reality, even if it is neither humorous nor 'a laughing matter'.

L. MUSIC THERAPY

Music therapy is a general name for different ways of using music for helping the patient cope, or more specifically, for providing a feeling of satisfaction and harmony (Bruscia 1991), facilitating relaxation, moderating physical symptoms, such as pain and nausea and reducing anxieties, loneliness and stress (Bunt 1998). Music is particularly adapted to attain goals of this kind because of its harmonious structure, its use of components that are not found in their pure form in external reality (e.g., tones, melody) and its structural properties, manifested especially in its rhythm (Kreitler and Kreitler 1972). The major processes involved in music therapy are promoting nonverbal interaction, expressing repressed emotions, enabling diversion, providing fun and entertainment and facilitating indirectly the acceptance of the new reality. A great variety of means is available for exercising music therapy. The major means used most often at centers such as the Rambam Medical Center, the Ireland Cancer Center (University Hospital of Cleveland), and University Hospitals Rainbow Babies and Children's Hospital, include the following: exploring and stating one's musical preferences; listening to the desired music usually in the company of the therapist, nurses or other patients; listening to live music played or sung by an individual present (e.g., the therapist); engaging in relaxation exercises or anxiety-relieving fantasies with background music (Bonny and Savary 1990); using musical instruments or playing rhythm instruments, including improvisational drumming; learning to play instruments, such as the guitar, omnichord, shakers, bells and drums; composing original songs or melodies; drawing under the inspiration of musical pieces; playing music on the inspiration of a drawing (the child's own, another child's or a printed painting); listening to special musical tones or chords (e.g., electronic music, Indian gongs, or even vibrations produced by tones) (Lane 1996). The sessions may last from 15 minutes to one hour, and may be conducted in individual sessions, even at the patient's bedside, or in groups, which may be open also to family members and other visitors.

Music therapy was shown to be of great help in reducing the distress of children undergoing painful medical procedures (Hockenbery and Bologna-Voughan 1985, Malone 1996). A study with 65 pediatric hematology/oncology patients whose mean age was 7 years (range: birth to 17) showed significant improvement in the children's ratings of their mood in terms of the 'faces pain scale' (a pictorial scale of faces depicting various degrees of pain, including numbers, colours and definitions) from pre- to post-music therapy, whereas the parents perceived an improved play performance after music therapy in preschoolers and adolescents. Notably, 49% of the parents in this study said that the music therapy brought comfort to them and reduced their own anxiety (Barrera, Rykov and Doyle 2002). In children with myeloid leukemia music therapy was observed to promote the child's behavior from being 'just a patient' into playing temporarily a more active social role (Aasgaard 2001). Playing music for children in isolation (in the course of bone marrow transplantation) is of particular help and significance because it decreases their loneliness and sense of detachment from the world (Brodsky 1989, Kuttner 1996, Pfaff, Smith and Gowan 1989). It may even help reduce anxieties in terminally sick children (Fagan 1982, Garrison and McQuiston 1989). Music therapy was also observed to promote more engaging behaviors in the children than activities, such as unstructured play or reading taped storybooks with the therapist (Robb 2000).

Two examples may serve to illustrate the uses of music therapy. The first concerns K., a 13-year-old girl diagnosed with lymphoma, who suffered badly from the disease and the treatments. She became so distressed by the changes in her appearance caused by the treatments that she refused to have any contacts with others. In this case, one purpose of music was to provide the girl with diversion and relaxation in the course of chemotherapy. While listening to the music she loved (ballet music with clear rhythm and musical patterns) she was encouraged to make a fantasy voyage by using imagery. The voyage led her to distant worlds that opened a window to dreams and space. Another function of music in this case was to enable K. to meet with her friends at school. She agreed to meet them when they were all listening to their preferred music.

The second example concerns T., a 10-year-old girl diagnosed with sarcoma in the pelvis. Following the disease and the treatments T. ruptured all social contacts and became a withdrawn taciturn person, hardly reacting to the environment. She gradually emerged from this state only when she started learning to play the electric organ. She learned notes, chose songs she liked and then started to play them to others, first her family and then her friends. Playing music symbolized for her her ability to give something to others and be accepted again as a member of the children's social community.

M. SINGING AND CHORUS

Songs and singing as therapeutic means share a few elements with music therapy but also differ from it in basic respects. First, the elements of singing are more intrinsically human than musical components. Second, producing singing sounds involves activation of a bodily organ, unlike musical sounds whose production does not necessarily depend on the body. Due to the origin of singing in the human body, listening to singing sounds activates the listener's body in a way different from listening to musical sounds. Since singing is a product of the human voice, it may be expected to be related most intimately to the expression of emotions. Thus, it is natural for human beings to express their joy, suffering, pain, even despair through sounds, which are often not words but rather vowels or combinations of sounds mimicking the emotion (e.g., Aah, Ooh, Oiy, Rrrr). When combined and sounded in a kind of protracted melody (e.g., undulating sound, repetitive sounds in staccato) these moans and other sound combinations form the elements of singing. This affinity of sounds to emotions may constitute the understructure which promotes the therapeutic use of singing (Bailey 1984, Dileo 1999). Further, since singing and composing songs do not require accessories or even training (at least not on the basic level), singing provides a ready means for creative expression (Turry and Turry 1999). A highly specific property of singing which enhances its therapeutic potential is the fact that it uses the human voice in two capacities – expressive and communicative. Notably, the two functions may use nonverbal or verbal means or both, so that reactivity and interaction can be both verbal and nonverbal (Newham 1999). Thus, when singing the patient may use words or, for that matter, sounds or nonsense syllables at his or her discretion – all the time, part of the time or not at all.

Singing may be used with individual patients or with groups, in which case it may assume the form of a chorus. Singing in groups strongly enhances the community feeling of the sick children on the ward and greatly reduces the sense of loneliness. Family members, other patients, and friends may be invited to join the session. A child may be induced to listen to recorded singing or to singing by the therapist or an actual singer, and may be encouraged to join the singing to the extent that he or she wishes or is able to. Often children prefer to sing on their own. Of course, the quality of the singing plays no role at all. The singing may take place anywhere on the ward or outside it and often does not need any accessories (Logis and Turry 1999, O'Callaghan 1996).

N. DANCE AND MOVEMENT THERAPY

The American Dance Therapy Association defines dance or movement therapy as 'the psychotherapeutic use of movement as a process which furthers the emotional, cognitive and physical integration of the individual'. In recent years more specific goals were developed in regard to helping patients including oncology patients and children. Dance therapy relies almost exclusively on nonverbal expression and uses for therapy mainly muscular and kinesthetic responses. The special focus of dance therapy is *bodily movements*. This is of particular importance in the case of pediatric oncology patients whose body image may be impaired following surgery and oncological treatments. Therapeutic use of movements may restore the children's contact with the body and lead them to accepting their body despite the changes it has undergone temporarily or permanently (Levy, Fried and Leventhal 1995).

Dance therapy may be conducted for single patients or groups. When children dance in groups, there may or may not be coordination between them. When each child in a group dances for himself or herself without coordination in the movements of the children in the group, the outcome resembles 'a collective monologue' in the sphere of language (Piaget 1959). The extent of the movements may also vary greatly. Dance therapy may be enacted in space, with the child moving in space as much as the body enables or as minimally as the child is able and willing to move. Dance therapy may also not involve changing location in space but be focused only on bodily movements. Thus, dancing may involve the whole body or parts of it, so that sometimes only the fingers or eyelids dance. The dance may even be enacted only in fantasy, when the child is unable or unwilling to move, or simply too fatigued and exhausted to move. Hence, dance therapy may be done in the child's bed.

Dance therapy may use music as background or not. The dance may be performed according to the child's own rhythm and patterns or according to externally presented rhythm, with or without musical tones. When the melodious aspect of music is distracting for the child, rhythm alone may be used. Some children find it beneficial to move in time with rhythm that is familiar to them or precisely unfamiliar, even bizarre.

Dance therapy may be expressive to varying degrees. It is completely expressive when the movements are free, improvised by the child as he or she goes along, and do not conform to any code or style of motion taught to the child or agreed upon prior to the dance. More often at least some elements of diverse motional codes or styles are incorporated into the child's dance. Some therapies focus primarily on the performance of prescribed movements or postures, which may conform to specific dance styles (e.g., Latin American or Indian or local folk dancing) or specific movement codes reflecting a conceptual or symbolic tradition (e.g., yoga), a specific theory or a physiological conception (e.g., Alexander, Aikido, Feldenkrais, Hanna Somatic, Chi Kung and Tai Chi Chuan) (Behar-Horenstein and Ganet-Sigel 1999, Halprin 2000; Levy, Fried and Leventhal 1995, Newham 1999). Movement therapies of this kind provide the patient primarily with renewed contact and awareness of one's body and an enhanced sense of bodily control.

Possibly, movement therapy may include also the special practices of swimming or splashing in water, taking hot or cold baths, and massage (insofar as it is medically approved) which resembles passive movement. These motional practices may be enjoyable for the child and contribute to restoring his or her acceptance of the body and mastery over one's body following the changes in body image in the course of treatments.

O. ANIMAL-ASSISTED AND PET-FACILITATED THERAPIES

The psychological effects of contact with animals have been recognized already by the ancient Greeks. But the earliest documented reports of the use of animals in therapy date from the late 18th century from the UK and beginnings of the 20th century in the USA. The rapidly accumulating evidence shows the beneficial impact of contact with animals on patients with different diagnoses – psychiatric patients, geriatric patients, patients with Alzheimer or dementia, patients with spinal cord injuries, regardless of the place in which the patients stay – at home, in hospitals, in nursing homes and rehabilitation units. Animal-assisted therapy has been reported to be particularly effective with children and adolescents (Kale 1992).

There are various forms of practicing animal-assisted therapy. For example, the child may own a pet or actually help to take care of an animal, by himself or herself or as part of a team of children, usually under the guidance or active participation of an adult, who may be the therapist. The child may interact with the animal, touching it or talking to it, in the presence of the therapist. The child may simply watch the animal and learn about it and its behavior, for example, fish in an aquarium. A pet may be adopted by the ward as 'our animal' without the active participation of the children in taking care of it. The adopted pet must not be on the ward, but may stay somewhere else on the hospital grounds or at home with the child or children going to visit it.

The major observed effects of animal-assisted therapy were increased readiness of patients to communicate; increase in trust, social contacts, and cooperation; reduction of anxiety, depression, distress, loneliness, stress and the sense of threat; increase in relaxation; enhanced responsiveness to the sensory environment; increased physical activity; promotion of responsibility; and improvement in confidence, self-image and self-esteem (e.g., Carpenter 1997, Willis 1997).

Up to now there has been a relatively limited use of animal-assisted therapy in oncology, mainly because of fear of infection in patients with suppressed immune system function. However, even though the experience is limited, the results showed that contact with animals markedly decreased depression and distress in oncology patients in regular hospital units (Muschel 1984, Raveis *et al.* 1993) and hospices (Chinner and Dalziel 1991, Slavin 1996). There is an increasing number of anecdotal reports about the introduction of animals into pediatric oncology units while observing adequate precautions to prevent infections – for example, restricting contact with the animals merely to observing them, communicating with them without touching them, and in general avoiding any physical contact with the animals.

Animal-assisted therapy may be expected to be particularly effective in the context of pediatric oncology because it focuses on social interaction in its basic and simplest form. It offers the chance for forming and maintaining a simple companionship, a bond based on give and take without the damaging intervention of prior conceptions, biases, and emotions, such as shame, guilt and sense of inferiority. The contact with the animal is mostly nonverbal and consists in interaction for its own sake. One gives as much or as little as one can give and is appreciated for this. Hence, this kind of therapy provides the child the chance for feeling accepted despite limitations, such as one's fatigue, sadness, sense of restricted ability to give, and one's changed body image. The contact with the animal gives the children the feeling that they are needed and appreciated for what they are. The animal may become a friend indeed because it is a friend in need.

Further contributions of animal-assisted therapy are that through the animal the ward or the sick room gains an element of normality and everyday-life atmosphere, which may be important for children hospitalized for longer periods of time or whose daily routine has been ruptured in other ways. Last but not least, animals and pets may provide the sick child a theme to think about, possibly fantasize about, outside the range of the disease and the treatments. Being preoccupied with the animal even for limited periods of time enables dissociation from the painful and anxiety-evoking.

P. PARTIES AND OUTDOOR ENTERTAINMENT

It has become traditional in pediatric oncology wards around the world to organize for the children parties, balls, shows, picnics, outings, excursions, and other forms of entertainment, considering their state of health. Children who are confined to the bed or ward or hospital are entertained at the spot in which they have to stay, whereas others who may be freer to move are taken outside the hospital into the community, on trips and even to other countries. These entertainments are always planned in cooperation with and under the guidance of the medical staff. Moreover, members of the medical staff participate in these events mainly for medical reasons in order to make sure that the health of the children is not compromised in any way and to take care of any unusual medical occurrence.

Since such entertainment events are so common, it is likely that they contribute in some form to the wellbeing of the children. The reasons seem clear. First, the explicit goal of such events is to provide the children fun and entertainment, at least in partial compensation for the suffering they have been undergoing. Second, elements of different forms of art therapy are often incorporated into these events, such as play, humor, clowns, jesters, magicians, music, dance, singing and storytelling. These art therapeutic components exert their beneficial effect also in this setting. Third, since some of the restrictions and rules that govern the children's behavior are lifted on these occasions (e.g., one may scream, laugh loudly, throw things around, be impertinent), the children may enjoy a cathartic effect to counterbalance their frustrations and anger. Fourth, on these occasions the children get the opportunity to interact with the medical staff on a more day-to-day level, not necessarily with less distance, but often without the role-bound limitations of 'doctor' and 'patient'. This experience may help the children accept the need for compliance in the regular hospital routine. And last but not least, the entertainment occasions sound loud and clear the encouraging message that 'life goes on' and soon the child may perhaps be able to rejoin it.

CONCLUDING REMARKS

This chapter has presented a variegated colorful panorama of a great number of therapeutic modes and media, most of which go under the name of 'art therapy'. Though each of the therapies is unique, they share a great number of characteristics. The shared elements concern the goals, the therapeutic processes, and the manner of application or practicing.

A great variety of goals are listed by the different therapies, including mostly palliation of physical symptoms, improvement of mood, boosting of body image and increasing self-esteem. Despite differences in formulation, it is evident that all the goals boil down to improving the child's quality of life, and do not refer to survival or improving the recovery chances of the child.

The therapeutic processes involved in art therapeutic media were summarized aptly by Luzzatto and Gabriel (1998) as 'the six "C"'s': Catharsis by creating conditions for externalizing pent-up emotions; Creativity by promoting self-expression through artistic media; Communication by expressing for others what one feels and how one perceives reality; Containment by providing legitimacy to attitudes and emotions difficult to acknowledge as part of oneself; Connections by enabling integration between different forces within oneself and outside oneself; and Changing the image by facilitating transformations in meanings.

Finally, there are many similarities in the manner in which art therapies are practiced. First, the approach is mostly multidisciplinary and consists in applying several art therapeutic media conjoinedly in the same session or in a sequence with the same child or group of children. It seems to be the rare case when art therapy is focused on one medium exclusively. This seems to be rooted in the orientation of art therapies towards the person as a whole, including his or her emotional, cognitive, physiological, emotional and behavioral needs (Kreitler and Kreitler 1978). The holistic orientation may generate the desire to apply to as many of the child's needs as possible. Second, the application of art therapeutic means is more often tailored to the specific needs and problems of the patient as conceptualized in the 'here and now' rather than adhering to a strict structured protocol. There seems to be a great sensitivity in art therapists to changing situations, needs, interests and problems of the patient. Hence the tendency to use a variety of art therapeutic means for attaining basically the same goals. Third, the art therapies use artistic means for attaining goals other than art, without pretending to teach the arts for their own sake or to turn the children into artists at present or in the future. Fourth, in many of the art therapies there is an interplay between the more passive and more active forms of application, for example, between viewing films and producing films, between reading stories and inventing stories, between listening to songs and singing. This interplay introduces an element of tension into the practice of art therapy but widens immensely the potentiality of the medium to appeal to the child and awaken his or her response. Fifth, the art therapies focus on the use of nonverbal means, which are appropriate for children and promote their expressiveness. And last but not least, art therapies seem to be open to incorporating new media and widening the scope of the applied therapies. At present we are witnessing the expansion of art therapy into the domains of computerized art and video art. In the near future we may witness the incorporation of virtual reality media, electronic music, or installation art. However, in art therapy the message is *not* the medium. Rather, the message underlying and inspiring the diverse present and future forms of art therapy is that even though the child is sick, he or she is still a child and we have to do all in our power to keep it that way.

ACKNOWLEDGEMENTS

The authors would like to thank all those who have contributed to this chapter: Tlalit Asna, Ofra Levanoni, AnaLia Magen and Michal M. Kreitler.

The first paragraph of the Introduction, 'A report from the department of paediatric oncology, Institut Gustave Roussy, Villejuif, France' (in section C) and section J 'Clown therapy' were written by Daniel Oppenheim. Thanks are due to Lorna Saint Ange who helped with the translation.

Section B 'Guided imagery combined with computerized art therapy' and 'Focus on producing' (in section I) were written by AnaLia Magen, art therapist in the unit of paediatric hematology/oncology in the Meyer Children's Hospital, Rambam Medical Center, Haifa, Israel.

Section D 'Bibliotherapy' was written by Tlalit Asna (teaches bibliotherapy at the Haifa University, Tel-Aviv University, Gordon College Haifa, and Lewinsky College Tel-Aviv).

'A study with Arab patients in Israel' (in section E) was written by Elsa Segev-Shoham, Herzel Gavriel and Yoseph Horowitz, Medical Center Haemek Afula.

'Dramatic play therapy in the hospital setting' (in section H) was written by Elsa Segev-Shoham with the cooperation of Dina Soberano, Jennifer Zellas, Dr Yoseph Horovitz and Dr Herzel Gavriel from the Pediatric Oncology Unit, Haemek Medical Center, Afula, Israel.

Section L 'Music therapy' was written by Ofra Levanoni, music therapist in the unit of paediatric hematology/oncology in the Meyer Children's Hospital, Rambam Medical Center, Haifa, Israel.

Section O 'Animal-assisted and pet-facilitated therapies' was written by Michal Gressel, a certified animal therapist.

The second and third paragraphs of the Introduction, section A, in section C Introduction and Varieties, in section E Introduction, section F, section G, in section H the part on Drama Therapy and Psychodrama up to Dramatic Play Therapy in the Hospital Setting, in section I Focus on Viewing, section K, section M, section N, section P and Concluding Remarks were written by Shulamith Kreitler.

REFERENCES

Aasgaard, T. (2001) An ecology of love: Aspects of music therapy in the pediatric oncology environment. *Journal of Palliative Care* **17**, 177–181.

Achtenberg, J., Lawlis, G.F. (1984) *Imagery and Disease*. Champaign, IL: Institute for Personality and Ability Testing.

Ancelin-Schuetzenberger, A. (1991) The drama of the seriously ill patient: Fifteen years' experience of psychodrama and cancer. In Holmes, P., Karp, M. (Eds), *Psychodrama: Inspiration and technique*. New York: Tavistock/Routledge, pp. 203–224.

Bailey, L. (1984) The use of songs in music therapy with cancer patients and their families. *Music Therapy* **4**, 5–17.

Barrera, M.E., Rykov, M.H., Doyle, S.L. (2000) The effects of interactive music therapy on hospitalized children with cancer: A pilot study. *Psycho-Oncology* **11**, 379–388.

Behar-Horenstein, L.S., Ganet-Sigel, J. (1999) *The Art and Practice of Dance/Movement Therapy.* Boston, MA: Pearson Custom Publishing.

Boldt, S. (1996) The effects of music therapy on motivation, psychological well-being, physical comfort and exercise endurance of bone marrow transplant patients. *Journal of Music Therapy* **33**, 164–188.

Bonny, H., Savary, L. (1973 (reprint 1990)) *Music and your Mind: Listening with a new Consciousness.* New York: Harper & Row.

Booth, R.J., Petrie, K.J., Pennebaker, J.W. (1997) Changes in circulating lymphocyte numbers following emotional disclosure: Evidence of buffering? *Stress Medicine* **13**, 23–29.

Borden, W. (1992) Narrative perspectives in psychosocial intervention following adverse life events. *Social Work* **37**, 135–141.

Brodsky, W. (1989) Music as an intervention for children with cancer in isolation rooms. *Music Therapy* **8**, 17–34.

Bruscia, K.E. (1991) *Case Studies in Music Therapy.* Barcelona, Spain: Barcelona Publishers.

Buckman, E.S. (1994) *Handbook of humor: Clinical applications in psychotherapy.* Melbourne, FL: Krieger.

Bunt, L. (1998) *Music Therapy: An art beyond words.* London: Routledge.

Carpenter, S. (1997) Therapeutic roles of animals. *Journal of the American Veterinary Medical Association* **211**, 154–155.

Chinner, T.L., Dalziel, F.R. (1991) An exploratory study on the viability and efficacy of pet-facilitated therapy project within a hospice. *Journal of Palliative Care* **7**, 13–20.

Clayton, G.M. (1993) *Living Pictures of the Self: Applications of role theory in professional practice and daily living.* Victoria, Australia: ICA Press.

Collie, K. (1998a) Computer support for distance art therapy. Paper presented at Human Factors in Computing '98. CHI98, Los Angeles, CA, USA, April 18–24.

Collie, K. (1998b) Internet art therapy. Paper presented at Discipline and Deviance: Genders, Technologies, Machines. Duke University, Durham, NC, USA, October 2–4.

Cooper, S.E., Blitz, J.T. (1985) A therapeutic play group for hospitalized children with cancer. *Journal of Psychosocial Oncology* **3**, 23–37.

Cotanch, P., Hockenberry, M., Herman, S. (1985) Self-hypnosis, antiemetic therapy in children receiving chemotherapy. *Oncological Nursing Forum* **12**, 41–46.

Cothern, N. (1994) Healing with books: Literature for children dealing with health issues. *Ohio Reading Teacher* **28**, 8–15.

Cotton, M.A. (1985) Creative art expression from a leukemic child. *Art Therapy* **2**, 55–65.

Darrach, J. (1990) Send in the clowns – Clown Care Unit. *Life Magazine* August, 76–85.

Dileo, C. (1999) Songs for living: The use of songs in the treatment of oncology patients. In Dileo, C. (Ed.) *Music Therapy and Medicine: Theoretical and clinical applications.* Silver Spring, MD: AMTA, pp. 151–166.

Dowling, J.S. (2001) Sense of humor, childhood cancer stressors, and outcomes of psychosocial adjustment, immune function, and infection. *Dissertation Abstracts International, Section B: The Sciences and Engineering* **61**(7-B), 3506.

DuHamel, K.N., Johnson Vickberg, S.M., Redd, W.H. (1998) Behavioral interventions in pediatric oncology. In Holland, J.C. (Ed.) *Psycho-oncology.* New York: Oxford University Press, pp 962–977.

Dunne, P.B. (1992) *The Narrative Therapist and the Arts: Expanding possibilities through drama, movements, puppets, masks and drawings.* Los Angeles, CA: Drama Therapy Institute of Los Angeles.

Esterling, B.A., LaAbate, L., Murray, E., Pennebaker, J.W. (1999) Empirical foundations for writing in prevention and psychotherapy: Mental and physical health outcome. *Clinical Psychology Review* **19**, 79–96.

Fagan, T.S. (1982) Music therapy in the treatment of anxiety and fear in terminal pediatric patients. *Music Therapy* **2**, 1.

French, G.M., Painter, E.C., Coury, D.L. (1994) Blowing away shot pain: A technique for pain management during immunization. *Pediatrics* **93**, 384–388.

Gardner, A.R. (1986) *Therapeutic Communication with Children: The mutual storytelling technique.* Northvale, NC: Jason Aronson.

Garrison, W.T., McQuiston, S. (1989) *Chronic Illness during Childhood and Adolescence: Psychological aspects.* Newbury Park, CA: Sage.

Genuis, M.L. (1995) The use of hypnosis in helping cancer patients control anxiety, pain and emesis: A review of recent empirical studies. *American Journal of Clinical Hypnosis,* **37**, 316–325.

Géricot, C., Perrignon, J. (2000) *La Porte Bleue: Autoportraits d'enfants atteints de Cancer.* Paris: Institut Gustave Roussy/Les Arènes.

Goodman, R.F. (1999) Childhood cancer and the family: Case of Tim, age 6, and follow-up at age 15. In Webb, N.B. (Ed.) *Play Therapy with Children in Crisis: Individual, group, and family treatment* (2nd edn). New York: Guilford Press, pp. 380–404.

Halprin, A. (2000) *Dance as a Healing Art: Returning to health through movement and imagery.* Mendocino, CA: LifeRhythm.

Hilgard, J.R., LeBaron, S. (1982) Relief of anxiety and pain in children and adolescents with cancer: Quantitative measures and clinical observation. *International Journal of Clinical and Experimental Hypnosis* **4**, 417–442.

Hilgard, J.R., LeBaron, S. (1984) *Hypnotherapy of Pain in Children with Cancer.* Los Altos, CA: William Kaufmann.

Hockenberry, M.H. (1989) Guided imagery as a coping measure for children with cancer. *Journal of the Association of Pediatric Oncology Nurses* **6**, 29.

Hockenberry, M.J., Bologna-Voughan, S. (1985) Preparation for intrusive procedures using noninvasive techniques in children with cancer: State of the art vs new trends. *Cancer Nursing* **8**, 97–102.

Hockenberry-Eaton, M., Barrera, P., Brown M., Bottomley, S.J., O'Neill, J.B. (1999). Pain management in children with cancer. Texas Cancer Council, www.childcancerpain.org

Jay, S.M., Elliott, C.H., Woody, P.D., Siegel, S. (1991) An investigation of cognitive-behavior therapy combined with oral valium for children undergoing painful medical procedures. *Health Psychology* **10**, 317–322.

Jones, V.M. (1997) Mask making as art therapy with pediatric oncology patients. *Dissertation Abstracts International: Section B: The Sciences and Engineering* **57**(8-B), 5330.

Kale, M. (1992) Kids and animals: A comforting hospital combination. *Interactions* **10**, 17–21.

Katz, E.R., Kellerman, J., Ellenberg, L. (1987) Hypnosis in the reduction of acute pain and distress in children with cancer. *Journal of Pediatric Psychology* **12**, 379–394.

Kolko, D.J., Rickard-Figueroa, J.L. (1985) Effects of video games on the adverse corollaries of chemotherapy in pediatric oncology patients: a single-case analysis. *Journal of Consulting and Clinical Psychology* **53**, 223–228.

Kreitler, S., Drechsler, I., Kreitler, H. (1988) How to kill jokes cognitively? The meaning structure of jokes. *Semiotica* **68**, 297–319.

Kreitler, H., Kreitler, S. (1970) Dependence of laughter on cognitive strategies. *Merrill-Palmer Quarterly of Behavior and Development* **16**, 163–177.

Kreitler, H., Kreitler, S. (1972) *Psychology of the Arts*. Durham, NC: Duke University Press.

Kreitler, H., Kreitler, S. (1978) Art therapy: Quo vadis? *Art Psychotherapy* **5**, 199–209.

Kunzendorf, R.G. (Ed.) (1991) *Mental Imagery*. New York: Plenum Publishing.

Kuttner, L. (1996) *A Child in Pain: How to help, what to do*. Point Roberts, WA: Hartley & Marks.

Kuttner, L., Bowman, M., Teasdale, M. (1988) Psychological treatment of distress, pain and anxiety for young children with cancer. *Journal of Developmental Behavior Pediatrics* **9**, 374–382.

Lahad, M. (1992) *All Life Stretches before You*. Haifa, Israel: Nord (in Hebrew).

Lane, D. (1996) Music therapy interventions with pediatric oncology patient. In M.A. Froehlich (Ed.) *Music Therapy with Hospitalized Children, Creative Arts Child Life Approach*. Cherry Hill, NJ: Jeffrey Books.

LaRue, E., Zigler, E. (1986) Psychological adjustment of seriously ill children. *Journal of the American Academy of Child Psychiatry* **25**, 708–712.

LeBaron, S., Zeltzer, L.K. (1984) Behavioral intervention for reducing chemotherapy-related nausea and vomiting in adolescents with cancer. *Journal of Adolescent Health Care* **5**, 178–182.

Leedy, J.J. (Ed.) (1985) *Poetry a Healer: Mending the troubled mind*. New York: Vanguard Press.

Lefcourt, R.M. (2001) *Humor: The psychology of living buoyantly*. New York: Kluwer Academic/Plenum Publishers.

Lerner, A. (Ed.) (1994) *Poetry in the Therapeutic Experience* (2nd edn). St. Louis: MMB Music.

Levy, F.J. Fried, J.P., Leventhal, F. (Eds) (1995) *Dance and Other Expressive Art Therapies: When words are not enough*. London: Routledge

Lingnell, L., Dunn, L. (1999) Group play: Wholeness and healing for the hospitalized child. In Sweeney, D.S., Horneyer, L.E. (Eds) *The Handbook of Group Play Therapy: How to do it, how it works, whom it's best for*. San Francisco, CA: Jossey-Bass/Pfeiffer, pp. 359–374.

Logis, M., Turry, A. (1999) Singing my way through it: Facing the cancer pain and fear. In Hibben, J. (Ed.) *Inside Music Therapy: Client experiences*. Phoenixville, PA: Barcelona, pp. 97–117.

Luzzatto, P., Gabriel, B. (1998) Art psychotherapy. In Holland, J.C. (Ed.) *Psycho-oncology*. New York: Oxford University Press, pp. 743–757.

Magen, A., Ben Arush, M. (1999) Computerized art therapy and guided imagery for pediatric oncology and hematology. *Medical and Pediatric Oncology* **23**, 151.

Mair, M. (1989) Kelly, Bannister and a story-telling psychology. *International Journal of Personal Construct Therapy* **2**, 1–14.

Malchiodi, C.A. (2000) *Art Therapy and Computer Technology: A virtual studio of possibilities*. London: Jessica Kingsley.

Malone, A. (1996) The effects of live music on the distress of pediatric patients receiving intravenous starts, venipunctures, injections, and heel sticks. *Journal of Music Therapy* **23**, 19–33.

Manheimer, L. (2000) Harry: A 10-year-old's last summer. In Oremland, E.K., Oremland, J.D. (Eds) *Protecting the Emotional Development of the Ill Child: The essence of the child life profession*. Madison, CT: Psychosocial Press, pp. 59–71.

Manne, S., Bakeman, R., Jacobsen, P., *et al.* (1994) An analysis of an intervention to reduce children's distress during venipuncture. *Health Psychology* **13**, 556–566.

Martin, R.A. (2001) Humor, laughter and physical health: Methodological issues and research findings. *Psychological Bulletin* **127**, 504–519.

McCall, J. (2000) Dana: A 7-year-old girl with leukemia. In Oremland, E.K., Oremland, J.D. (Eds) *Protecting the Emotional Development of the Ill Child: The essence of the child life profession*. Madison, CT: Psychosocial Press, pp. 73–84.

McGrath, P.A., de Veber, L.L. (1986) The management of acute pain evoked by medical procedures in children with cancer. *Journal of Pain and Symptom Management* **1**, 145–150.

Moreno, J.L. (1994) *Psychodrama*, Vols 1–3 (4th edn) McLean, VA: ASGPP.

Muschel, I.J. (1984) Pet therapy with terminal cancer patients. *Social Casework* **65**, 451–458.

Newham, P. (1999) *Using Voice and Movement in Therapy: The practical application of voice movement therapy*. London: Jessica Kingsley.

Noonan, W. (1992) Healing tales: The metaphors of folktales help cancer patients in their therapy. *Creation Spirituality* **4**, 28–30.

O'Callaghan, C. (1996) Pain, music creativity and music therapy in palliative care. *The American Journal of Hospice and Palliative Care* **13**, 43–49.

O'Connor, K.J., Schaeffer, C.E. (1994) *Handbook of Play Therapy*, Vol. 2: *Advances and innovations*. San Francisco, CA: Jossey-Bass.

Olness, K. (1981) Imagery (self-hypnosis) as adjunct therapy in childhood cancer: clinical experience with 25 patients. *American Journal of Pediatric Hematology/ Oncology* **3**, 313–321.

Oppenheim, D., Simonds, C., Hartmann, O. (1997) Clowning on children's wards. *Lancet* **350**, 1838–1840.

Pennebaker, J.W., Kiecolt-Glaser, J., Glaser, R. (1988) Disclosure of traumas and immune function: Health implications for psychotherapy. *Journal of Consulting and Clinical Psychology* **56**, 239–245.

Pfaff, V., Smith, K.E., Gowan, D. (1989) The effects of music assisted relaxation on the distress of pediatric cancer patients undergoing bone marrow aspirations. *Children's Health Care* **18**, 232–236.

Piaget, J. (1959) *The Language and Thought of the Child* (Trans. Marjorie and Ruth Gabain). New York: Humanities Press.

Prager, A. (1995) Pediatric art therapy; strategies and applications. *Art Therapy* **12**, 32–38.

Raveis, V.H., Mesagno, F., Karus, D., Gorey, E. (1993) Pet ownership as a protective factor supporting the emotional well-being of cancer patients and their family members. Memorial Sloan–Kettering Cancer Center, Department of Social Work Research Unit (mimeograph).

Redd, W.H., Jacobsen, P.B., Die-Trill, M., Dermatis, H., McEvoy, M., Holland, J. (1987) Cognitive-attentional distraction in the control of conditioned nausea in pediatric cancer patients receiving chemotherapy. *Journal of Consulting and Clinical Psychology* **55**, 391–395.

Remen, R.N. (1996) *Kitchen Table Wisdom: Stories that heal*. New York: Putnam.

Robb, S.L. (2000) The effect of therapeutic music interventions on the behavior of hospitalized children in isolation: Developing a contextual support model of music therapy. *Journal of Music Therapy* **37**, 118–146.

Rudloff, L. (1985) Michael: An illustrated study of a young man with cancer. *American Journal of Art Therapy* **24**, 49–62.

Schneider, J., Smith, C. S., Whitcher, S. (1983) The relationship of mental imagery to white blood cell (neutrophil) function: Experimental studies of normal subjects. Memo. Michigan State University, East Lansing, MI.

Slavin, P. (1996) A sense for who needs them. *Hospice* **7**, 21–26.

Sourkes, B. M. (1991) Truth to life: Art therapy with pediatric oncology patients and their siblings. *Journal of Psychosocial Oncology* **9**, 81–96.

Tacata, J. (2000) Brief encounters. In E.K. Oremland, J.D. Oremland (Eds) *Protecting the Emotional Development of the Ill Child: The essence of the child life profession.* Madison, CT: Psychosocial Press, pp. 85–91.

The Hamptons Comedy Festival (2002) http://hamptonscomedyfestival.com/2002.

Turry, A., Turry, A.E. (1999) Creative song improvisations with children and adults with cancer. In Dileo, C. (Ed.) *Music Therapy and Medicine: Theoretical and clinical applications.* Silver Spring, MD: AMTA, pp. 85–91.

Vaillant, G.E. (2001) Adaptive mental mechanisms: Their role in a positive psychology. *American Psychologist* **55**, 89–98.

Walker, C. (1989) Use of art and play therapy in pediatric oncology. *Journal of Pediatric Oncology Nursing* **6**, 121–126.

Wall, V.J., Womack, W. (1989) Hypnotic versus active cognitive strategies for alleviation of procedural distress in pediatric oncology patients. *American Journal of Clinical Hypnosis* **31**, 181–190.

Willis, D.A. (1997) Animal therapy. *Rehabilitation Nursing* **2**, 78–81.

Zeltzer, L., LeBaron, S. (1982) Hypnosis and nonhypnotic techniques for reduction of pain and anxiety during painful procedures in children and adolescents with cancer. *Journal of Pediatrics* **101**, 1032–1035.

16

Psychological Intervention with the Dying Child

SHULAMITH KREITLER

*Psychooncology Unit, Tel-Aviv Medical Center
and Department of Psychology, Tel-Aviv University, Israel*

ELENA KRIVOY

*Pediatric Hematology Oncology Department, Meyer Children's Hospital, Rambam
Medical Center, Faculty of Medicine, Technion, Haifa, Israel*

PSYCHOLOGICAL INTERVENTION AS A COMPONENT OF PALLIATIVE CARE

Psychological intervention with the dying child has not yet become a standard element in the treatment of the child with cancer. But there is little doubt that there is a great need for it. In our view, psychological intervention is to be considered as a major means of palliative care with sick child facing the terminal stage of cancer. Notably, discussions of quality of care at the end of life include references to psychological state, for example, the patient's emotional symptoms, autonomy, and satisfaction (Morrison and Siu 2000). As will be seen, there are unique features characterizing the population of patients, the issues, the means, the restrictions and the setup of this kind of psychological intervention. Therefore we suggest calling it *Pediatric Psychological Palliative Care* to distinguish it from psychological intervention practiced in other stages of pediatric oncology.

The concept of Pediatric Psychological Palliative Care (PPPC) has several implications. A major implication concerns the goals. PPPC is not designed to

Psychosocial Aspects of Pediatric Oncology. Edited by S. Kreitler and M. Weyl Ben Arush
© 2004 John Wiley & Sons Ltd: ISBN 0 471 49939 0

cure any psychological ailment or disorder but to improve the child's state, overall or any particular aspect, and sometimes prevent, moderate or delay any adverse effects of physical or psychological state. The palliative aspect indicates that we should regard the child's welfare in a holistic manner, be attentive to multiple domains and help wherever we can, but stay within the boundaries of palliative care, that is to say, let ourselves be guided primarily by concerns of the here-and-now rather than promoting the emergence or resolution of problems that have significance mainly for the future.

A major characteristic of PPPC is that it enables and encourages the child to express himself or herself in whatever form he or she prefer (without harming themselves or others) by creating a safe atmosphere and offering an empathic and maximally permissive listening. No prescriptions, criticism or instructions accompany the listening. The psychologist is equally receptive to an adolescent who spends the sessions discussing Buber's I–Thou conception, another who may prefer to sit silently, and still another who may fill up pages with colored lines.

As a component of palliative care, PPPC is primarily a client-centered *responsive* kind of intervention. This indicates that it is initiated and functions mainly in response to the needs and possibilities of the child at a given time and place and adapts its tools in line with these needs and possibilities, rather than in accordance with some preconceived scheme or theory about the needs of a dying child. For example, it is not advisable to approach the dying child with the preconception that a dying individual should resolve previously unresolved issues ('close up circles', so to say). Some children may express the wish or need to do so, whereas others may shy away from it or not be at all aware of such issues. Whereas there may be a justification for promoting the resolution of unresolved issues within the framework of some psychotherapeutic conceptions, within the framework of palliative care it is justified only if the patient herself or himself is aware of the need to do so.

In line with the general approach of palliative care which deals primarily with symptoms, PPPC is also focused on specific issues, in an attempt to resolve particular problems or conflicts so as to reduce distress as much as possible. For example, when a patient is anxious or depressed, PPPC is geared to identify the particular source of the anxiety or depression in the here-and-now and resolve it, without necessarily attempting to provide the patient with tools to deal with anxiety and depression in general and without expecting that the problem that has caused the anxiety or depression will not recur.

As noted, PPPC advocates the adaptation of tools to the needs and possibilities of the child. A whole variety of tools stands at the disposal of the PPPC practitioner. Rather than starting, for example, with the common assumption that play or drawing are the major vehicles of communication with children in therapy, PPPC advocates the use of whatever tool is adequate at a given time for a particular child handling a specific issue. In the framework of

PPPC it is legitimate to use drawing at the beginning of a therapeutic session with the child, then switch over to verbal discussion, and finish with dance-like movements enacted by both therapist and child.

Similarly, in regard to other rules and routines concerning therapy. It is usual in psychological interventions to set fixed times and even locations for the therapy. PPPC does not necessarily abide by these conventions. It does not make sense to strictly limit the psychological intervention sessions to the routine of a fixed number of times per week or to conduct the therapy only in the therapist's room. Rather, if necessary, PPPC may take place twice a day on some days and at the child's bedside when the child so prefers or is unable to move.

The same goes for the convention of treating the child alone, without the presence of others. This convention too may be set aside in favor of treating the child with other close persons (e.g., a parent, a sibling), if the child expresses the need or the wish to do so.

Further, PPPC considers the child within the framework of the whole family system, including whoever is actively involved in or affected by the child's disease, namely, the parents in the first place, but also grandparents and siblings and in exceptional cases also other relatives. Their involvement may range all the way from active participants to observers.

In general, palliative care is mostly based on team work. Hence, PPPC should be viewed as part of the total palliative care of the patient, and its practice is to be coordinated with the other palliative care measures administered to the sick child. Beyond coordination, PPPC requires coopera-tion with the rest of the palliative team. Implementing the cooperation may vary with the specific patient. Sometimes it entails mainly getting information from the other team members and providing them information about the patient's psychological state; in the case of other patients it may entail mobilizing the whole team for the attainment of a goal that has come up in the framework of the PPPC, such as making up with a sibling, or fulfilling the child's wish for a leave-taking party; in still other cases it may imply providing the child opportunities to raise the bothering issues with any member of the team preferred by the child.

Finally, since PPPC is designed for children in advanced disease stages, it is to be initiated only when the child enters the terminal phase. However, the child and the parents may be dismayed and scared if they are suddenly exposed to PPPC. Therefore, it may be advisable to let the child and family meet the person or team of PPPC earlier, in an informal manner, maybe as part of getting acquainted with the ward and hospital services. If the child and family have at least had a chance of meeting the person or team of the PPPC before it is launched as a full-fledged intervention, they may be better able to respond to it and benefit from it without being threatened or embarrassed.

DEATH AWARENESS

A lot of what would go on in the framework of PPPC depends on the child's awareness of death and dying. This issue has been studied from two major perspectives: the cognitive one, focusing on children's conceptions of death in general, and the experiential one, focusing on children's construction of their state. The two perspectives complement each other. We will deal with both in turn.

Children's Conceptions of Death

The construction of death is a theme of paramount importance in life and may start at a very early age. The major approaches to studying the development of death conceptions in children either adopt the 'comprehensive stages' approach or follow the developmental sequence of specific themes that make up the conception of death.

The 'comprehensive stages' approach is based on the assumption that the child's conception of death is some kind of an integrated conceptualization that depends primarily on the child's cognitive abilities and changes in an orderly sequence. Though the rate at which one moves from one stage to another may differ across children, the sequence stays consistent. The developmental sequence has been described as following closely the Piagetian model. The empirical data has been collected in different countries and by means of different research tools (e.g., Anthony 1972, Gartley and Bernasconi 1967, Koocher 1973, Nagy 1948, Schilder and Wechsler 1934, Wass, Guenther and Towry 1979). In the sensorimotor stage of infancy (0–2 years), dominated by sensory and motor actions, babies below 6 months of age have no understanding of death because it requires a grasp of the constancy and identity of objects which are still missing. Hence, they react to death only as the absence of familiar persons (i.e., separation, loss), demonstrated sometimes by stranger anxiety. Toddlers identify objects but are limited by their inability to assume a frame of reference other than their own, which is being alive. In the pre-operational stage (2–7) of early childhood, marked by magical thinking and egocentricity, there is no real understanding of the universality and irreversibility of death. Death is conceived as a state similar to sleep, characterized by the activities of the living, e.g., eating, going fishing. At the stage of concrete operations (7–11/12) of middle childhood, marked by concrete naturalistic thinking, children will personify death, often in evil images (e.g., devil, bogeyman) and will tend to regard death as punishment for evil deeds. By the age of 9 or 10 years, most children have an adult conception of death as universal and irreversible, further influenced by the religious conceptions of their culture. In the stage of formal operations (over 12 years), marked by propositional and deductive thinking, the adolescents have a good understanding of death. Hence, the possibility of non-being poses for them a great anxiety-provoking threat, which religious beliefs may mitigate to some extent.

The above presentation of stages, which the conception of death is assumed to undergo until it reaches maturity, is highly common. It has generated the conclusion that, up to the age of 10, terminally ill children are not concerned with their possible death and has served as basis for the recommendation not to discuss this theme with them (Rando 1984, Spinetta 1974). Needless to mention, both the conclusion and the recommendation have been proven wrong. One major fault of this approach is that it is concerned mainly if not exclusively with verbal expression of concepts by the children and hence captures only partial, possibly distorted aspects of the phenomenon. Moreover, it expects consistency across children where there may be none. It is, however, important insofar as it reveals the situation when one focuses on verbal expression which may be the preferred mode of communication by specific psychotherapists or children.

The 'specific themes' approach starts with identifying particular aspects of the death conception and follows their development separately. It developed mostly after the stage approach. The major most frequently examined aspects are non-functionality (i.e., death ends all life-sustaining functions), irreversibility, universality, causality (i.e., what causes death) and personal mortality. Kenyon's (2001) excellent review shows that each of the five themes develops differently and separately. For example, conceptualizing causality changes in the sense that the causes to which death is attributed shift from non-natural causes (e.g., violence, accident) in 5–6 year-olds to natural causes (e.g., illness) in 8-year-olds, to spiritual causes (e.g., invocation by God) in 11-year-olds (Reilly, Hasazi and Bond 1983). Awareness of personal mortality follows more closely the binary developmental track: from denial in 3–4-year-olds to confirmation in 8- and 11-year-olds (Atwood 1984). This suggests that there are no stages defined by a bundle of features but different developmental trajectories following individual tracks. Further, each of the themes of the death concept is affected differently by major factors, such as age, gender, cognitive ability, and culture.

Most important in our context is the effect of experience on the development of death concepts. Studies of children from 5 to 12 years showed that having lost a loved one through death was related to less accurate death scores (especially in regard to causality and universality) (Cotton and Range 1990), or was not correlated with death concept scores at all (Jenkins and Cavanaugh 1985–6, Mahon 1993, McIntire, Angle and Struempler 1972). However, being oneself sick with a life-threatening disease does affect death concepts. Jay *et al.* (1987) found that children with cancer differed from matched healthy children in their concepts about personal mortality and death-as-justice. Pediatric oncology patients did not necessarily have more advanced death concepts but different ones. They more often acknowledged personal mortality and less often viewed death as a punishment. Moreover, within the oncology group, those who had experienced the death of a close friend or relative had a deeper understanding of personal mortality, universality and irreversibility of death, irrespective of age. Also Clunies-Ross and Lansdown (1988) found that leukemic children (4–9 years old) did not differ from healthy children in their overall death scores, but had better understanding of the irreversibility and non-functionality of death. It is of interest to note that independently of disease, anxiety was found to lower scores of understanding different death aspects, notably universality, irreversibility and non-functionality (Orbach *et al.* 1986) as well as personal mortality (Candy-Gibbs, Sharp and Petrun 1984–5). These findings suggest that personal experience with death in the form of a life-threatening disease like cancer may override the effects of death anxiety observed in healthy children, that may cause distortions or denial.

It is advisable for any health professional planning psychological intervention with dying children to be aware of the research findings about children's conceptions of death. But he or she should be aware no less of the fact that these findings are to be complemented by findings about the awareness of death in dying children.

Children's Awareness of Dying

Different authors who have had therapeutic or research experience with dying children have reached the conclusion that dying children are aware of their state. Kübler-Ross, a pioneer in this domain, writes that 'small children, even three- and four-year-olds, can talk about their dying and are aware of their impending death' (Kübler-Ross 1981, p. 51). The issue was studied from the early 1950s, relying first on clinical observations and semi-structured interviews with children and their parents (Cobbs 1956, Richmond and Weisman 1955, Solnit and Green 1959), then on the accounts of parents and hospital staff (Morrissey 1963, Natterson and Knudson 1960) and later on examining directly the terminally ill children, for example, by means of projective techniques (Waechter 1971, 1987). All studies showed unequivocally that children were aware of the seriousness of their condition and their impending death.

Some children actually express their awareness in words (e.g., J., a 4-year-old, said one week prior to his death of leukemia: 'Mommy, I don't want you to cry when I die, I want to see your smile'), but others do it in a symbolic form, using images, drawings, toys and other objects. Thus, G., an 8-year-old with retinoblastoma, had an imaginary rabbit whom she treated for weeks until one day she declared that it was going to die on Wednesday 'because when rabbits get that sick they cannot live much longer'. On Friday of that same week she died. Kübler-Ross (1983) cites many examples of stories, poems and dreams of dying children who clearly express their awareness of their own impending death (see also Jampolsky and Taylor 1978). Similar conclusions are supported by the drawings of dying children (Bach 1975, Bertoia and Allen 1988, Furth 1988). The anthropologist Bluebond-Langner (1978) also found that terminally ill children understand their prognosis and know that they will die, even if no one tells them, but in conformity with the social rules of 'mutual pretense' which they somehow surmise, they often conceal this knowledge from their own parents and the medical staff. Kübler-Ross (1983) believes that all terminally ill children are aware that they are dying but only those whose awareness is conscious and intellectual express it verbally whereas those whose awareness is preconscious express it symbolically. In contrast, we believe that form of expression has more to do with form of experience and habitual forms of expression by the child than with level of awareness (Kreitler 1965).

One of the most widely known descriptions of the development of awareness of death in sick children has been offered by Bluebond-Langner (1978). Stage 1, defined as 'seriously ill', reflects the children's experiences of admission to the hospital for diagnostic tests, the ensuing medical treatments and the changed caring attitude assumed toward them by the adults. Most of their fears at this stage are of the unknown rather than of the prognosis. The children pass into stage 2 defined as 'seriously ill and will get better' after they have experienced a remission and a few rapid recoveries of disease-related symptoms, such as nosebleeds. After having got drugs which make them feel better and noticing that most people treat them in a normal way again, they conclude that eventually they will get better. Stage 3, defined as 'always ill and will get better', sets in after they have been through the relapse–remission cycle and have noticed the uneasy avoidance response of the adults around them. The fears focus on recurrence but there is still the belief that despite it one can still recover. Stage 4, defined as 'always ill and will never get better', sets in after more relapses, pain and drug complications. At this stage the children become aware that they are getting weaker, that they can plan only for very short terms and they start grieving about all those things of the future that they will most probably not do. They get used to the sickness staying always with them. Children move to stage 5, defined as 'dying', following an event such as the death of another child on the ward. The similarity in disease and treatments between themselves and the dead child may spur the sick children to integrate all their knowledge about the disease and treatments and get to the startling disastrous conclusion that they themselves are dying. The pace at which they reach this conclusion varies from one child to another, but eventually they all get to that awareness. It is then that they begin expressing their awareness of impending death verbally and symbolically. The awareness may be accompanied by decreased communication with adults, from whom the dying children tend to hide their new awareness, and by lowered cooperation with different medical procedures that have not helped in the past. Slowly their world starts narrowing down in terms of themes, activities and interests: they play less, they move around less, and they are concerned more with death. Gradually death comes to permeate their minds and thinking.

The detailed description provided by Bluebond-Langner demonstrates that the awareness of one's death is a slowly developing process, fed, on the one hand, by the child's personal experiences of disease and treatments, and, on the other hand, by information obtained from the adults, mostly indirectly through eavesdropping and observing their behaviors toward oneself or among themselves (e.g., special caring, crying surreptitiously).

In parallel to the gradually growing awareness of one's death, there occurs another process – gradual dying in a psychological sense. As noted, the children lose interest in many things, give up plans for the future, do not look forward to holidays, refer to the shortness of time they have, prepare less for the future ('you don't have to work hard for becoming a ghost' said a 5-year-old two weeks prior to his death).

Reconciling the Findings on Death Concepts and Awareness of One's Death

We are confronted here with two traditions of research. Though one can identify a variety of themes on which they agree, it is no less evident that there are large gaps between them. One source for the disparity may be traced back to methodological issues, mainly the research tools used predominantly in each of these research traditions (i.e., verbal expression and questionnaires versus drawings, stories, semi-structured interviews and observations). Lonetto (1980, p. 176) has aptly summarized the situation as follows: 'The evidence suggests, then, that relying solely on the terminally ill child's overt expressions of anxiety yields incomplete or misleading information'. However, there may be more to it. The disparities may arise out of the basic difference there may be between talking or thinking about death in general or the death of others and confronting the issue of one's own death. Kastenbaum (1992, p. 88) analyzed in detail what goes into the apparently simple proposition 'I will die'. It presupposes, for example, awareness of being a person with a life of one's own, of belonging to a class of beings one of whose attributes is mortality, of awaiting the certain occurrence of death at an uncertain timing, accepting the finality of the event of death as the ultimate separation of oneself from the world and from existing as a human being at least on this earth. In particular, it requires bridging the gap between what one has actually experienced of life and a hypothetical construct of life's negation, when we have absolutely nothing on which to build. To this, one should add the emotional component of sadness about not being any more, which compounds the situation further. What all this amounts to is that when one deals with providing PPPC to a dying child, one is well advised to use all available channels of communication – verbal and nonverbal – keeping in mind what children may be expected to know or understand of death, without losing sight of the important distinction between death in general and one's own death.

CONCERNS OF THE DYING CHILD AND HOW TO DEAL WITH THEM PSYCHOLOGICALLY

In this section we will deal with different issues and problems that often come up in the treatment of children in the terminal phase and what to do about them in the framework of PPPC. However, it is necessary to emphasize that these issues do not always come up, nor are they the only ones. The basic principle of PPPC is to be attentive to the child's needs without enforcing the discussion of any theme according to a preordained scheme.

Fear of Abandonment and Separation

The dying child may have fears. Some of the more characteristic fears are fears of abandonment, of being left alone, or simply of loneliness. Some sick children or adolescents are even scared of falling asleep for fear that precisely then they will be left alone. The physical presence of others, especially family members, provides them with reassurance that nothing evil will happen to them. Some children may even need recurrent physical contact in order to feel reassured. In some cases this fear is manifested as fear of the dark, because in the darkness one is less certain of the presence of others. In other cases the fear of abandonment or of loneliness is explicitly expressed as fear of being separated from one's family. For example, Rachel, a 7-year-old leukemic girl, is quoted as saying: 'I am so worried because . . . I think I may die and I don't want to leave my family . . . Promise me that if I die before you and Daddy that you and Daddy will be buried beside me' (Bertoia 1993, p. 30).

This fear, or rather family of fears, may be an expression of the child's fear of separation, of leaving its family and friends, of being lost (as noted, for example, by Rochlin (1967, p. 58)). Hence, it is possible that this fear expresses fear of death. Indeed, fear of annihilation, fear of separation, and fear of vanishing are identified components of death anxiety (e.g., Lifton 1979, Stern 1968). However, it could also express the child's sense of helplessness and weakness as compared with the tasks of confronting forces partly known to be strong and evil (e.g., pain) and partly not yet experienced. It is only natural for the child to feel the need of support, reinforcement through the presence of others who may be a great help when things get tough. Some children deal with the fear of loneliness and separation by invoking the presence of imaginary figures, as for example, Rachel (Bertoia 1993, p. 30) who could feel the presence of her guardian angel, but only when she was alone. PPPC would not try to allay the fears or tell the child 'there is nothing to fear'; on the contrary, it would encourage the child to ask for the presence of others and encourage others to stay with the child. Indeed, it would even praise the child for asking for help and for preparing in this way to face the hardships in store.

The described complex of fears seems to be related to anticipatory reactions to impending separation from mother, family, or friends that have been widely documented in children, for example, in the course of a mother's temporary hospitalization or before being transferred to a new school (Field 1985). The response to separation is typically biphasic, including a first phase of agitation with increased behavioral and physiological activation, followed by a second phase of depression, apathy and withdrawal. The manifestations may be observed in play behavior, activity level, sleep and eating patterns, heart rate, body temperature and immune functions (Reite, Harbeck and Hoffman 1981). Similar reactions were noted in preschool children sick with cancer who were treated with chemotherapy (Hollenbeck *et al.* 1980). The inborn source of these reactions is suggested by their occurrence in primates (Reite *et al.* 1978). Of particular interest in this context is the observation that the two phases of anticipatory separation reaction resemble active and passive coping, respectively (Schneiderman and McCabe 1985). The phase of agitation reflects the child's attempts to master the situation and minimize the evil, whereas the phase of depression expresses despair or giving up in view one's helplessness. Notably, this double-pronged interpretation parallels the two aspects of separation fear emphasized by us.

Fears of Leaving the Familiar and of Confronting the Unfamiliar

Fear of leaving the familiar was already mentioned above, as part of the fear of separation. Yet, this pair of fears seems to us sufficiently important to deserve a separate section. Leaving the familiar means not only leaving parents, siblings, family at large and friends. It may mean in addition leaving one's clothes, familiar objects, one's bed and desk, one's home, in short all those things one has learned over the years to love, to use, to call 'my own'. Indeed, it may mean leaving behind, being disconnected from everything on which one's sense of pride, security and even identity had been based. Confronting the unfamiliar represents a different complex. It may indicate being in a strange, bizarre environment, completely different from anything one has known before, possibly experiencing things one has never experienced before and of which no one has ever told you, acting in a setting of which one knows nothing and for which no one has ever prepared the child in any way. Whereas leaving the familiar may evoke in the child fear, anger and sorrow, confronting the unfamiliar may evoke plain terror, regardless of how self-confident the child may be. Children deal with these in different ways. Studying examples of children's coping may help the PPPC practitioner devise means of helping other children.

Here are some examples concerning leaving the familiar. Naama, a 6-year-old, dying of a brain tumor, organized a set of rituals for taking leave of her things, each in turn, for example, kissing it, whispering to it, touching it. Joseph, a 9-year-old with leukemia, started to wrap up his beloved things as presents, and stuck on each a note indicating to whom he wanted the object to be given. He had to stop because this procedure evoked great anxiety in his mother. She blamed him for 'robbing' her of his things, which she wanted to keep. In the framework of PPPC the mother was led to understand that Joseph wanted to make sure his things would not grieve for him but be happily used by other children. Older children may assume the attitude of 'I have outgrown these things, like an old pair of pants; they are of no use to me any more'.

The examples concerning confronting the unfamiliar are different. Moshe, a 12-year-old, with Ewing's sarcoma, 'populated' the hereafter with many different individuals whom he expected to help him. He started out with saying that he knew his grandfather, who had recently died, would wait for him. A few days later he wondered about whether his grandpa would look in the hereafter for his pals who had previously died. Then he said he thought this is the thing his grandpa would do 'and this is a good thing 'cause they would all be like my friends'. Gila, a 15-year-old with leukemia dealt with the question of whether one kept one's body after death. She hoped not because this meant all children would have to start from scratch, no one would have an advantage due to previously acquired skills. Some children try to construct an imaginary world based on movies they have seen and stories they had read. Preparing for the unknown may be one reason why children in this state were reported to be eager to read books about death (Bluebond-Langner 1978, p. 186; Ross 1967, Wass 1984).

Fear of Punishment

Another class of fears focuses on being punished. Sometimes children talk of being attacked, hit, molested, beaten or incarcerated by other people or forces, familiar or unfamiliar, which may appear to the children in the form of monsters, 'bad people', witches, ghosts, skeletons or other symbolic figures. Personifications of death which assume these forms were found to be common in children in the middle years of childhood, 6–8 years (Lonetto and Templer 1986, pp. 61–62). This fear may reflect the child's fear of the unknown that lies ahead. It may also arise out of the child's feeling that there may be tasks to handle in the future which it may not be able to master. PPPC would lead us to strengthen the child by reminding him or her of all the tasks in the past which they were afraid they could not handle but eventually handled successfully. Memories of past successful coping are designed to lead to the conclusion that there is no reason to assume the child would not be able to do in the future as well as it had done in the past. Also, there is no reason to assume at all that there would be tests, hardships and bad things to experience. The monsters and other symbolic evil figures may be overcome by means of guided imagery which may be taught to the child or performed with it (see Chapter 15).

However, fear of punishment may also have to do with the children's past – with the sense of guilt or remorse about 'bad' things the children think they have done in the past or 'good' things they have failed to do. For example, some children and adolescents are guilt-ridden because they have not been good to their parents, have not treated their siblings well, have lied, taken things that do not belong to them, have evaded their duties, had forbidden thoughts, and so on. The therapeutic attitude of PPPC would stress that such and similar things may be bad, but doing bad things is part of being human, all children do things of this kind, and adults know that children do them. The bad that human beings do is offset by the good things that one does. PPPC would urge the child to recall as many good things that it had done in the past, recount them and dwell on them. Some children and adolescents may express the tendency to re-evaluate conceptions of good and evil. It would be advisable to help them along this route. But if the child shows no such tendency, it would not be advisable at this stage to plunge into a process of checking one's values which might contribute to undermining the child's sense of security.

Fear of punishment and the sense of guilt may be related to the child's religious beliefs and concern with the afterlife (Kavanaugh 1977). The child's conception of life after death may focus on punishments meted out to the evil human beings by superior powers, on suffering and hell. PPPC would focus on humanizing the scene in afterlife, complementing the conception by elaborating on the concepts of paradise and good angels, mitigating the child's sense of guilt and self-blame, dwelling on the good deeds the child had done, and reminding the child of the suffering it had already suffered through the illness and the treatments which may obviate the need for further suffering.

Fear of Pain and Suffering

Some children and adolescents may have fears of pain and suffering. It would be natural for them to have those fears both because of what they have already undergone themselves and because of what they may have observed in other children on the ward or in the clinic. Sometimes the fears refer to specific symptoms, such as being immobilized, suffocating, losing control over bowel movements, losing a limb, or not being able to see. Fears of this kind may reflect the child's fear of the unknown lying ahead, focused on one's body rather than on the external environment (as in fear of the unfamiliar). But they may also reflect distrust of the physicians and nurses taking care of them. Some children develop with time a growing distrust when they become aware of the fact that although the physicians do for them the utmost, there are limits to what they can do. Nevertheless, it is of utmost importance that the child stay convinced that the doctors really do the utmost for him or her, and even when they cannot heal, they can alleviate pain and suffering. Maybe a good way to put it is that the child patient has to make the shift from curative to palliative medicine, just as the doctors had done. In this context, PPPC often consists in helping the child express his or her fears, communicate them to the doctor and be courageous enough to insist on getting all the help medicine can offer. Quite a number of children still need to be convinced that they are not to blame for feeling pain, that they do not have to feel ashamed for confessing they feel pain, and that it is not a sign of weakness not to want to feel pain. Some are not even sure that pain can be controlled to a large if not full extent.

A Note on the Fear of Death

In the literature on death at least three basic approaches to conceptualizing the issue of death anxiety can be detected. One approach maintains that there is no true death anxiety. That which appears to be death anxiety is in fact anxiety displaced from other unresolved conflicts and problems, such as between love and hate, aggression and its suppression. This approach is rooted in Freud's (1953/1913) reasoning that our own death is completely unimaginable because on the conscious level we have never experienced it and on the unconscious level it is completely inconceivable since the unconscious knows no negation. Hence, we cannot fear something which we do not at all know. A second approach views death anxiety as basic. It is rooted in the awareness of our mortality, is an inalienable aspect of our existence and dominates every aspect of our lives (Becker 1973). The only reason why we are not constantly aware of it is that its sheer intensity calls for repression. Finally, a third approach maintains that we are actually not afraid of death itself but of a variety of things that have come to be associated with death, such as pain, suffering, separation, loneliness, punishment, or destruction (Hinton 1967, pp. 21–30, Ryle 1941). The proponents of this view maintain that many of these fears are based on mistakes, misinformation, and ignorance. Actually, death is often free of distress and may seem more horrifying to the spectators, who dread the approaching bereavement and loss, than to the dying individual who is protected by diminished consciousness. In sum, we suggest calling the three approaches to death anxiety 'the displacement theory', 'the existential theory' and 'the pragmatic theory', respectively.

What do the three approaches imply in regard to reducing death anxiety? The displacement theory would advocate resolving unconscious conflicts; the existential theory would advocate confronting the existential issues involved in living and dying, fulfilling our roles in life as we conceive them and applying denial to the remnants of anxiety; the pragmatic approach would advocate easing the process of dying as much as possible and allaying the fears that relate to the different real or imagined connotations of death. Hence, the solutions are psychological, philosophical and medical-palliative, respectively. As described in this chapter, PPPC applies mainly the medical-palliative treatment, rooted in the pragmatic approach, but is open to deal with the philosophical existential aspects, and also with the psychological dynamic ones if the child is bothered by an unresolved conflict and is in need of its resolution.

Being Told the Truth

For children in the terminal phase, being told the truth reduces to being told about impending death. As noted above, many of the young patients are aware of this eventuality on a certain level of consciousness. This section is devoted to discussing the issue of impending death, rather than whether children are aware of death. Some children and adolescents do not raise the issue at all with the doctors or parents. The reason may be denial, desire to deal with this issue on one's own terms (i e., with oneself alone, with one's peers or with the psychotherapist), or safeguarding one's parents.

Denial is not an all-or-nothing phenomenon. Weisman (1972) defined three levels of denial in terminally ill adults: denial of the facts, denial of the worst implications, and denial of one's own extinction. There are many more forms (Kreitler 1999) not to mention the fact that denial is subject to fluctuations and change due to circumstances, mood and new information (Lazarus 1981). In the framework of PPPC awareness is not considered as an asset in its own right. Hence, as long as the child cooperates with the basic medical requirements, PPPC respects the child's right to denial.

Some children and adolescents in the terminal phase may feel more comfortable discussing death and dying with individuals other than their doctors and parents. PPPC respects the right of children to choose the person with whom they want or do not want to discuss their own death. Respecting their right may entail helping the adults understand, tolerate and accept this behavior, which may not always be easy, particularly not for parents.

Sometimes more complex situations occur. Nir, a 17-year-old adolescent suffered from a recurrence of ALL (leukemia) after 13 years. He knew very soon that he was dying, but his father, who assumed complete and exclusive control of Nir's treatment, was not ready to accept the fact and refused to talk about it. Nir pressured him to discuss it but to no avail. The psychologist had a few sessions with the father. When finally the father was able to tell his son that he knew he was dying, Nir calmed down and died peacefully 48 hours later.

Dov was a 12-year-old patient who had a similar problem with his father. The father cried a lot (in fact, so much that the children on the ward called him 'a water source') but did not talk. Only after he met the psychologist a few times he was able to talk with his son who said 'now that my father knows I can go to paradise'.

These examples demonstrate that discussing death with the parents may sometimes be important for the children for reasons, such as getting confirmation that the parent respects them sufficiently to be able to accept them as mature partners, or being reassured that the parent is not angry with them for dying, that the parent knows they have done everything in order to stay alive but may not succeed in this venture.

On several occasions dying children who knew of their impending death explained to the psychologist that they wanted nevertheless to be 'told the truth' as a sign that they are sufficiently respected to be considered as worthy and able to get the right information.

Protecting One's Parents

Concern over one's parents is an issue that may bother quite a number of children in the terminal phase. They are concerned about the suffering and pain of their parents and try to hide from them how much they suffer. Dalia was a 10-year-old girl with sarcoma who stayed on the ward for five months, almost continuously. When she went home, mostly over the weekend, she developed high fever and other complications (e.g., neutropenia, low magnesium level) which necessitated her return to the hospital. Her mother stayed with her most of the time, despite the fact that there was another 3-year-old boy at home. Dalia felt that her mother suffered because she had to neglect the small brother. Dalia started gently communicating to her mother that she felt better, had no pain, was in good mood and could take care of herself. She even said 'I am not a 3-year-old baby that you have to look after all the time'. Notably, the mother was persuaded to go home and leave Dalia alone for periods that grew longer until the psychologist succeeded in improving communication between the mother and daughter so that Dalia could tell her mother what she had been doing.

Protecting one's parents may take diverse forms. Sometimes the child would simply hide from the parent his or her pain, sometimes the child would deceive the parent by enacting a gay play or appearing to be immersed in some trivial task. Adams and Deveau (1986, p. 91) tell of Mary who chose to stay in the hospital because she believed that care at home would be too difficult for her parents. Dan, an 11-year-old boy with sarcoma, told the psychologist 'my mother need not suffer for me; it does not help me but it harms her, she will live after I die'. However, Zehava who was only 8 years old, disclosed another surprising insight: 'mummy and daddy when they come here don't cry, they cry when they are not in the room, but outside, in the corridor; it is better to cry alone, I also cry alone when they don't see, I don't want them to cry because of me'. Thus, it is possible that a child may imitate the parent in hiding one's grief.

PPPC indicates the need for improving communication between parents and children so that, if they wish, they can openly discuss the issue of whether to share one's pain and suffering with each other. It is through communication that they may find out, for example, as Itay the 8-year-old did, that when his parents spoke of being strong they did not mean not complaining about pain, or, as Tami the 5-year-old did, that her parents suspected she was dissimulating and it pained them that she did not trust them enough to share her pain with them. In both these cases the improved communication led to increased sharing on the part of the children. Increased communication can also lead initially to decreased sharing as, for example, in the case of Avi, who found out that his disease reminded his mother of the Holocaust. Following several common sessions with the psychologist, Avi and his mother understood how misleading it was to equate their predicament with the Holocaust.

Guilt in Regard to One's Parents

A dying child may feel guilty for letting down its parents by dying before the child could realize their wishes and expectations of him or her. 'My father wanted me to be an officer in the army, now I will only be a dead child' said Gil, a 7-year-old with sarcoma. A girl on the ward wrote a note to her parents asking them for forgiveness 'because all you put into me is going down the drain'. This girl felt guilty because she could not give her parents back what she thought they deserved in return for everything they had given her.

There are several ways to deal with this issue in the framework of PPPC. One way is to let the child see that its parents did not bring it into the world in order to fulfill their expectations; they created life for life's sake. Another way is to let the child perceive that the future is only one aspect of life, complementing the present and the past but not replacing them and not outweighing them in importance. Still another way is to let the child perceive all the happiness it had given its parents and let the parents tell the child how happy it had made them all through. Which one or more of these different ways is adequate for any specific child depends on the child.

Loss of Respect for Authorities

Children and adolescents in the last phases of terminal disease sometimes suffer from a crumbling respect for authorities. It may have its roots in the gradually emerging awareness that the doctors are unable to provide the means for full recovery, cannot promise full recovery, do not always know what the next step in the disease would be, sometimes cannot even help in fully controlling pain. This awareness is all the more disconcerting because it has come to replace the complete trust that the child and its family had in the medical institution. In addition, there is the growing recognition on the part of the child that even the all-powerful parents, who have always shielded the child from all evil and have satisfied all its needs, are unable to prevent impending death in the future and all of the suffering at present. These are very difficult and painful insights because parents and doctors are mainstays of one's sense of security and confidence in the benevolence of life and reality. Instead of the shielded security of childhood and teenage, the patient stays with 'a tattered cloak' of make-beliefs, half-truths, and uncertainties. The 13-year-old boy with sarcoma who used this metaphor added 'this cloak gives you no warmth'.

It is difficult to evaluate for whom these insights are harder: for the smaller child who up to the occurrence of the disease has lived in a state of complete trust in one's parents, or for the adolescent who has already started his or her exploration of reality and has had a chance 'to see through the veil of certainty', to use another metaphor of a sick teenager. For the younger children the collapse of trust may be more extensive, but for the adolescents it is no less vital because it is precisely the trust in their parents that gives them the courage to explore.

The insights about the inability of doctors and parents to avoid the evil bring in their wake disappointment, frustration, enhanced sense of helplessness and weakness. As far as the parents are concerned, various feelings may be evoked, starting with anger for their having misled the child, through guilt about feeling that way, to pity which generates the desire to protect the parents since 'they are not stronger than I am' (in the words of the boy who produced 'the tattered cloak' metaphor).

PPPC tries to help the patient recognize that having limits on one's capacity does not mean the absence of all ability and effectiveness. The extreme all-or-nothing approach is to be complemented by the realistic approach which takes into account abilities, knowledge and goodwill, coupled with the recognition of limitations to what one can achieve. From one child we have learned 'that sometimes my math teacher gives me a good grade because I tried hard even though I did not have the solution'. In other words, it is justified to respect people for what they are trying to achieve and for the effort they put into it even if they fail. Also, not all failures are identical. Some failures are closer to success than others.

Loss of Control

Loss of control at present and in the future bothers some of the children and teenagers in the terminal phase. Due to their experiences in previous stages of the disease and treatments, the patients have noticed the gradual loss of their control over the body, appearance, actions, feelings and behaviors. Since control is tightly bound with the sense of identity, diminished control indicates a threat to one's self-identity and comfort of being in the world.

PPPC concentrates in these cases on constructing the sense of control both from bottom up and from top to bottom. Examples of the bottom-up approach include insisting on the child deciding about small or concrete things, such as where to put objects in his or her room, what to wear, where to sit, who would visit and when. Examples of the top-down approach include discussing with the child the issue of control in general, the limitations on control, the illusion of having control even when one has little or no control, and 'respect for reality' which has not been constructed so as to enable each and everyone to have control over most things. Helping the child remember events and situations when it felt it had control or no control provides examples that help the child gain insight about how control functions and its limitations.

Sadness and Sorrow

The terminal phase of illness is often the period when the child or adolescent starts the process of grieving and mourning over oneself. PPPC enables the children to express their sadness. One child said, 'Look at me, so young and such a pretty body, what a pity'. Dying children and adolescents may become poignantly aware of all the things in the present and especially in the future which they would miss by being no more. They may think of careers, of getting married and having kids, of traveling in the world, of participating in parties, of having fun, of loving and being loved. The more they know of the world and of life the deeper the potential sorrow. In the framework of PPPC there are a variety of ways to deal with this important issue. One way consists in elaborating on moments of joy and happiness from the child's past. This serves not only to raise the mood at present but also communicates the message that 'life has been wonderful and has had its exquisite moments even if they belong to the past' or 'no one can take from me wonderful moments I have experienced'. Another way we have learned from one of our patients. Silvia was an 11-year-old girl when it became evident that she would die from Wilms' disease. Her physical suffering was intense. She expressed a wish to have a party. A party was organized for her on the ward and many of her friends participated. Silvia enjoyed the party enormously and a few days later she asked for another party. 'I know we had a party but that was long ago, like "last year".' A series of six parties was organized for Silvia, which she experienced as if they stretched over a time period of years. In the last party she asked to be dressed in a white dress 'like a bride', and insisted on video photos to be taken of her all in white, to show everyone 'next year'. What Silvia attempted to do was to compress the future as much as possible, reduce it to fun and parties and live as many of its delightful moments as she could. Silvia acted out in reality or quasi-reality what many others do in fantasy and daydreams. A similar insight was expressed by Avi, a 15-year-old, who drew 'a bird's song', consisting only of different colored dots and lines. He explained that life was the dots and lines, which in the case of some people were strewn around over a larger space and in the case of some over a much smaller space.

Anger

Anger often appears in the process of coping with the awareness of death. It is generally known and expected after Kübler-Ross (1969) identified it as one of the five stages of dying, occurring as second, following denial and preceding bargaining. Although we have not observed that it appears always or as a definite stage, there is little doubt that it often occurs and recurs in the course of confronting death. It may appear in varied forms. Sometimes it takes the form of envy of others in general or of specific others (e.g., a sibling or a schoolmate) who are not sick and stay alive. In others it may appear as rebellion or refusal to cooperate with the medical treatment ('anyway it does not help at all'). It often accompanies the complaint of injustice ('Why me?' or 'It is not fair that I should die, I have done so little . . .'). It may also take the form of a desire to destroy, to vent out the anger ('I want to see everyone dead when I am dead', said one 4-year-old). A 15-year-old girl dying of leukemia was full of rage to such an extent that she could not tolerate anything living in her vicinity, no animal, no flower, no picture of an animal, not even anything that moves of its own accord. Indeed, she put herself into a world of total death, as a kind of protest against her fate.

PPPC provides a framework for expressing the anger. It enables the child or adolescent to externalize the anger by using the variety of expressive means suggested by the psychologist (e.g., words, enacted movements, drawings, fantasy). The mere expression may already be helpful. Once released, the emotion may be more manageable. PPPC turns the anger into a legitimate emotion and thus frees the patient of the need to hide it or fight it, and encourages him or her to devote these energies instead to confronting the situation that had produced the anger. Some of the patients get into a fierce dialogue with life, fate or God in their efforts to overcome the anger. Some find within themselves an answer that brings with it some comfort; others find in themselves the courage to face the silence. In the context of this confrontation not a few seek solace in faith and religion.

Wish Fulfillments

As illustrated above (see the section on 'Sadness and sorrow'), some children use wish-fulfillments in order to solve problems they have when facing death. Fulfilling wishes which it is possible to fulfill at this stage is a most important and potent means of PPPC. For many children it is an exhilarating experience to find out that their wishes may not only be fulfilled, but often without delay and without compromising. The fulfillment of some of these wishes may get to be reported in the media, as for example, the visit of a famous artist or entertainer in the children's ward because a sick child wanted to meet him or her. Some wishes are touchingly modest, as to own some object, see a certain picture, wear a certain piece of jewelry, listen to a particular music and so on. One 10-year-old girl on the ward had a wish to kiss her mother's breasts (in a kind of regression to early infancy); another boy (a 12-year-old dying of a brain tumor) wanted to have in his room in the hospital many different colored balloons; another older boy (a 14-year-old) wanted to have privacy because 'I am not a public ground where everyone can come and go when they want'.

Some wish-fulfillments require special effort on the part of the parents, such as the wish of one dying girl to see her recently divorced parents staying together at least in her room, or the wish of another girl to spend the last weeks of her life at home rather than in the hospital. PPPC tries to create an atmosphere in which the children can express wishes and makes a point of promoting the fulfillment of the patients' wishes as promptly as possible. Fulfilling the patients' wishes may require a close cooperation between the parents, the medical staff and the psychologist.

Hope and Self-comforting

Dying children and adolescents often seek hope, comfort, or consolation openly. Some may beg for it ('tell me something that will give me hope'), others may tell of their success in finding it ('I saw an angel and he was smiling at me' or 'I dreamt I went to heaven and then came back and was all healthy; I know this can happen to you'). In their effort to get hope they often turn to faith and religion, even if their upbringing has not been strictly orthodox and even if they do not know too much about religion. Contact with higher powers (e.g., God, angels), high-ranking individuals (e.g., Rabin, the prime minister) or close people who had died before (e.g., the child's grandmother) may be very comforting to some children. To the question that is sometimes asked 'Will they help me?', the psychologist can only answer, 'I hope so'. No doubt, the belief itself is helpful.

Search for Meaning

Although children and adolescents are generally not expected to deal with abstract issues of this kind, some nevertheless do and raise questions, such as 'Who am I?', 'What is the meaning of my life?', 'What was my role in life and did I fulfill it?', 'Why was I born?', and 'Why do I die?' PPPC considers it as its function to help young patients confronting death to explore these issues and chart for themselves some kind of answer. Help in this domain does not mean by any means indoctrination, persuasion, or providing answers; rather it means encouraging the child to look for himself or herself, explore optional answers, provide information when the child asks for it, sometimes rephrasing clearly what the child has been trying to say or conceptualize. The major characteristic feature of the approach of PPPC is that meaning resides in the act of assigning meaning. Hence, meaningfulness is the product of the meaning or meanings the human being assigns to the facts rather than of the facts or events as such. Assigning meaning may be a laborious process that may lead to unexpected results. Sometimes it reveals that events which seemed in the past highly meaningful lose some of their meanings, whereas others which had been hardly noticed assume great significance. Some young people draw a lot of comfort from the discovery that by relating events to one another and by exploring interactions among components one may discover meanings which had not been evident in considering other relations or partial sections of the past. Other children find comfort in realizing that 'no one can finish the whole job, and others will go on with the job in the future', e.g., 'my younger sister will make nice drawings for my mother because she loves them' and 'my older brother said that he will not go to the army and help my father because I cannot help him'. The search may end with the conclusion 'I don't know' or 'I will find out only after I die'. It may, however, also end with the realization that there is no sense in anything. The psychologist may then help in avoiding the subsequent emergence of despair.

Sometimes the search for meaning focuses on concern with self-identity. This issue may be of enhanced importance in adolescence, the period when a child is focused on developing his or her identity and individuality. With a curtailed life expectancy that greatly limits the options for actions and experiences, the youngster may feel that he or she has missed out on developing their self-identity. PPPC would promote the child's enhanced sense of uniqueness and individuality by encouraging the child to dwell at length on behaviors, experiences, daydreams, friendships that demonstrate how special he or she is, how different from anyone else they know. Further, PPPC would encourage the child to express his or her individuality also in the context of the terminal phase in the hospital in a variety of ways, such as through clothing, choice of objects to be placed around, and so on. It is of special importance, particularly in the case of adolescents, to promote cultivation of their external appearance, for while 'dying does not remove the desire to be attractive' (Adams and Deveau 1986, p. 82), attractiveness may be one of the earmarks of individuality.

GENERAL ISSUES IN PROVIDING PPPC

As noted earlier, two major principles of PPPC are considering the child patient within the context of the whole family system and considering PPPC within the total context of palliative care provided to the sick child.

The Dying Child and the Family

Providing PPPC to a sick child in the terminal phase means treating the child *and* his or her family, that is to say, together with the family, within the family, sometimes through the family. The family consists naturally first and foremost of the parents, but includes also grandparents and siblings insofar as they are involved with the treatment of the sick child. In practice this entails, for example, dealing with the anxieties of the parents that may transfer to the child (Papadatou, Yfantopoulos and Kosmidi 1996); helping the parents and the child talk openly, especially about their emotions (Sourkes 2000); and promoting mutual communication of needs and desires.

Often taking care of the family may require improving communication also within the family, for example, between the two parents who may not be communicating openly concerning their sick child or in general, as well as between the parents or the sick child and a sibling who may suffer from anger, envy or guilt in regard to the dying child. Tension-laden situations of this kind call for the attention of the psychologist because they may project on the sick child and even interfere with satisfying the child's needs. PPPC advocates adopting a flexible approach and treating the family as a whole, or in pairs or each member individually, as required for a speedy resolution of the problems.

The parents are not only the primary care-takers of the child in the hospital no less than at home, they are also the prime decision-makers in regard to anything that concerns the child. While this in no way restricts the responsibility of the medical treatment and palliation team in the hospital, it increases the child's sense of security, belongingness and identity.

However, treating the child in the context of the family does not mean that the psychologist is free to communicate to the parents everything that has taken place in the therapeutic session with the child. The child's right to privacy has to be defended no less than the parents' rights. It is also important that the therapeutic session provides a safe haven for the child to express thoughts and feelings that he or she finds difficult to express elsewhere. However, the psychologist may ask the child's permission to share with the parents any theme that came up in therapy and which it may be important to communicate to the parents so as to improve the child's state or quality of life. Involving the parents is important all along, but in particular in regard to themes that have any operational implications. Asking the child for permission is one way to empower the child and help him or her resume control of their life. More importantly, the psychologist will encourage, enable and help the child and the parents to discuss among themselves themes that were discussed in therapy as well as others. Further, with the consent of both parties, in some or all PPPC sessions both child and parents may participate.

PPPC and the Treatment Team

Workers in the field have noted how difficult it may be to produce cooperation between the treatment team, the family and the child, coordinating their sometimes different needs (Schlebush and du Plessis 1992). Communication and cooperation between the nursing staff and the family may sometimes require psychological intervention (Lipton 1978). When PPPC has become a part of the palliative therapy in a specific ward or clinic, the treating teams are trained in the specific techniques and issues of PPPC and may only need adjustment or focused intervention for particular cases.

PPPC advocates treatment of the therapeutic staff both in general and in regard to cases of specific patients. The purpose is double – both to help in providing PPPC to the dying child and to keep burnout of the staff as low as possible. Treatment of the staff includes providing understanding of the psychological setup of the child and his or her family, analyzing and – if necessary – improving communication and cooperation with the child's family, working through one's reactions and difficulties in the course of treating the child, and resolving the pain and shock after the child's demise.

The involvement of the staff in PPPC may sometimes require imparting information about the child's psychological needs and state. In view of the child's right to privacy and in order to enhance the child's sense of security, it is advisable that no information be imparted without prior discussion with the child and his or her fully informed consent.

Issues of Time and Place

There are two emotionally highly difficult issues with which PPPC may be concerned and which involve the child, the parents and the staff. These have to do with the decision about palliative sedation and with the location in which the child will stay in the last period of his or her life. These issues are both operational and concrete and loaded with heavy emotional connotations (see also Chapters 3 and 5). They are mentioned here primarily because they may fulfill a central role in PPPC. The decision of palliative sedation is all the more difficult because it is a decision for another human being who is one's own child. To hold on to life, not to relinquish the smallest chance of hope, is strengthened further by the belief in a just world when a child is involved (Stillion and Papadatou 2002). One of the hard tasks of PPPC is to help the parents confront their inner attitudes and decide or express the decision they have already undertaken.

Determining the location for the child to spend the terminal period requires a decision of a different order. The desire of the parents to protect their child and provide the warmest and most comfortable environment is of prime importance, but it is necessary to consider also the child's desire and needs as well as the logistics of treatment at home that may be difficult (Martinson 1978). The home is also for many children the most favorable environment, but not for all. It is of paramount importance to find out what the child's desires in this respect really are. For example, some children, perhaps the youngest, would prefer home at all costs, but others may feel safer and more protected medically in the hospital. Again, some children would like to take leave of their beloved objects at home or perform symbolically important acts like bathing in their own bathtub or extend as much as possible the illusion of normal daily routine at home. Other children, however, may prefer to forgo the pain of leave-taking of places and objects or may already be at a stage where these symbolic acts have already become meaningless. PPPC means that special means and care are applied for helping in clarifying or identifying the child's desires in this as in other respects and encouraging their expression so that they may be implemented with all possible promptness, care, devotion and love.

REFERENCES

Adams, D.W., Deveau, E. (1986) Helping dying adolescents: needs and responses. In Corr, C.A., McNeil, J.N. (Eds) *Adolescence and Death*. New York: Springer, pp. 79–96.

Anthony, S. (1972) *The Discovery of Death in Childhood and After*. New York: Basic Books.

Atwood, V.A. (1984) Children's concepts of death: A descriptive study. *Child Study Journal* **14**, 11–29.

Bach, S. (1975) Spontaneous pictures of leukemic children as an expression of the total personality, mind and body. *Acta Paedopsychiatrica* **41**, 86–104.

Becker, E. (1973) *The Denial of Death*. New York: The Free Press.

Bertoia, J. (1993) *Drawings from a Dying Child: Insights into death from a Jungian perspective*. London: Routledge.

Bertoia, J., Allen, J. (1988) Counselling seriously ill children: Use of spontaneous drawings. *Elementary School Guidance and Counselling* **22**, 206–221.

Bluebond-Langner, M. (1978) *The Private Worlds of Dying Children*. Princeton, NJ: Princeton University Press.

Candy-Gibbs, S.E., Sharp, K.C., Petrun, C.J. (1984–5) The effects of age, object and cultural/religious background on children's concepts of death. *Omega: Journal of Death and Dying* **15**, 329–346.

Clunies-Ross, C., Lansdown, R. (1988) Concepts of death, illness and isolation found in children with leukemia. *Child Care, Health, and Development* **14**, 373–386.

Cobbs, B. (1956) Psychological impact of long-term illness and death of a child on the family circle. *Journal of Pediatrics* **49**, 746–751.

Cotton, C.R., Range, L.M. (1990) Children's death concepts: Relationship to cognitive functioning, age, experience with death, fear of death, and hopelessness. *Journal of Clinical Child Psychology* **19**, 123–127.

Field, F. (1985) Coping with separation stress by infants and young children. In Field, T.M., McCabe, P.M., Schneiderman, N. (Eds) *Stress and Coping*. Hillsdale, NJ: Erlbaum, pp. 197–219.

Freud, S. (1953/1913) Thoughts on the times on war and death. In *Collected Works of Sigmund Freud* Vol. 4. London: Hogarth Press, p. 288–317.

Furth, G. (1988) *The Secret World of Drawings: Healing through art.* Boston: Sigo Press.

Gartley, W., Bernasconi, M. (1967) The concept of death in children. *Journal of Genetic Psychology* **110**, 71–85.

Hinton, J. (1967) *Dying.* Harmondsworth, UK: Penguin Books.

Hollenbeck, A.R., Sussman, E.J., Nannis, E.D., Strope, B.E., Hersh, S.P., Levine, A.S., Pizzo, A.S. (1980) Children with serious illness: Behavioral correlates of separation and isolation. *Child Psychiatry and Human Development* **11**, 3–11.

Jampolsky, G.G., Taylor, P. (1978) *There is a Rainbow behind Every Dark Cloud.* Tiburon, CA: Celestial Arts.

Jay, S.M., Green, V., Jonson, S., Caldwell, S., Nitschke, R. (1987) Differences in death concepts between children with cancer and physically healthy children. *Journal of Clinical Child Psychology* **16**, 301–306.

Jenkins, R.A., Cavanaugh, J.C. (1985–6) Examining the relationship between the development of the concept of death and overall cognitive development. *Omega: Journal of Death and Dying* **16**, 193–199.

Kastenbaum, R. (1992) *The Psychology of Death* (2nd edn). New York: Springer.

Kavanaugh, R.E. (1977) *Facing Death.* New York: Penguin Books.

Kenyon, B.L. (2001) Current research in children's conceptions of death: a critical review. *Omega: Journal of Death and Dying* **43**, 63–91.

Koocher, G.P. (1973) Childhood, death, and cognitive development. *Developmental Psychology* **9**, 369–375.

Kreitler, S. (1965) *Symbolschöpfung und Symbolerfassung: Eine experimental-psychologische Studie.* Munich: Reinhardt.

Kreitler, S. (1999) Denial in cancer patients. *Cancer Investigation* **17**, 514–534.

Kübler-Ross, E. (1969) *On Death and Dying.* New York: Macmillan.

Kübler-Ross, E. (1981) *Living with Death and Dying.* New York: Macmillan.

Kübler-Ross, E. (1983) *On Children and Death.* New York: Macmillan.

Lazarus, R. S. (1981) The costs and benefits of denial. In Spinetta, J.J., Deasy-Spinetta, P. (Eds) *Living with Childhood Cancer.* St. Louis: Mosby, pp. 50–67.

Lifton, R.J. (1979) *The Broken Connection.* New York: Simon & Schuster.

Lipton, H. (1978) The dying child and the family: The skills of the social worker. In Sahler, O.J.Z. (Ed.) *The Child and Death.* St. Louis: Mosby, pp. 52–71.

Lonetto, R. (1980) *Children's Conceptions of Death.* New York: Springer.

Lonetto, R., Templer, D.I. (1986) *Death Anxiety.* New York: Hemisphere.

Mahon, M. (1993) Children's concept of death and sibling death of trauma. *Journal of Pediatric Nursing* **8**, 335–344.

Martinson, I.M. (1978) Alternative environments for care of the dying child: hospice, hospital, or home. In Sahler, O.J.Z. (Ed.) *The Child and Death.* St. Louis: Mosby, pp. 83–91.

McIntire, M., Angle, C., Struempler, L. (1972) The concept of death in mid-western children and youth. *American Journal of Diseases of Children* **123**, 527–532.

Morrissey, J.R. (1963) Children's adaptations to fatal illness. *Social Work* **8**, 81–88.

Morrison, S., Siu, A.L. (2000) The hard task of improving the quality of care at the end of life. *Archives of Internal Medicine* **160**, 743–747.

Nagy, M. (1948) The child's theories concerning death. *Journal of Genetic Psychology* **73**, 3–27.

Natterson, J.M., Knudson, A.G., Jr. (1960) Observations concerning fear of death in fatally ill children and their mothers. *Psychosomatic Medicine* **22**, 456–465.

Orbach, I., Gross, Y., Glaubman, H., Berman, D. (1986) Children's perceptions of various determinants of the death concept as a function of intelligence, age and anxiety. *Journal of Clinical Child Psychology* **15**, 120–126.

Papadatou, D., Yfantopculos, J., Kosmidi, H.V. (1996) Death of a child at home or in hospital. *Death Studies* **20**, 215–235.

Rando, T. (1984) *Grief, Dying and Death: Clinical interventions for caregivers.* Champaign, IL: Research Press.

Reilly, T.P., Hasazi, J.E., Bond, L.A. (1983) Children's concepts of death and personal mortality. *Journal of Pediatric Psychology* **8**, 21–31.

Reite, M., Harbeck, R., Hoffman, A. (1981) Altered cellular immune response following separation. *Life Sciences* **29**, 1133–1136.

Reite, M., Short, R., Kaufman, I.C., Stynes, A.J., Pauley, J.D. (1978) Heart rate and body temperature in separated monkey infants. *Biological Psychiatry* **13**, 91–105.

Richmond, J.B., Weisman, H.A. (1955) Psychologic aspects of management of children with malignant disease. *American Journal of Diseases of Children* **89**, 42–47.

Rochlin, G. (1967) How younger children view death and themselves. In E.A. Grollman (Ed.) *Explaining Death to Children.* Boston: Beacon Press, pp. 51–85.

Ross, E.S. (1967) Children's books relating to death: A discussion. In Grollman, E.A. (Ed.) *Explaining Death to Children.* Boston: Beacon Press, pp. 249–271.

Ryle, J.A. (1941) *Fears May Be Liars.* London: Allen & Unwin.

Schilder, P., Wechsler, D. (1934) The attitudes of children toward death. *Journal of Genetic Psychology* **45**, 406–451.

Schlebush, L., du Plessis, W.F. (1992) Psychological issues in the management of the terminally ill child. *South African Journal of Child and Adolescent Psychiatry* **4**, 60–63.

Schneiderman, N., McCabe, P.M. (1985) Biobehavioral responses to stressors. In Field, T.M., McCabe, P.M., Schneiderman, N. (Eds) *Stress and coping.* Hillsdale, NJ: Erlbaum, pp. 13–61.

Solnit, A.J., Green, M. (1959) Psychologic considerations in the management of death on pediatric hospital services. *Pediatrics* **24**, 106–112.

Sourkes, B.M. (2000) Psychotherapy with the dying child. In Chochinov, H.M., Breitbart, W. (Eds) *Handbook of Psychiatry in Palliative Medicine.* New York: Oxford University Press, pp. 265–272.

Spinetta, J.J. (1974) The dying child's awareness of death. *Psychological Bulletin* **4**, 256–260.

Stern, M.M. (1968) Fear of death and neurosis. *Journal of the American Psychoanalytic Association* **16**, 3–31.

Stillion, J.M., Papadatou, D. (2002) Suffer the children: An examination of psychosocial issues in children and adolescents with terminal illness. *American Behavioral Scientist* **46**, 299–315.

Waechter, E.H. (1971) Children's awareness of fatal illness. *American Journal of Nursing* **71**, 1168–1172.

Waechter, E.H. (1987) Children's reactions to fatal illness. In Krulik, T., Holaday, B., Martinson, I.M. (Eds) *The Child and Family Facing Life-threatening Illness.* Philadelphia, PA: Lippincott, pp. 108–119.

Wass, H. (1984) Books for children: An annotated bibliography. In Wass, H., Corr, C.A. (Eds) *Helping Children Cope with Death: Guidelines and resources* (2nd edn). New York: Hemisphere, pp. 151–207.

Wass, H., Guenther, Z.C., Towry, B.J. (1979) United States and Brazilian children's concepts of death. *Death Education* **3**, 41–55.

Weisman, A.D. (1972) *On Dying and Denying: A psychiatric study of terminality.* New York: Behavioral Publications.

17

Education of the Sick Child: Learning and Reintegration into the School

CIPORAH S. TADMOR AND MYRIAM WEYL BEN ARUSH

Pediatric Hematology Oncology, Rambam Medical Center, Technion Faculty of Medicine, Haifa, Israel

INTRODUCTION

Recent advances in the treatment of childhood cancer have dramatically improved the prognosis of children diagnosed with cancer. Childhood cancer has gradually evolved from a rapidly progressing fatal disease to a life-threatening chronic illness (Varni *et al.* 1995). Today, most children survive for five years or longer (e.g., Bleyer 1990) and achieve long-term disease-free survival. With the increase in long-term survival of pediatric cancer patients, quality of life issues have come to assume a more prominent role in their comprehensive treatment. This trend has led to a shift from psychological emphasis on crisis intervention confronting imminent death to facilitating coping with a serious life-threatening disease (Varni and Katz 1987) to primary prevention of emotional dysfunction (Tadmor and Weyl Ben Arush 2000). In this chapter, the risk of protective factors with respect to the mental health of children with cancer is discussed, and a survey of a representative sample of school intervention programs is presented. The preventive intervention program implemented in the school at Rambam Medical Center in Haifa, Israel, is discussed and evaluated, and an illustrative case study is presented.

Psychosocial Aspects of Pediatric Oncology. Edited by S. Kreitler and M. Weyl Ben Arush
© 2004 John Wiley & Sons Ltd: ISBN 0 471 49939 0

THE RATIONALE FOR PREVENTIVE INTERVENTION IN THE SCHOOL

Risk Factors that Endanger the Mental Health of Children with Cancer

School absenteeism

The underlying rationale for preventive intervention is derived from empirical and clinical studies that report excessive absenteeism from school for pediatric cancer patients. In spite of a general consensus with respect to the significance of school in a child's life, it is well reported in the literature that cancer creates educationally related barriers for children with cancer, which may contribute to school problems (e.g., Adamoli *et al.* 1997), to school absenteeism (Lansky and Cairns 1979), and even to school phobia (Lansky *et al.* 1975). Research has shown for at least 30 years that children with chronic diseases are likely to have 50% more school absences a year than other children. Among these, children diagnosed with cancer have three to six times more school absences a year than do chronic or orthopedic conditions (91, 29, 15 days per year, respectively). Indeed, the only significant factor associated with the number of absences caused by treatment was the type of illness, namely cancer (Charlton *et al.* 1991). Pediatric cancer patients appear to have very high absence rates, even after their return to school (Lansky and Cairns 1979, Cairns *et al.* 1982, Lansky, Cairns and Zwartjes 1983). The absence rate decreases but still remains considerably high for two (Stehbens, Kisker and Wilson 1983) or three years after diagnosis, not necessarily related to treatment (Eiser 1980).

As early as 1979, Lansky and Cairns reported that the average school absence after diagnosis was 41.1 days, 35 days in the first year post-diagnosis, 29.1 days in the second year, and 28.3 days in the third year. Fourteen years later, the absence rate is strikingly similar at 45–21 days per year (Brown and Madan-Swain 1993).

Concern regarding the academic achievement and psychological adjustment of children with cancer is advanced by findings that suggest that children who miss 20 or more days per year are liable not to maintain their pre-illness academic level of achievement. School absenteeism of 20 days or more a year is associated with other significant school difficulties, such as a decline in grades, behavioral problems, inattention and acting out. These problems are serious obstacles that interfere with rehabilitation and reintegration into the school setting (Lansky and Cairns 1979).

School phobia

School phobia is seen in 1% of the general population and in 10% in a large sample of school-age children with cancer (Lansky *et al.* 1975). School phobia is characterized by a refusal to attend school due to fear of separation and somatic complaints (Klopovich *et al.* 1981), and fear of social rejection and teasing due to altered physical appearance (Ross and Ross 1984). The latter holds true in particular for adolescents whose impaired self-image and loss of autonomy and control, coupled with fear of peer reactions and loss of academic work, may lead to absenteeism and, consequently, to social isolation (Klopovich *et al.* 1981). Even in children who are not school phobic, absenteeism is a significant problem. In a study conducted in 1975 in Kansas, the authors found that 67% of their large study population were absent from school for more than four weeks per year for no apparent reason (Lansky *et al.* 1975).

Academic Achievement of Survivors of Childhood Cancer

Further support for the significance of preventative intervention designed to facilitate the re-entry of children with cancer into the school is derived from studies that investigate the academic achievement of survivors of childhood cancer. Although, in general, findings are quite optimistic and suggest that there are no overall differences in self-esteem of young adult survivors of childhood cancer as compared to their siblings (e.g., Evans and Radford 1995) and matched controls (e.g., Sloper, Larcombe and Charlton 1994), and although, in general, the survivors of childhood cancer were coping well in their adult life, 75% of survivors of childhood cancer reported that their education had suffered as a result of their illness. Some traced the difficulties of their re-entry into the school to the lack of communication between teachers, parents and the medical staff (Evans and Radford 1995). Furthermore, survivors of childhood cancer were significantly less likely to go on to higher education (16 years plus) than their siblings (Evans and Radford 1995) and were more likely to be placed in special education classes than their siblings (Haupt *et al.* 1994).

Factors that Interfere with the Successful Return to School of Children with Cancer

There are many factors that interfere with the child's successful return to school. Some of the problems are associated with parents, teachers, peers and the child (e.g., Ross and Scarvalone 1982).

Problems associated with parents

Problems associated with parents stem from their own fears about separation and about the child's safety and health (McCarthy, Williams and Plumer 1998). Some parents have a tendency to ignore problems related to the child's absenteeism and may even encourage it. Others are very concerned about the child's poor school attendance, but have difficulty in enforcing discipline. They feel helpless, frustrated and in constant conflict with the child due to their own unresolved guilt feelings about the child's disease (McCarthy, Williams and Plumer 1998). Other parents are reluctant to share information about the nature of the disease with school personnel and the child's classmates (Ross and Scarvalone 1982). They fear that exposing the child's disease may arouse negative reactions from peers and teachers (McCollum 1975). Parents, overwhelmed and burdened by the illness, its treatment and the threat to the child's life in the present, do not focus on the child's potential to achieve in the future. Children sense their parents' lack of confidence in their ability and react with disillusionment, helplessness and anger (Katz *et al.* 1977). The end result is overprotection by the parents and a discriminatory or preferential attitude by school personnel (McCollum 1975).

Problems associated with teachers

Problems associated with teachers derive from their misconceptions, their lack of knowledge about childhood cancer, and their own personal biases. The teacher is expected to share responsibility for the child's care upon his return to school; however, the teacher is neither trained nor emotionally prepared to deal with this responsibility. In many cases, the teacher has little knowledge about childhood cancer, its treatment and prognosis, and can neither understand nor accept the frequent absences and changes in physical appearance of the child (Kaplan, Smith and Grobstein 1974). Teachers may struggle with their own personal biases and experiences with cancer which, at times, evoke images of death and the futility of treatment. This pessimistic outlook may affect the teacher's ability to successfully manage the child's return to school, becoming overly lenient with the child's academic performance, sending the message that s/he does not have to make an effort, lowering expectations and performance, and reinforcing the already impaired self-image. The teacher, burdened by the responsibility of caring for the child and insecure about how to deal with medical emergencies, feels trapped and overwhelmed. The teacher's lack of knowledge of what to expect of the child physically and academically can lead to the child's exclusion from class activities, leading to social isolation (Ross and Scarvalone 1982).

Problems associated with peers

Problems associated with peer reactions stem from their lack of knowledge about their classmate's illness. They often have myths and misconceptions about cancer which can affect their reactions to their sick friend (Sach 1980). Data suggest that children and adolescents with cancer are more likely to be perceived by their peers as more socially isolated, sick, fatigued, and often absent from school even after treatment has ended (Noll *et al.* 1990, 1991, 1993).

The teacher, unable to deal with his/her own insecurities and misconceptions, is unable to reassure the classmates, to help them to understand the long absences from school and the changes in physical appearance. If the teacher is lenient with the child with cancer, peers may react negatively, isolating and alienating the child even further (Ross and Scarvalone 1982).

Problems associated with the child

There are also difficulties associated with the child which may interfere with a smooth return to school. Firstly, there are medical factors that contribute to absenteeism, such as: (a) chemotherapy regimens, (b) hospitalization, (c) routine follow-up, (d) stage of the disease, (e) infection, and (f) chicken pox in the classroom (Ross and Scarvalone 1982). Other factors are associated with invisible side effects of chemotherapy, such as nausea, fatigue and neutropenia, visible side effects, such as hair loss or weight fluctuations (Katz *et al.* 1992, Varni *et al.* 1994), or treatment-induced learning disabilities, such as a reduced level of concentration or memory deficits (Rubenstein, Varni and Katz 1990). In addition, there are psychosocial factors that contribute to the child's refusal to attend school. The child is burdened by the threat of a recently diagnosed cancer, heightened by an impaired self-image. The low self-image is derived from the side effects of chemotherapy which alter physical appearance, such as hair loss, weight fluctuations or loss of limb through amputation. These emotional difficulties are aggravated by a fear of being rejected and teased by peers (Ross and Ross 1984) and by a loss of academic work and fears that s/he cannot keep up with schoolmates (Ross and Scarvalone 1982).

The possible stigma associated with children with cancer highlights the risk of a self-fulfilling prophecy placing them at risk for social isolation and alienation even after treatment has ended (Vannatta *et al.* 1998). In line with concerns that children with cancer are perceived by peers as having psychological problems and of being socially isolated, children with cancer, especially those who have a higher level of behavioral problems, are more likely to view themselves as having lower levels of scholastic competence, lower levels of close, confiding friendships and lower levels of social acceptance from peers (Sloper, Larcombe and Charlton 1994), perceiving themselves as more socially isolated and exhibiting more shy and anxious behavior patterns (Noll *et al.* 1993). The end result is that the child may dislike school, resort to absenteeism (Lansky and Cairns, 1979a) or drop out of school to avoid situations that heighten feelings of insecurity. All these misconceptions may lead to negative personality changes, low motivation, underachievement, social isolation, negative attitudes toward school, excessive absenteeism and, eventually, school phobia (Lansky *et al.* 1975, Klopovich *et al.* 1981).

Protective Factors that Enhance Mental Health

Recent studies investigating the psychosocial adjustment of pediatric cancer patients have resulted in mixed findings. Some studies suggest that these children are at high risk for psychosocial problems both during and after treatment (e.g., Vannatta *et al.* 1998), while other studies have reported no such effect (e.g., Kazak and Meadows 1989). Discrepant findings among studies addressing the adaptation of youth with cancer may be the result of methodological and design variables: (a) source of information – self, teacher or peers – and (b) the specific instrument employed – questionnaires or clinical interviews. While self-reporting questionnaires are likely to yield a remarkable positive picture (Puukko *et al.* 1997) due to social desirability and/or defensive denial (Gray *et al.* 1992), clinical interviews suggest impairments in the psychological wellbeing of survivors of childhood cancer (Fritz and Williams 1988). Another interpretation that may explain the observed variability in the individual adaptation of pediatric cancer patients is mediating or protective factors, such as self-esteem and social support (Varni and Wallander 1988, Varni *et al.* 1994, Varni and Katz 1997).

Peer support

Empirical findings identify mainly two protective factors that buffer children from the negative emotional sequelae of cancer. The first, most consistent predictor of the psychological adaptation of children with cancer is perceived classmate support. Peer support was consistently and significantly associated with psychological adjustment measures at a greater magnitude than other perceived social support domains, namely that of parents and teachers. Higher perceived social support was associated with fewer depressive symptoms, lower state, trait and social anxiety, higher general self-esteem, and lower acting-out behavior (Varni *et al.* 1994), and a lower perception of stressors associated with cancer and the side effects of chemotherapy yielding a lower negative affectivity score (Varni and Katz 1997). These empirical findings are in line with theoretical works that identify peer relations as playing a central role in children's social and emotional development (e.g., Sullivan 1953). Peer relations are viewed as fundamental for the development of adequate social skills and for the emergence of a healthy self-concept (Bukowski and Hoza 1989). These notions hold true for children and adolescents in general and for pediatric cancer patients in particular. The ability to maintain social relationships during the illness was identified as an important factor in the long-term adjustment of survivors of childhood cancer (O'Malley, Foster and Koocher 1979).

School attendance

The second protective factor identified by empirical findings as an excellent predictor for psychological adjustment of children with cancer is school attendance. Children who missed more school days had a lower adjustment rate and more stressors associated with cancer. The more integrated into the school setting the child with cancer, the more likely that s/he will perceive as less stressful cancer-related stressors, such as hair loss, nausea, fatigue, pain, and weight fluctuations, and the more likely to keep up with school assignments, have more friends, share feelings, be happy and content, and display positive thinking and enhanced self-image (Hockenberry-Eaton, Manteuffel and Bottomley 1997).

These findings highlight the significance of interventions designed to facilitate the return of children with cancer to school to prevent psychological maladjustment. School represents the work of children and the opportunity for socialization and social support. For the child newly diagnosed with cancer, continuation of social and academic activities as early as is medically feasible provides an important opportunity to normalize as much as possible an ongoing stressful experience by focusing on the healthy aspects of life. These findings suggest that peer support is not only critical in the psychosocial adjustment of the child but it also facilitates return to school. When the perceived social support of the classmates is low, not only may the child feel depressed and exhibit low self-esteem, but he may also avoid school altogether. Children who are poorly accepted by their peers are more likely to manifest school adjustment problems and are at a greater risk for long-term maladjustment (Parker and Asher 1987).

The implications of these findings cannot be overstated. Peer support and school attendance are the two most important facets of preventive intervention since they are crucial for the child's normal socialization and positive adaptation. In this context, preventive intervention designed to facilitate the smooth return of pediatric cancer patients to school and the opening of channels of communication between children with cancer, their classmates and teachers is of the utmost importance.

Preventive intervention for pediatric cancer patients in the school falls into the realm of primary prevention designed to promote emotional wellbeing and psychological adjustment (Joint Commission on Mental Illness and Health 1961, Caplan 1964), and to promote their mental health and quality of life. Implications of these findings are two-fold: (a) the significance of intervention in the school to promote academic and psychosocial adjustment of children with cancer is highlighted, and (b) preventive intervention designed to facilitate the return to school must be comprehensive and address the concerns of children with cancer, their parents, teachers and classmates.

SURVEY OF SCHOOL INTERVENTION PROGRAMS FOR CHILDREN WITH CANCER

Introduction

School is an important facet of children's lives. It is a critical psychological goal for children in general and for children with cancer in particular. Consequently, school is a crucial area of concern in the comprehensive treatment of children with cancer for many reasons. Firstly, it is important for these children to maintain their pre-illness level of academic achievement to become productive adults. Secondly, children with cancer, like all children, need normal peer contacts and a social life to help them become mature adults (Bukowski and Hoza 1989). Finally, regular school attendance and participation in regular intellectual and social activities counterbalance anxiety and depression in children diagnosed with cancer (Noll et al. 1991).

Regular school attendance by children with cancer is considered to be the primary measurable parameter of rehabilitation (Hockenberry-Eaton, Manteuffel and Bottomley 1997). It is an anchor emphasizing the healthy aspects of children's lives; it instates hope and enables planning for the future. Klopovich et al. (1981) enumerated the following contributions of school attendance to the wellbeing of children with cancer: (a) provides social contacts with peers, (b) boosts morale, (c) counterbalances boredom, (d) maintains dignity, and (e) normalizes life. All these assets are facilitating factors which promote the quality of life of children with cancer and enhance their mental health. Children who are denied continued school participation are denied a major opportunity to engage in age-appropriate goal-oriented behavior, which may lead to hopelessness, learned helplessness and despair (Katz 1980, Deasy-Spinetta and Spinetta 1981, Lansky, Cairns and Zwartjes 1983). The accompanying social isolation experienced by children with cancer has been related to problems in adaptation to the disease (Varni and Katz 1987, Katz, Dolgin and Varni 1990, Katz et al. 1992, Hockenberry-Eaton, Manteuffel and Bottomley 1997).

In the 1980s, realizing the significance of regular school attendance by children with cancer, the American Cancer Society funded research projects designed to develop school intervention programs to ease the return of children with cancer to school and to identify cognitive dysfunction that might be due to treatment. This explains the abundance of school intervention programs, each with its unique characteristics, throughout the USA and Europe (Deasy-Spinetta 1993). However, in 1997, realizing that return to school of children with cancer could not be taken for granted, the Leukemia Society of America made the development of school re-entry programs a top priority (McCarthy, Williams and Plumer 1998).

Survey of School Intervention Programs

The objectives of most intervention programs are: (a) to open channels of communication between the child, parents, hospital staff, school personnel and peers, (b) to safeguard academic progress and peer relations, (c) to facilitate a smooth return to school, and (d) to prevent delayed psychosocial difficulties. Table 17.1 describes a representative sample of school programs to date.

As soon as the child is diagnosed as having cancer, the child's teacher is contacted and a school conference is scheduled with school personnel, either in the hospital (Klopovich *et al.* 1981, Ross and Scarvalone 1982, Deasy-Spinetta 1993, Gregory, Parker and Craft 1994, Evans and Radford 1995, Larcombe and Charlton 1996) or in the school (Katz *et al.* 1992, Baysinger *et al.* 1993, Häcker, Klemm and Böpple 1995, McCarthy, Williams and Plumer 1998, Whitsett, Pelletier and Scott-Lane 1999). The scheduled school conference is conducted, in general, between a hospital interdisciplinary team, such as the hospital teacher, pediatric oncology nurse and team psychologist, and school personnel, such as the school nurse, teacher counselor and principal (e.g., Evans and Radford 1995). The pediatric oncology nurse (e.g., McCarthy, Williams and Plumer 1998) or the pediatric hematologist (Deasy-Spinetta 1993) provides information about the child's specific disease, treatment options, expected side effects and realistic prognosis. The hospital psychologist suggests how to deal with peer reactions and encourages maintaining contact with the child during prolonged absences (e.g., Evans and Radford 1995).

Some school intervention programs identified liaison professionals to play a central role in the implementation of school intervention. Deasy-Spinetta (1993) identified the classroom teacher, the school psychologist and the school counselor as playing a pivotal role in facilitating the school intervention program. Klopovich *et al.* (1981) preferred the school nurse to play a valuable role in the reintegration of the child with cancer into the school for three reasons: (a) the school nurse is the source of information for health-related issues, (b) the authors report findings which suggest that the school nurse is the most pessimistic with respect to the child's prognosis, and (c) the school nurse is the best trained to deal with medical problems that may occur, such as bleeding, fever and chickenpox exposure. Other authors have designated the hospital teacher as the liaison between the hospital and the school (e.g., Häcker, Klemm and Böpple 1995). The liaison person is in charge of setting up the school conference and periodic follow-up visits to the school. Katz *et al.* (1992) identified the hospital pediatric psychologist as the one to open channels of communication between the hospital and the school. S/he is in charge of setting up the conference in the child's school with the teacher, focusing on the child's medical and psychosocial concerns, such as school attendance, grades and discipline. Other authors delegated this role to the pediatric oncology nurse (e.g., Baysinger *et al.* 1993, McCarthy, Williams and Plumer 1998), while

Table 17.1 School intervention programs for pediatric cancer patients in the USA, Canada and Europe

Authors	Mode of intervention			Focus of intervention				Location of intervention		Liaison personnel	Evaluation
	School conference	Class presentation	Day seminar	Child	Parent	School personnel	Peers	Hospital	School		
Lansky and Cairns (1979)	×			×	×	×				Educational counselor	
Sach (1980)			×								Overall improvement in school attendance
Klopovich et al. (1981)	×					×	×	×		School nurse, nurse clinician	Increased knowledge, dispelled fears, increased confidence, positive feedback
Ross and Scarvalone (1982)			×			×		×		Social worker	
Katz et al. (1992)	×	×		×	×	×	×		×	Hospital pediatric psychologist	Positive feedback from children, parents and teachers
Deasy-Spinetta (1993) Adamoli et al. (1997)	×	×		×	×	×	×	×	×	School teacher, counselor or psychologist	Regular school attendance
Baysinger et al. (1993)	×			×	×	×	×	×	×	Pediatric oncology nurse	Positive feedback from children, parents, peers and teachers
Gregory, Parker and Craft (1994)			×		×	×		×		Community nurses and social workers	Smooth reintegration into the school
Häcker, Klemm and Böpple (1995)	×			×	×	×	×		×	Hospital teacher	Enhanced confidence and knowledge of teachers and peers
Larcombe and Charlton (1996)		×	×			×		×			Enhanced knowledge and confidence
Cleave and Charlton (1997)			×			×		(University)			Enhanced teacher confidence
McCarthy, Williams and Plumer (1998)	×	×		×	×	×	×		×	Pediatric oncology nurse	Positive feedback, some original concerns resolved, new emerged
Whitsett, Pelletier and Scott-Lane (1999)		×		×	×	×	×		×		

still others identified the teacher counselor (e.g., Sach 1980, Deasy-Spinetta 1993) or social worker (Ross and Scarvalone 1982) as the one to implement school intervention, whether at home or in the school.

Some school intervention programs focus not only on the child and school personnel but also on the concerns of parents and siblings. A school re-entry program implemented in Alberta Children's Hospital in Alberta, Canada, includes, in addition to school conferences with teachers, workshops for parents and siblings to facilitate the return of the child with cancer to school (Whitsett, Pelletier and Scott-Lane 1999).

Some comprehensive school intervention programs not only address the concerns of the child, parents and teachers, but also focus on the needs of the child's classmates (Katz et al. 1992, Baysinger et al. 1993, Häcker, Klemm and Böpple 1995, Adamoli et al. 1997, McCarthy, Williams and Plumer 1998, Whitsett, Pelletier and Scott-Lane 1999). The presentation in the child's classroom begins with discussing the classmates' experiences with cancer, followed by information about childhood cancer according to the developmental phase of the children. Emphasis is placed on some basic facts, such as that the disease is treatable and not contagious. The peers are encouraged to keep in touch and support their sick friend (Katz et al. 1992). Häcker, Klemm and Böpple (1995) and Adamoli et al. (1997) reported that a physician visits the child's school and provides information about childhood cancer to the classmates. Whitsett, Pelletier and Scott-Lane (1999) relate that, because of recent budget constraints, their visits to schools have been discontinued and, instead, a handbook entitled 'Childhood Cancer, School Re-Entry' is sent to each school to assist teachers in managing the child with cancer safely back to school.

All school intervention programs are implemented after permission is received from the parents and the child with cancer. The child with cancer is involved in some intervention programs (Katz et al. 1992) and, although they are encouraged to attend the class presentation, most abstain (McCarthy, Williams and Plumer 1998).

Instead of a school conference, a few school intervention programs entail a one-day seminar conducted for school personnel in the hospital. One such program was initiated as early as 1978 by Ross and Scarvalone. The authors identified the social worker to play a principal role in the implementation of the one-day seminar. The objectives of the seminar were to (a) increase the participants' knowledge about childhood cancer, (b) to increase their confidence to deal with the child with cancer upon his return to school, and (c) to increase their ability to share information with classmates. The one-day seminar consisted of frontal lectures followed by small-group discussions and a tour of the pediatric cancer facility.

Larcombe and Charlton (1996), like Ross and Scarvalone (1982), have conducted study days for teachers. The first part of the seminar consisted of information about childhood cancer provided by hospital staff, and the second part consisted of small-group discussions on either the teachers' personal experiences with cancer or on relevant topics dealing with prevention of cancer, such as smoking, sun exposure, etc.

All the authors conducting school intervention programs report favorable outcomes. Some studies report positive feedback from parents, children and teachers (Katz *et al.* 1992, Baysinger *et al.* 1993, McCarthy, Williams and Plumer 1998). Other studies suggest an increase in the teacher's confidence (Häcker, Klemm and Böpple 1995, Cleave and Charlton 1997) and knowledge (Ross and Scarvalone 1982, Larcombe and Charlton 1996), and increased optimism and alleviation of fears (Ross and Scarvalone 1982). The most significant finding of school intervention programs is the smooth reintegration of the child with cancer back into the school (Gregory, Parker and Craft 1994) and improved school attendance (Klopovich *et al.* 1981, Adamoli *et al.* 1997).

PREVENTIVE INTERVENTION IN THE SCHOOL FOR CHILDREN WITH CANCER: THE RAMBAM MEDICAL CENTER EXPERIENCE

Theoretical Background

The Perceived Personal Control Crisis Model

Preventive intervention is based on a theoretical model of crisis that has received empirical and theoretical verification (Tadmor 1984, Tadmor and Brandes 1984, Tadmor, Brandes and Hofman 1987). The theoretical crisis model is a synthesis derived from Lazarus' (1968) notion of idiosyncratic perception of the stressor and Caplan's (1964) notion of availability of a coping response that mediates between the individual's appraisal of the event and his response to it. The theoretical crisis model, denoted as the Perceived Personal Control (PPC) Crisis Model, explains the locus and intensity of crisis as a function of the PPC of the individual. It is assumed that the potential benefit of the PPC is derived from a combination of perceived control on the cognitive, emotional and behavioral levels. The PPC model has significant implications for crisis intervention. It calls for manipulation of situational variables, such as natural and organized support systems, information, anticipatory guidance, and the person's share in the decision-making process, as well as task-oriented activity geared to enhancing emotional, cognitive and behavioral control of the individual, respectively.

The PPC model adheres to the goals of primary prevention, namely preventing emotional dysfunction in a population free of psychiatric symptomatology, and implies intervention on two distinct but complementary levels: (a) preventive intervention administered by a network of natural and organized support systems, denoted as Personal Interaction, and (b) introduction of changes in policies, structures and allocation of resources and services in the relevant departments conducive to positive mental health, referred to as Social Action (Caplan 1964).

The PPC Preventive Intervention Model has been implemented at Rambam Medical Center in Haifa, Israel, since 1980, and has been successfully applied to the following populations at risk from a mental health point of view: (a) caesarean birth mothers (Tadmor 1984, 1988, Tadmor and Brandes 1984, Tadmor, Brandes and Hofman 1987); (b) mothers of premature infants (Tadmor and Brandes 1986); (c) mothers encountering neonatal death (Tadmor 1986); (d) medical staff dealing with terminally ill patients (Tadmor 1987); (e) children undergoing elective surgery and their parents (Tadmor *et al.* 1987), and (f) children with leukemia (Tadmor and Weyl Ben Arush 2000). In 1986, the PPC Preventive Intervention Model for caesarean birth population and pediatric surgery patients was selected by the American Psychological Association (APA) Task Force on Promotion, Prevention and Intervention Alternatives in Psychology as an exemplary model with another 13 primary prevention models and published in 1988 in a casebook for practitioners (Price *et al.* 1988).

Preventive intervention based on the PPC model for children with cancer and their parents

Preventive intervention based on the PPC model is one of the emerging preventive technologies (Gullotta 1987, Swift and Levin 1987). It empowers people by increasing control over their lives by either competence building or by modifying institutional practices that contribute to dysfunctional outcomes for the target population that is the focus of the preventive intervention. Thus, the PPC preventive intervention is both preventive and empowering, since mental health promotion activities are clearly empowering as well as preventive (Swift and Levin 1987). In this chapter, a comprehensive preventive intervention on both counts for pediatric cancer patients is presented, with particular emphasis on preventive intervention in the school. Preventive intervention is implemented by an interdisciplinary staff designed to answer the specific concerns of children with cancer, their parents, siblings, teachers and peers. The interdisciplinary staff consists of psychologists, social workers, art and music therapists, hospital teachers, teacher counselor and volunteers who empower the child and parents, each in his/her area of expertise to deal with the threatening disease and its emotional sequelae.

The content of preventive intervention is to enhance emotional, cognitive and behavioral control of pediatric cancer patients. Emotional control is achieved by convening a network of support systems around the pediatric cancer patient, consisting of natural supports, such as the parents and peers, and organized supports, including an interdisciplinary staff and survivors of childhood cancer. Cognitive control is achieved by the provision of information with respect to diagnosis, treatment options and medical tests, anticipatory guidance with respect to expected side effects of chemotherapy and a share in the decision-making process with respect to timing medical tests, starting treatment, preferred ways of induction of anesthesia, etc. Behavioral control is attained by task-oriented activities, making the child an active participant in his/her treatment and recovery process. Activities include caring for the Broviac catheter, taking the medication, patient-controlled analgesia, employing relaxation, guided imagery and problem-solving techniques, and reintegration into the school system as soon as is medically feasible.

Mental health services consist of crisis intervention and supportive counseling. In most instances, the psychologist attends the session when the pediatric hemato-oncologist imparts the diagnosis to the child. In the initial phase of diagnosis, a considerable amount of time is spent with the parents and the child and siblings to assist them in assimilating and coping with the threatening situation. In addition, a series of 6–8 workshops are conducted for parents and children by an interdisciplinary staff on relevant topics such as: (a) childhood cancer and treatment options; (b) expected side effects of chemotherapy; (c) psychological coping with cancer; (d) siblings' coping; (e) significance of school attendance; (f) nutrition; (g) innovative treatments, such as bone marrow transplantation, and (h) encounters with pediatric cancer survivors.

Follow-up of the child and his/her parents is conducted during hospitalization and day-care treatment, as well as during the maintenance phase and the medical follow-up in the outpatient clinic. Psychological intervention is more intensive during the initial phase of diagnosis and the induction phase, and as needed during continuation of treatment. At times of crises, relapse or the terminal phase, psychological intervention is considerably more intensive.

Preventive intervention is complemented by a series of changes in policies in the Department of Pediatric Hemato-Oncology, designed to promote the mental health of pediatric cancer patients. Great care is taken to differentiate between necessary pain and unnecessarily painful procedures. In order to reduce pain and ameliorate fears associated with invasive medical procedures, such as bone marrow transplantation (BMT), bone biopsy (BB) and lumbar puncture (LP), a combination of psychological preparation and pharmacological agents is employed. The psychological preparation consists of anticipatory guidance coupled with relaxation and guided imagery techniques and parental presence. The pharmacological preparation employed consists of conscious sedation by administration of Midazolam through the Broviac or Port catheter by the pediatric hemato-oncologist for LP, and deep sedation administered by a pediatric anesthesiologist for BMA and BB. Changes in the policies of the departments catering to pediatric cancer patients to foster positive mental health are discussed elsewhere (Tadmor and Weyl Ben Arush 2000).

Preventive Intervention in the School

Historical perspective

Preventive intervention in the school is one facet of a comprehensive preventive intervention approach for pediatric cancer patients. The general objective of preventive intervention in the school is to open channels of communication between hospital staff, parents, children, school personnel and classmates. As early as 1982, a school conference was scheduled in the hematology outpatient clinic between an interdisciplinary hospital staff consisting of a pediatric oncology nurse, a hospital-based psychologist and a social worker, and school personnel which included the child's teacher, school nurse and guidance counselor. The conference was initiated with the permission of the parents and the child. The purpose of the school conference was to exchange information about the child. The school personnel updated the hospital staff about the child's academic and social status, while the hospital team imparted information about leukemia, its treatment and side effects. School personnel were made aware that the child would be absent from school for some six to seven months because of the side effects of chemotherapy, such as immunosuppression and aggressive treatment regimens. In light of these constraints, a coordinated plan of action was set in motion to care for the child's academic and psychosocial needs. Subsidized interim tutoring at home or in the hospital was initiated. This service was enabled by a series of laws enacted to safeguard the scholastic achievements of pediatric cancer patients. The Ministry of Education makes it mandatory for each school to provide from three to four hours weekly of homebound instruction. Additional interim instruction in computers is provided by a private organization subsidized by the Ministry of Education, and an additional six weekly hours of tutoring are supplemented by the Israel Cancer Association. The teachers are encouraged to reinforce continuous peer contact and support while the hospital staff see to it that the child attends class as soon as medically feasible. An ongoing follow-up system was established, keeping channels of communication open between the hospital staff and school personnel.

By 1986, the pediatric oncologist conducted occasional presentations in the class of the sick child. However, only in 1995, when a teacher counselor joined the pediatric hemato-oncology unit, did preventive intervention in the school become institutionalized and systematic, benefiting every pediatric cancer patient.

The following are the specific objectives of preventive intervention in the school for children with cancer, their parents, school personnel and peers:

Objectives of preventive intervention for children with cancer

1. Promote mental health and enhance quality of life
2. Promote a positive educational experience and facilitate the child's reintegration into the school setting (Baysinger *et al.* 1993)
3. Enhance peer support (Sloper, Larcombe and Charlton 1994, Varni *et al.* 1994, Hockenberry-Eaton, Manteuffel and Bottomley 1997)
4. Reduce stress associated with cancer and its treatment (Varni and Katz 1997)
5. Safeguard academic achievements
6. Master the environment and develop positive attitudes about themselves and their future (Polland 1985)
7. Prevent alienation and social isolation
8. Encourage regular school attendance
9. Encourage the child's confidence to deal with peer reactions
10. Assess the child's specific academic needs and assist in their implementation (Katz *et al.* 1992)

Objectives of preventive intervention for parents

1. Increase their knowledge about childhood cancer
2. Increase their confidence about their child's safety in the school (Baysinger *et al.* 1993, McCarthy, Williams and Plumer 1998)
3. Encourage parents to disclose child's illness
4. Encourage parents to allow children to return to school
5. Encourage parents to focus on the child's future potential (Evans and Radford 1995)
6. Alleviate parents' guilt and empower them to enforce discipline and regular school attendance (Evans and Radford 1995)

Objectives of preventive intervention for school personnel

1. Enhance their knowledge about childhood cancer
2. Encourage teachers to have realistic expectations about the child's prognosis
3. Increase sensitivity in dealing with the academic, emotional and physical reactions of the child with cancer (Häcker, Klemm and Böpple 1995)
4. Increase confidence to deal with issues such as discipline, grades and absenteeism
5. Encourage realistic expectations with respect to the child's academic abilities and performance
6. Increase confidence to deal with reactions and issues raised by classmates

7. Increase awareness of the teachers' personal experiences and biases regarding cancer (Larcombe and Charlton 1996)

Objectives of preventive intervention for classmates

1. Enhance peer empathy and support
2. Enhance knowledge about childhood cancer, clarify misconceptions (Sach 1980)
3. Dispel myths and alleviate fears (Ross and Scarvalone 1982)
4. Dissipate rumors
5. Allow peers to express their feelings

Preventive Intervention for School Personnel

When the child is initially diagnosed as having cancer, his/her teacher is contacted by the teacher counselor and a meeting is scheduled in the pediatric hemato-oncology department. The conference is attended by the pediatric hemato-oncologist, the psychologist, social worker and teacher counselor. The school personnel includes the child's teacher, school counselor, school nurse and, occasionally, the school principal.

The school conference focuses on an exchange of information about the child's academic, medical and psychological status. Topics such as childhood cancer, treatment options and expected side effects are discussed. Teachers are made aware of the realistic challenges associated with the child's reintegration process, as well as the dangers entailed in school absenteeism for the mental health of the child with cancer. Issues such as discipline, grading, peer reactions and management of typical situations that may be encountered when the child returns to school are raised. Furthermore, a realistic expectation about the child's progress is provided. This issue is particularly important since teachers who have a pessimistic outlook about the child's chances to survive are likely to refrain from making any demands on attendance and performance. This attitude will be internalized by the child, impairing his/her chances for continued academic progress. In this context, teachers are encouraged to be aware of their own biases, to treat the child as a regular child and to have realistic expectations about academic performance. Teachers are encouraged to maintain ongoing contact between the child and the classmates, and emphasis is placed on the significance of continuous peer support and regular school attendance, not only on the academic aspects of the child's life but also on his/her psychosocial adjustment in the long run. At the same time, we impress upon teachers that children should be reintegrated into their original classes. At the end of the conference, the school personnel receive written material about relevant topics and a date is set for a class presentation in the school. The duration of the school conference is about an hour and a half.

Preventive Intervention for Classmates

At the scheduled date, the interdisciplinary hospital team, consisting of a pediatric hemato-oncologist, a pediatric oncology nurse, a mental health expert and the teacher counselor arrive at the child's school for a class presentation. The child is involved in the class presentation and encouraged to attend with his parents and siblings. The class discussion begins with an airing some of the peer concerns about childhood cancer, allowing the peers to express their feelings and to ask relevant questions. The pediatrician provides information about childhood cancer, differentiating it from adult cancer. Topics such as treatment procedures and expected side effects such as hair loss, weight fluctuations, immunosuppression, and the Broviac catheter are discussed. The mental health expert deals with the children's death fears, and dispels rumors and misconceptions associated with cancer, such as it being contagious, and the threat of imminent death. The children are encouraged to express their concern and are encouraged to keep in touch with the sick child by frequent visits and telephone calls. At times, the child him/herself will express concerns, such as infrequent visits by friends and the fear of being abandoned. S/he may be willing to show his/her Broviac catheter to friends and answer some of their questions. A videotape on the experiences of a childhood cancer survivor is screened. In the last session of the class presentation, the teacher counselor asks the classmates to organize into groups and to draw pictures or write poems for their friend to take home. The sick child is also involved in this informal creative endeavor. At the end of the session, s/he receives the finished products made by his/her friends. The duration of the class presentation is about two hours. The teacher counselor who serves as a liaison between the hospital and the school maintains periodic follow-up concerning the child's school attendance record and scholastic progress.

EVALUATION OF PREVENTIVE INTERVENTION IN THE SCHOOL FOR CHILDREN WITH CANCER

Introduction

In the last five years, we have conducted 70 systematic school conferences and class presentations, from kindergarten to high school. We have received positive feedback from everyone involved – children, parents, school personnel and classmates. Moreover, class presentations are perceived as a positive and rewarding experience by the hospital staff involved in their implementation. Systematic follow-up conducted by the teacher counselor who serves as a liaison between the hospital and the school reveals regular school attendance by all children with cancer who can attend school, except for one girl who insisted on joining a lower grade and had social difficulties initially.

We have witnessed a remarkable evolutionary process in which various segments of the Israeli community have opened up and are willing to deal with cancer facts, thereby reducing the stigma associated with cancer and fostering more positive attitudes toward survivors of childhood cancer. We have reached Arab and orthodox Jewish populations who, traditionally, were reluctant to disclose issues that were considered secret and private. This openness in the Israeli community facilitates not only a smoother reintegration of children with cancer back into the school system, it gradually fosters more positive and optimistic cancer-related attitudes.

An Illustrative Case Study

A case study of a 17-year-old Christian Arab boy can serve as an illustrative evaluation of preventive intervention in the school. M. was 8 years old when he was diagnosed in 1990 as having acute lymphoblastic leukemia (ALL). He received the Berlin-Frankfurt-Munster (BFM) protocol for pediatric ALL patients (Reiter *et al.* 1994), attained remission and within six months, during the maintenance phase, returned to his original class. When M. was initially diagnosed as having ALL, the bibliotherapist contacted his school and met with the head nun and principal of the school, updating them with respect to M.'s diagnosis and treatment, and encouraged maintaining open channels of communication between the school and the hospital. M. received intermittent tutoring at home and had no difficulties returning to his class. He was a bright and sensitive boy who established good rapport with the hospital-based psychologist. He freely and openly discussed his feelings of anger, hope and belief in God. At the end of 1992, he encountered a testicular relapse. He received intensive chemotherapy and radiation therapy that lasted for about one year. At this time he visited school less frequently due to treatments, hospitalization, fatigue, nausea and immunosuppression. Yet, all this time he received homebound instruction and maintained relationships with his peers. In December 1995, at the age of 13, M. encountered bone marrow relapse and underwent allogeneic bone marrow transplantation. Due to the bone marrow transplantation and follow-up treatments, M. was absent from school throughout 1996. During all this time, however, he continued studying at home with a teacher assigned by the Ministry of Education and he passed the exams with his classmates. Periodic telephone and written communications with the head nun were maintained. It was during this period of time that M. started writing poems, expressing his fears and hopes. In September 1996, although he had missed a year of schooling, he joined his original classmates in the 9th grade, doing well in school, keeping up with the educational assignments in the classroom and continuing tutorial services at home. M. was loved by friends who kept in touch with him throughout his illness, relapse and treatment.

In May 1998, at the age of 16, M. encountered a third relapse in the bone marrow. This time, in contrast to previous relapses, he became depressed and anxious, refusing to see his friends and to attend school even when it was medically feasible. The social and emotional isolation that he encountered mirror research findings that suggest that cancer is a more difficult challenge for adolescent patients than for school-age children. It apparently interferes less with the psychological tasks of infancy than with those of adolescence (Koocher *et al.* 1980). These studies highlight the significance of physical appearance as a predictor for depressive symptoms, social anxiety being mediated by self-esteem in adolescence (Varni *et al.* 1995, Pendley, Dahlquist and Dreyer, 1997). Adolescence is a developmental phase where autonomy, control and self-identity are valued. The adolescent is likely to be concerned with body image, peer relations, emerging sexuality and vocational plans for the future, all complicated by cancer and its treatment. In line with these notions, M. became extremely self-conscious and embarrassed by his physical appearance, due to visible body changes such as loss of hair and eyebrows. He was thin, pale and short for his age. He felt lonely, stigmatized, threatened by the aggressive nature of leukemia and saddened that his life was again disrupted. M. was irritable and depressed. His belief in God was unshattered, but he felt abandoned. He felt he was losing control and becoming dependent and helpless. He feared emotional and social isolation and expressed death fears. Valuing learning more than anything else, he feared that a loss of scholastic achievement endangered his vocational plans for the future. He expressed lower self-worth and impaired self-image. He felt different and lost confidence in interpersonal relationships. He gradually withdrew from all social activities and became isolated from his life-long friends. He became overburdened by his increased dependency on his parents and concerned that he was a source of continued worry for them, fearing for their own wellbeing. He revealed uncertainty and ambiguity about the future and resented the restrictions and limitations imposed on him.

In order to counterbalance the psychosocial difficulties encountered by M., in September 1998, a class presentation was scheduled at his school with the permission of M. and his parents. An interdisciplinary team, consisting of a pediatric oncology nurse, the hospital-based psychologist and a social worker attended the session with two 10th grade classes and their teachers. M. refused to attend the class presentation. The pediatric oncology nurse discussed leukemia, its treatment and expected visual and invisible side effects. She discussed the relapse of leukemia in M. and the treatment options for him. The psychologist discussed the psychological reactions typical during adolescence, such as body image, self-esteem affected by physical appearance, loss of autonomy, increased dependency needs and the threat of loss of academic standing and friends. Peers were encouraged to express their fears and concerns about M.'s health status and possible death, as well as their own psychological reactions. The social worker revealed M.'s affection toward his friends and encouraged them to keep in touch with him, and jointly discussing ways in which their assistance could be valuable, such as home visits, telephone calls, bringing homework, inviting him to parties and field trips. He encouraged them to accept M. the way he was although he may look different externally. At the end of the session, the classmates divided into groups of 3–4 students, drawing pictures and writing messages and letters to M.

A group of children took it upon themselves to bring the products of the creative endeavor to M. that very day. In the afternoon, his friends visited M. at home and shared information with him about new students and teachers in class. They discussed study material and M. felt that they treated him as an ordinary fellow. Before leaving, they assured him that if he did not show up in school the next day, they would come to fetch him. The next day, after an absence of six months, M. returned to school. His friends prepared a welcoming party for him. They sat in a circle and briefly discussed his ongoing treatments, then went on with their studies in an ordinary fashion. From that day on, M. attended classes for the rest of the 1998–1999 academic year.

The transformation was remarkable and instantaneous. Although he continued throughout 1998–1999 to receive chemotherapy once a month and his physical appearance remained the same, he attended school even on days that he did not feel well. Being a perfectionist, he studied hard and passed all exams with high marks. His spirits were high and he started writing love poems. He felt relieved that he had returned to school. He maintained that the class presentation gave him the necessary strength to confront his friends and he was relieved that they knew what he looked like without having to explain to each and every one of them separately. Consequently, there was nothing to separate him from his friends, allowing him to love and appreciate them, and to involve them in his subsequent treatments. He sat next to his friend in class and, from day one, had no more problems attending school. At first, he remained in class during recess, fearing the reaction of smaller children at school but, gradually, he overcame his shyness and embarrassment and he joined his friends in the schoolyard. M. attended field trips and parties where he read his poems to a cheering crowd. He walked the streets of his town and dared to enter the neighborhood store for the first time in many months. He felt free, confident and relieved. He felt that returning to school and to his friends had a positive effect not only on his morale, but also on his relationships with his siblings. He felt that teachers treated him as a regular student, with realistic expectations about his capabilities. With the approval of the Ministry of Education, matriculation exams were scheduled in chemistry and civil studies. M. passed with excellent grades.

His parents were also relieved that he had returned to school on a regular schedule. They saw the miraculous change in him after he returned to school and were appreciative and grateful. His peers felt that the provision of information about his illness answered their questions, alleviated their fears, enhanced their confidence and counterbalanced their guilt feelings, allowing them to be genuinely helpful.

In July 1999 during summer vacation, M. encountered a fourth bone marrow relapse. He accepted the situation surprisingly well, hoping that by September he would be able to resume his studies in the 11th grade. It was at that time that he drew a picture of a shining sun in the right-hand corner over a wavy blue sea. He explained that he was in the middle of the sea and his illness proceeded as waves, remission–relapse, remission–relapse, and so on. By August 1999, he knew that the chemotherapy was not being effective and that he would not be able to return to school in September. He expressed death fears that were addressed frankly and directly, alleviating his fears, comforting him and strengthening his belief in God and in the afterlife. He spent most of his time at home, and he and the hospital-based psychologist planned to publish a second volume of poems entitled 'Love Songs'.

M. died on September 27, 1999. After his death, the social worker returned to his classroom and discussed with his peers and teachers his unavoidable death since, this time, M. had not responded to treatment. He informed them that M. had died peacefully and painlessly, surrounded by his loved ones, at peace with himself, his family and his God.

CONCLUSIONS

Paradoxically, the improved survival of children with cancer has brought into focus new problems affecting their psychosocial adjustment, problems such as absenteeism, school performance, school anxiety, social isolation and the misconceptions of teachers and peers. Consequently, it is becoming increasingly evident that successful rehabilitation of the child with cancer demands comprehensive preventive intervention, focusing on all aspects of the child's life and not only on medical control of the disease as s/he moves on the continuum from diagnosis to subsequent school reintegration and rehabilitation.

Recent studies have suggested that school attendance, participation in school activities and peer support are mediating, buffering factors that affect the perception of the stressors associated with cancer and the child's psychosocial adjustment. The implications of these studies cannot be overstated. The more integrated the child is in the school setting, the more friends s/he has, the more likely that his/her quality of life and mental health are enhanced. These findings hold true not only in the short run but, indeed, in the long run; the adjustment of survivors of childhood cancer is affected by the extent to which the child was able to maintain social relationships during the illness (O'Malley et al. 1979). This data makes preventive intervention in the school an important facet of comprehensive preventive intervention designed to promote the mental health of children with cancer. Indeed, school attendance is both a marker and an etiological factor. In both cases, preventive intervention is indicated (Caplan, personal communication, April 2000).

School re-entry programs are, thus, cost-effective preventive interventions because they can prevent future scholastic and psychosocial problems for children with cancer. Consequently, it is recommended that preventive intervention in the school should be an integral part of the comprehensive treatment plan of pediatric hemato-oncology centers and should be provided to all newly diagnosed children with cancer. The preventive intervention program must be initiated as early as possible in the treatment. Clinical and empirical findings indicate that children who do not return to school early in their treatment find it increasingly difficult to be reintegrated at a later date (Katz, Dolgin and Varni 1990). This holds true for pediatric oncology patients in general, and for pediatric leukemia patients in particular. The former are more likely to attend school between treatments, while the latter, because of intensive and aggressive treatment regimens, are more likely to be absent from school and return only during the maintenance phase, 6–7 months after initiation of treatment, as in our pediatric hemato-oncology center, somewhat sooner in Monza, Italy (Adamoli et al. 1997). Consequently, pediatric leukemia patients may be at a higher risk for social isolation and academic difficulties.

It is possible to differentiate two kinds of preventive intervention programs in the school for newly diagnosed children with cancer: (a) programs such as annual seminars and workshops designed to enhance communication skills for school personnel to deal more effectively with cancer-related crises (e.g., Cleave and Charlton 1997), and (b) interventions targeted specifically for teachers and peers who currently have a child with cancer in the classroom (e.g., Katz, Dolgin and Varni 1990). Although the former generic intervention may have a valuable educational purpose within a primary prevention realm, it may not be as effective as more individualized, targeted presentations to teachers and students who currently have in the classroom a child recently diagnosed with cancer (Chekryn, Deegan and Reid 1987). Given limited resources, targeted interventions are more feasible and cost-effective. Yet, incorporating systematic presentations on cancer facts into the regular curriculum may increase cancer knowledge among all children and may facilitate the acceptance of a specific child with cancer (Mabe, Riley and Treiber 1987) as well as alleviate fears associated with cancer in the community. Both kinds of preventive interventions are complementary and examples of primary intervention at its best.

ACKNOWLEDGEMENTS

The authors express their thanks and appreciation to the interdisciplinary staff members of the Miri Shitrit Department of Pediatric Hemato-Oncology for their dedication and active involvement in the implementation of preventive intervention in the school for children with cancer: Dr R. Elhasid and Dr A. Ben-Barak, Nurse L. Sweetat, Clinical Psychologist E. Krivoy, Social Workers J. Eid and N. Perets-Salton, Educational Counselor R. Rosenkrantz, Art Therapist A. Magen and Music Therapist O. Levanoni. The authors also thank Mrs M. Perlmutter for her assistance in the preparation of this chapter.

REFERENCES

Adamoli, L., Deasy-Spinetta, P., Corbetta, A., Jancovic, M., Lia, R., Locati, A., Fraschini, D., Masera, G., Spinetta, J.J. (1997) School functioning for the child with leukemia in continuous first remission: Screening high-risk children. *Pediatric Hematology and Oncology* **14**(2), 121–131.

Baysinger, M., Heiney, S.P., Creed, J.M., Ettinger, R.S. (1993) A trajectomy approach for education of the child/adolescent with cancer. *Journal of Pediatric Oncology Nursing* **10**(4) 133–138.

Bleyer, W.A. (1990) The impact of childhood cancer on the United States and the world. *Ca: A Cancer Journal for Clinicians* **40**, 355–367.

Brown, R.T., Madan-Swain, A. (1993) Cognitive, neuropsychological and academic sequelae in children with leukemia. *Journal of Learning Disabilities* **26**, 74–90.

Bukowski, W.M., Hoza, B. (1989) Popularity and friendship: Issues in theory, measurement, and outcomes. In Berndt, T., Ladd, G. (Eds) *Contributions of Peer Relations to Children's Development*. New York: Wiley, pp. 15–45.

Cairns, N.U., Klopovich, P., Hearne, E., Lansky, S.B. (1982) School attendance of children with cancer. *Journal of School Health* **52**, 152–155.

Caplan, G. (1964) *Principles of Preventive Psychiatry*. New York: Basic Books.

Charlton, A., Larcombe, I.J., Meller, S.T., Morris Jones, P.H., Mott, M.G., Potton, M.W., Tranmer, M.D., Walker, J.J. (1991) Absence from school related to cancer and other chronic conditions. *Archives of Diseases in Childhood* **66**(10), 1217–1222.

Chekryn, J., Deegan, M., Reid, J. (1987) Impact on teachers when a child with cancer returns to school. *Children's Health Care*, **15**, 161–165.

Cleave, H., Charlton, A. (1997) Evaluation of a cancer-based coping and caring course used in three different settings. *Child: Care, Health & Development* **23**(5), 399–413.

Deasy-Spinetta, P. (1993) School issues and the child with cancer. *Cancer* **71**(10), 3261–3264.

Deasy-Spinetta, P., Spinetta, J.J. (1981) Educational issues in the rehabilitation of long-term survivors. In Pizzo, P.A. & Poplack, D.G. (Eds) *Principles and Practice of Pediatric Oncology* (2nd edn). Philadelphia, PA: Lippincott.

Eiser, C. (1980). How leukemia affects a child's schooling. *British Journal of Social and Clinical Psychology* **19**, 365–368.

Evans, S.E., Radford. M. (1995) Psychological adjustment and achievements of survivors of childhood cancer. *Archives of Diseases in Childhood* **72**(5), 423–426.

Fritz, C.K., Williams, J.R. (1988) Issues of adolescent development for survivors of childhood cancer. *Journal of the American Academy of Childhood and Adolescent Psychiatry* **27**, 712–715.

Gray, R.E., Doan, B.D., Shermer, M.A., Fitzgerald, A.V., Berry, M.P., Jenkin, D., Doherty, M.A. (1992) Psychological adaptation of survivors of childhood cancer. *Cancer* **70**, 2713–2721.

Gregory, K., Parker, L., Craft, A.W. (1994) Returning to primary school after treatment for cancer. *Pediatric Hematology and Oncology* **11**(1), 105–109.

Gullotta, T.P. (1987) Prevention's technology. *The Journal of Primary Prevention* **8**(1&2), 4–24.

Häcker, W., Klemm, M., Böpple, E. (1995) Heimatschulbesuche bei krebskranken Schülerinnen und Schülern während und nach der Therapie (Local school attendance by students with cancer during and after therapy). *Klinische Pädiatrie* **207**(4), 181–185.

Haupt, R., Fears, T.R., Robinson, L.L., Mills, J.L., Nicholson, H.S., Zeltzer, L.K., Meadows, A.T., Byrne, J. (1994) Educational attainment of long-term survivors of childhood acute lymphoblastic leukemia. *Journal of the American Medical Association* **272**(18), 1427–1432.

Hockenberry-Eaton, M., Manteuffel, B., Bottomley, S. (1997) Development of two instruments examining stress and adjustment in children with cancer. *Journal of Pediatric Oncology Nursing* **14**(3), 178–185.

Joint Commission on Mental Illness and Health (1961) *Action for Mental Health*. New York: Basic Books.

Kaplan, D.M., Smith, A., Grobstein, R. (1974) School management of the seriously ill child. *Journal of School Health* **44**, 250–254.

Katz, E.R. (1980) Illness impact and social reintegration. In Kellerman J. (Ed.) *Psychological aspects of cancer in children*. Springfield, IL: Thomas, pp. 14–45.

Katz, E.R., Dolgin, M.J., Varni, J.W. (1990) Cancer in children and adolescents. In A.M. Gross & R.S. Drabman (Eds) *Handbook of Clinical Behavioral Pediatrics*. New York: Plenum, pp. 129–146.

Katz, E.R., Kellerman, J., Rigler, D., Williams, K.O., Siegel, S.E. (1977) School intervention with pediatric cancer patients. *Journal of Pediatric Psychology* **2**, 72–76.

Katz, E.R., Varni, J.W., Rubenstein, C.L., Blew, A., Hubert, N. (1992) Teacher, parent and child evaluative ratings of school reintegration intervention for children with newly diagnosed cancer. *Child Health Care* **21**(2), 69–75.

Kazak, A.E., Meadows, A.T. (1989) Family of young adolescents who have survived cancer: Social-emotional adjustment, adaptability and social support. *Journal of Pediatric Psychology* **14**, 175–191.

Klopovich, P., Vats, T.S., Butterfield, G., Cairns, N.U., Lansky, S.B. (1981) School phobia: Interventions in childhood cancer. *Journal of Kansas Medical Society* **82**, 125–127.

Koocher, G.P., O'Malley, J.E., Gogan, J.L., Foster, D.J. (1980) Psychological adjustment among pediatric patients. *Journal of Child Psychology and Psychiatry* **21**, 165–173.

Lansky, S.B., Cairns, N.U. (1979a) Poor school attendance in children with malignancies. *Proceedings of the American Association for Cancer Research* **20**, 390.

Lansky, S.B., Cairns, N.U. (1979b) The family of the child with cancer. *Proceedings of the American Cancer Society National Conference on the Care of the Child with Cancer*. New York: American Cancer Society, pp. 156–162.

Lansky, S.B., Cairns, N.U., Zwartjes, W. (1983) School attendance among children with cancer: A report from two centers. *Journal of Psychosocial Oncology* **12**, 75–82.

Lansky, S.B., Lowman, J.T., Vats, T.S., Gyulay, J.E. (1975) School phobia in children with malignant neoplasms. *American Journal of Diseases in Children* **129**, 42–46.

Larcombe, I., Charlton, A. (1996) Children return to school after treatment for cancer: Study days for teachers. *Journal of Cancer Education* **11**(2), 102–105.

Lazarus, R.S. (1968) Emotions and adaptations conceptual and empirical relations. In Arnold W.J. (Ed.) *Nebraska Symposium on Motivation*. Lincoln, NE: University of Nebraska Press.

Mabe, P.A., Riley, W.T., Treiber, F.A. (1987) Cancer knowledge and acceptance of children with cancer. *Journal of School Health* **57**, 59–63.

McCarthy, A.M., Williams, J., Plumer, C. (1998) Evaluation of school re-entry nursing intervention for children with cancer. *Journal of Pediatric Oncology Nursing* **15**(3), 143–152.

McCollum, A.T. (1975). *Coping with Prolonged Health Impairment in Your Child.* Boston: Little Brown.

Noll, R.B., Bukowski, W.M., Rogosch, F.A., LeRoy, S., Kulkarni, R. (1990) Social interactions between children with cancer and their peers: Teacher ratings. *Journal of Pediatric Psychology* **15**, 43–53.

Noll, R.B., LeRoy, S., Bukowski, W.M., Rogosch, F.A., Kulkarni, R. (1991) Peer relationships and adjustment in children with cancer. *Journal of Pediatric Psychology* **16**(3), 307–326.

Noll, R.B., Bukowski, W.M., Davies, W.H., Koontz, K., Kulkarni, R. (1993) Adjustment in the peer system of adolescents with cancer: A two-year study. *Journal of Pediatric Psychology* **18**(3), 351–364.

O'Malley, J.E., Foster, D., Koocher, D., *et al.* (1979) Psychiatric sequelae of surviving childhood cancer. *American Journal of Orthopsychiatry* **137**, 94–96.

Parker, J.C., Asher, S.R. (1987) Peer relations and later personal adjustment: Are low-accepted children at risk? *Psychological Bulletin* **102**, 357–389.

Pendley, J.S., Dahlquist, L.M., Dreyer, Z. (1997) Body image and psychological adjustment in adolescent cancer survivors. *Journal of Pediatric Psychology* **22**(1), 29–43.

Polland, A. (1985) School and the child with cancer. A program to assist school personnel. *Journal of Pediatric Oncology Nursing* **2**, 7–10.

Price, R.H., Cowen, E.L., Lorion, R.P., Ramos-McKay, J. (Eds) (1988) *14 Ounces of Prevention: A casebook for practitioners.* Washington, DC: American Psychological Association.

Puukko, L.R., Sammallahti, P.R., Siimes, M.A., Aalberg, V.A. (1997) Childhood leukemia and body image: Interview reveals impairment not found with a questionnaire. *Journal of Clinical Psychology* **53**(2), 133–137.

Reiter, A., Schrappe, M., Ludwig, W.D. *et al.* (1994) Chemotherapy in 998 unselected childhood acute lymphoblastic leukemia patients: Results and conclusions of the multicenter trial. ALL-BFM.86. *Blood* **84**, 3122–3133.

Ross, D.M., Ross, S.A. (1984) Teaching the child with leukemia to cope with teasing. *Issues in Comprehensive Pediatric Nursing* **7**, 59–66.

Ross, J.W., Scarvalone, S.A. (1982) Facilitating the pediatric cancer patient's return to school. *Social Work* **27**(3), 256–261.

Rubenstein, C.L., Varni, J.W., Katz, E.R. (1990) Cognitive functioning in long-term survivors of childhood cancer: A prospective analysis. *Journal of Developmental and Behavioral Pediatrics* **11**, 301–305.

Sach, M.B. (1980) Helping the child with cancer go back to school. *Journal of School Health* **50**, 328–331.

Sloper, J., Larcombe, I.J., Charlton, A. (1994) Psychological adjustment of five-year survivors of childhood cancer. *Journal of Cancer Education* **9**(3), 163–169.

Stehbens, J.A., Kisker, C.T., Wilson, B.K. (1983) School behavior and attendance during the first year of treatment for childhood cancer. *Psychology in the Schools* **20**, 223–228.

Sullivan, H.S. (1953) *The Interpersonal Theory of Psychiatry.* New York: W.W. Norton.

Swift, C., Levin, G. (1987) Empowerment: An emerging mental health technology. *The Journal of Primary Prevention* **8**(1&2), 71–94.

Tadmor, C.S. (1984) The perceived personal control crisis intervention model: Training of and application by physicians and nurses to a high risk population of Caesarean birth in a hospital setting. Doctoral dissertation, Hebrew University, Jerusalem.

Tadmor, C.S. (1986) A crisis intervention model for a population of mothers who encounter neonatal death. *Journal of Primary Prevention* **7**(1), 17–26.

Tadmor, C.S. (1987) Preventive intervention for medical staff dealing with terminally ill patients. *Journal of Preventive Psychiatry* **3**(4), 393–409.

Tadmor, C.S. (1988) The perceived personal control preventive intervention for a caesarean birth population. In Price, R.H., Cowen, E.L., Lorion, R.P., Ramos-McKay, J. (Eds) *14 Ounces of Prevention: A casebook for practitioners.* Washington DC: American Psychological Association, pp. 141–152.

Tadmor, C.S., Brandes, J.M. (1984) The perceived personal control crisis intervention model in the prevention of emotional dysfunction for a high risk population of Caesarean birth. *The Journal of Primary Prevention* **4**, 240–251.

Tadmor, C.S., Brandes, J.M. (1986) Premature birth: A crisis intervention approach. *The Journal of Primary Prevention* **6**, 244–255.

Tadmor, C.S., Brandes, J.M., Hofman, J.E. (1987) Preventive intervention for a Caesarean birth population. *Journal of Preventive Psychiatry* **3**(4), 343–364.

Tadmor, C.S., Weyl Ben Arush, M. (2000) Changes in the policies of the department of hematology, 1982–1998, designed to promote the mental health of children with leukemia and enhance their quality of life. *Pediatric Hematology and Oncology* **17**, 67–76.

Tadmor, C.S., Bar-Maor, J.A., Birkhan, J., Shoshany, G., Hofman, J.E. (1987) Pediatric surgery: A preventive intervention approach to enhance mastery of stress. *Journal of Preventive Psychiatry* **3**(4), 365–392.

Vannatta, K., Garstein, M.A., Short, A., Noll, R.B. (1998) A controlled study of peer relationships of children surviving brain tumors: teachers, peer and self-ratings. *Journal of Pediatric Psychology* **23**(5), 279–287.

Varni, J.W., Katz, E.R. (1987) Psychological aspects of cancer in children: A review of research. *Journal of Psychosocial Oncology* **5**, 93–119.

Varni, J.W., Katz, E.R. (1997) Stress, social support and negative affectivity with newly diagnosed cancer: A prospective transactional analysis. *Psycho-oncology* **6**(4), 267–278.

Varni, J.W., Wallander, J.L. (1988) Pediatric chronic disabilities. In Routh, D.K. (Ed.) *Handbook of Pediatric Psychology.* New York: Guilford, pp. 190–221.

Varni, J.W., Katz, E.R., Colgrove, R.J., Dolgin, M. (1994) Perceived social support and adjustment of children with newly diagnosed cancer. *Journal of Developmental & Behavioral Pediatrics* **15**(1), 6–20.

Varni, J.W., Katz, E.R., Colegrove, R., Dolgin, M. (1995) Perceived physical appearance and adjustment of children with newly diagnosed cancer: A path analytic model. *Journal of Behavioral Medicine* **18**, 261–278.

Whitsett, S.F., Pelletier, W., Scott-Lane, L. (1999) Meeting impossible psychosocial demands in pediatric oncology: Creative solutions to universal challenges. *Medical and Pediatric Oncology* **32**, 289–291.

Index

Page numbers in *italics* indicate figures and tables.